MELLONI'S ILLUSTRATED DICTIONARY OF

MEDICAL
ABBREVIATIONS

D0885010

MEDICAL
ABBREVIATIONS

B. John Melloni, PhD
and
June L. Melloni, PhD

The Parthenon Publishing Group
International Publishers in Medicine, Science & Technology

NEW YORK   LONDON

Published in the USA by
The Parthenon Publishing Group Inc.
One Blue Hill Plaza, PO Box 1564
Pearl River, New York 10965, USA

Published in the UK by
The Parthenon Publishing Group Limited
Casterton Hall, Kirkby Lonsdale
Carnforth, Lancs LA6 2LA, UK

Library of Congress Cataloging-in-Publication Data
    Melloni, Biagio John.
    Melloni's illustrated dictionary of medical abbreviations /
    by B. John Melloni and June L. Melloni.
       p.   cm.
    ISBN 1-85070-708-1
    1. Medicine -- Abbreviations -- Dictionaries. I. Melloni. June L.
    II. Title. III.Title: Illustrated dictionary of medical
    abbreviations. IV. Title: Medical abbreviations.
      [DNLM: 1. Medicine abbreviations dictionaries. W 13 M527m 1998]
    R121.M539 1998
    610'.1'48--DC21
    DNLM/DLC
    for Library of Congress   98–11886
                                    CIP

British Library Cataloguing in Publication Data
Melloni, Biagio John, 1929–
    Melloni's illustrated dictionary of medical abbreviations
    1.Medicine – Abbreviations 2.Medicine – Terminology – Dictionaries
    I.Title II.Melloni, June L. III. Illustrated dictionary of medical
    abbreviations
    610.1'48
    ISBN 1-85070-708-1

Printed and bound by The Bath Press, Bath, UK

Preface

The growing reservoir of medical content, together with the increasing need to convey information quickly, have led to the importance of the abbreviated term. Although many abbreviations have multiple possibilities, such as AA (acute appendicitis, Alcoholics Anonymous, Australia antigen) most have become so familiar that we use them in preference to the full term, such as ECG, TB, OB/GYN, MRI, PDR, NIH, DNA, RNA, ICU, OR, IV, SIDS, and MS. Abbreviations actually have become a unique language. Thousands of abbreviations have become more commonly used than the full terms. The universal acceptance of MRI is so evident that to use its complete meaning, 'magnetic resonance imaging' over and over in an article or medical record would create a hindrance to smooth reading.

Many abbreviations have become a permanent part of the common vocabulary of the scientific language of medicine. Abbreviations effectively shorten speech and text for both convenience and better communication. Used properly, they significantly improve the written and spoken word, used carelessly, they can cause confusion and misunderstanding. To minimize confusion, most publications define abbreviations when they first appear in the text, which produces a more readable text and saves print space.

The medical abbreviations in this book were compiled from leading medical books such as Harrison's *Principles of Internal Medicine* (McGraw Hill), as well as from professional journals such as *The Journal of the American Medical Association* (JAMA) and *The New England Journal of Medicine* (NEJM). They represent the most commonly used abbreviations in both the medical literature and in the spoken language of medicine and therefore appear frequently in the medical records of patients, as well as in lectures to health science students.

While compiling the material for this book, we leaned heavily on current usage to determine format. For the most part, periods are not included except in the abbreviations of foreign words. Also, some abbreviations appear in both upper and lower case letters; there are variations among the different disciplines and within regions of the country. In alphabetizing the abbreviations, numbers are ignored and lower case letters follow the upper case letters.

As new abbreviations surface and become viable within disciplines, we intend to include them as new entries in future editions of this book. Suggestions from readers would be greatly appreciated and should be sent to B. John Melloni, PhD, 9308 Renshaw Dr., Bethesda, MD 20817 USA.

BJM

JLM

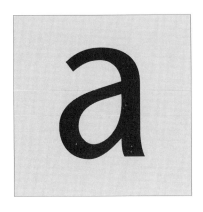

A	A-band
	abnormal
	absolute temperature
	accommodation
	acetabulum

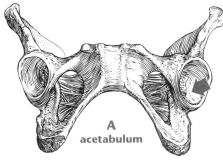

A
acetabulum

acetate
acne
acromion
adenine (a purine base constituent of DNA and RNA)
adenoma
adenosine (a nuceloside)
admittance
adult
age
allergic asthma
alveolar
ambulatory
amnion
ampere (a unit of electric current)
androgen (a substance that stimulates the development of male sex characteristcs)
angioplasty
angstrom unit (0.1 nm)
anode (the positive electrode of a galvanic battery)
anterior
area
artery
ascites (accumulation of fluid in the peritoneal cavity)
assessment
asthma (disorder marked by paroxysms of difficult breathing, wheezing and coughing)
atlas
atrium
auricle
axis
blood type A+, A−
dominant allele

A⁻	anion (an ion carrying a negative charge)
A̲	alveolar gas (as a subscript)
ˣA	mass number (the number of protons and neutrons in the atom of a nuclide)
A₁	aortic first heart sound
	major blood group
A₂	aortic second heart sound (aortic valve closure)
	major blood group
A₂₋ₒₛ	aortic second heart sound, opening snap
A I	angiotensin I
A II	angiotensin II
A III	angiotensin III
a	accommodation
	recessive allele
a.	*ante* [Latin] before
	arteria [Latin] artery
AA	abdominal auscultation
	acetic acid
	achievement age
	active alcoholic
	active assistive (range of motion)

active avoidance
acupuncture analgesia
acute abdomen (an
  incapacitating condition
  characterized by intense
  abdominal pain)
acute appendicitis
acute asthma
Addicts Anonymous
African American
Albert achillodynia
alcohol abuse
Alcoholic Anonymous
allergic angiitis
allergic asthma
alopecia areata (complete
  loss of hair in patches,
  chiefly on the scalp)
alveolar abscess
amino acid
aminoacyl (an amino acid
  acyl radical)
amplitude of
  accommodation
analgesic abuse
antacid
anticipatory avoidance
aortic arch
aplastic anemia
  (aregenerative anemia)
arachidonic acid (an
  unsaturated fatty acid
  essential for human
  nutrition)
ascending aorta
ascorbic acid (vitamin C)
audiologic assessment
Australia antigen (hepatitis
  B surface antigen)
automobile accident
nonimmunologic amyloid

A & A   acid and alkaline
arthrotomy & arthroscopy
awake and aware
aa.   *arteriae* [Latin] arteries
AAA   abdominal aortic
  aneurysm
aceto-acetic acid
acquired aplastic anemia

acute anxiety attack
alpha-adrenergic agonist
American Academy of
  Actuaries
American Association of
  Anatomists
anti-anginal agent
anti-anxiety agent
antisperm agglutinating
  antibodies
aaa   amalgam (an alloy of
  mercury and other
  metals)
AAAE   amino acid activating
  enzyme
AAAHC   Accreditation Association
  for Ambulatory Health
  Care
AAALAC   American Association for
  Accreditation of
  Laboratory Animal Care
AAAOM   American Association of
  Acupuncture and
  Oriental Medicine
AAAS   American Association for
  the Advancement of
  Science
AAAs   Area Agencies on Aging
AAB   alpha-adrenergic blocker
aminoazobenzene
AABA   American Anorexia
  Bulimia Association
AABB   American Association of
  Blood Banks
AABD   alpha-adrenergic
  blocking drug
AABS   automobile accident,
  broadside
AAC   Adrenalin, atropine, and
  cocaine
antibiotic-associated colitis
antigen-antibody complex
antimicrobial agent and
  chemotherapy
antimicrobial agent-
  associated colitis
AACAP   American Academy of
  Child and Adolescent
  Psychiatry

AACC American Association for Clinical Chemistry

AACCN American Association of Critical-Care Nurses

AACE American Academy of Clinical Electroencephalographers
American Association of Clinical Endocrinologists

AACG acute angle closure glaucoma (third phase of narrow-angle glaucoma with consequences if intraocular pressure is not reduced)

AACHP American Association for Comprehensive Health Planning

AACIA American Association for Clinical Immunology and Allergy

AACME Accreditation Council for Continuing Medical Education

AACN American Association of Critical-Care Nurses
American Academy of Clinical Neurophysiology
antibody-antigen complex nephritis

AACP American College of Chest Physicians

AACSA atlantoaxial cervical spine arthritis

AACSH adrenal androgen corticotropic stimulating hormone

AAD acid-ash diet (a diet intended to produce acidification of the urine for preventive treatment of urinary stones)
acute agitated delirium
acute amebic dysentery
American Academy of Dermatology
antibiotic-associated diarrhea
atypical Alzheimer's disease

AaDO₂ alveolar-arterial oxygen tension difference

AADS American Academy of Dental Schools

AAE active assistive exercise (voluntary exercise of specific muscle groups assisted by a therapist)
acute allergic encephalitis
American Association of Endodontists

AAEE American Association of Electromyography and Electrodiagnosis

AAEM American Academy of Environmental Medicine
American Association of Electrodiagnostic Medicine

AAF acetylaminofluorene (a carcinogenic compound)

AAFA Asthma and Allergy Foundation of America

AAFG Al-Anon Family Group (800) 356-9996

AAFP American Academy of Family Physicians

AAFPRS American Academy of Facial Plastic and Reconstructive Surgery

AAFS American Academy of Forensic Sciences

AAGP American Association for Geriatric Psychiatry

A-a gradient alveolar-arterial gradient

AAH acute alcoholic hepatitis
atypical adenomatous hyperplasia

AAHE Association for the Advancement of Health Education

AAHM American Association for the History of Medicine

AAHPM American Academy of Hospice and Palliative Medicine

AAHS American Association for

	Hand Surgery
AAI	American Association of Immunologists
AAIM	American Academy of Insurance Medicine
AAJ	atlantoaxial joint (a joint between the first and second vertebrae)
AAL	acute axial load (slamming in child abuse)
	anterior axillary line (a vertical line passing through the anterior fold of the axilla)
AALAS	American Association of Laboratory Animal Science
AAM	acute aseptic meningitis
	American Academy of Microbiology
AAMA	American Academy of Medical Acupuncture
AAMC	Association of American Medical Colleges
AAMD	antitissue antibody-mediated disease
AAMI	age associated memory impairment
AAMIH	American Association for Maternal and Infant Health
AAMRA	American Association of Medical Record Administrators
AAMRS	automated ambulatory medical record system
AAMS	acute aseptic meningitis syndrome
AAMSI	American Association for Medical Systems and Informatics
AAMT	American Association of Medical Transcription
AAN	AIDS-associated nephropathy
	AIDS-associated neutropenia
	American Academy of

	Neurology
	American Academy of Nursing
	analgesic abuse nephropathy
	analgesic-associated nephropathy
	attending's admission notes
AANA	American Association of Nurse Anesthetists
AANB	alpha-amino-butyric acid
AANM	American Association of Nurse Midwives
AANOS	American Academy of Neurological and Orthopaedic Surgeons
AANS	American Academy of Neurological Surgery
	American Association of Neurological Surgeons
AAO	American Academy of Ophthalmology
	American Academy of Osteopathy
	American Academy of Otolaryngology
	awake, alert, and oriented
AA of A	Ambulance Association of America
AAOC	antacid of choice
AAOM	American Association of Oral Medicine
	American Association of Orthopaedic Medicine
AAOP	American Academy of Oral Pathology
	American Academy of Orthotists and Prosthetists
AAOPCC	American Association of Poison Control Centers
AAOS	American Academy of Orthopaedic Surgeons
AAP	air at atmospheric pressure
	American Academy of Pediatrics
	American Academy of

Pedodontics

American Academy of Periodontology

American Academy of Psychoanalysis

American Academy of Psychotherapists

American Association of Pathologists

assessment adjustment pass

Association of Academic Physiatrists

Association of American Physicians

AAPA American Academy of Physician Assistants

AAPB American Association of Pathologists and Bacteriologists

AAPC American Association for Protecting Children (303) 792–9900

antibiotic-acquired pseudomembranous colitis

AAPCC American Association of Poison Control Centers

AAPM American Academy of Pain Medicine

AAPMC antibiotic-associated pseudomembranous colitis

AAPMR American Academy of Physical Medicine and Rehabilitation

AAPOS American Association for Pediatric Ophthalmology and Strabismus

AAPS American Association of Plastic Surgeons

Association of American Physicians and Surgeons

AAR active avoidance reaction

acute aortic regurgitation

acute articular rheumatism

against all risks

alpha-adrenergic receptor (receptor that responds to norepinephrine and to

some blocking agents)

amino acid replacement

antigen-antibody reaction

antigen-antiglobulin reaction (the reversible binding of an antigen to a homologous antibody)

aar against all risks

AARB alpha-adrenergic receptor blocker

AARC American Association of Respiratory care

AARE automobile accident, rear end

AARP American Association of Retired Persons

AARS atlantoaxial rotatory subluxation

AART American Association for Rehabilitation Therapy

American Association for Respiratory Therapy

AAROM active-assertive range of motion

active-assistive range of motion

AAS acute abdominal series

alcoholic abstinence syndrome

American Analgesia Society

American Association of Suicidology

anabolic androgenic steroids

androgenic-anabolic steroid

aortic arch syndrome

atomic absorption spectrometry

AASCD ampulla of anterior semicircular duct (duct in the inner ear that contains the ampullar crest with endings of the vestibular nerve)

AASD American Academy of Stress Disorders

AASeq amino acid sequence

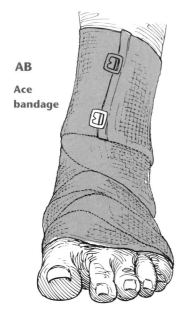

AB

Ace bandage

AASH   adrenal androgen-stimulating hormone

AASP   acute atrophic spinal paralysis

AAST   American Association for the Surgery of Trauma

AAT   academic aptitude test
activity as tolerated
adrenaline acid tartrate (epinephrine bitartrate)
alanine aminotransferase
alpha antitrypsin
at all times
aspartate aminotransferase (formerly SGOT)
atypical antibody titer
auditory apperception test
automatic atrial tachycardia

AATB   American Association of Tissue Banks

AATM   American Academy of Tropical Medicine

AATS   American Association of Thoracic Surgery

AAU   acute anterior uveitis

AAV   adeno-associated vector
adeno-associated virus

AAVMC   Association of American Veterinary Medical Colleges

AAVV   accumulated alveolar ventilatory volume

AB   abdominal
abdominal bloating
abductor
abnormal
abortion
Ace bandage (nonadhesive elastic bandage)
achillobursitis (inflammation of the bursa in front of the calcaneal tendon)
acute bronchitis
adaptive behavior
afterbirth
antibiotic
antigen binding
apical beat
Aschoff bodies (Aschoff's nodules)
aspiration biopsy
asthmatic bronchitis
blood type AB+, AB–

A/B   acid-base ratio

A₁B   major blood group

A₂B   major blood group

A & B   apnea and bradycardia

Ab   abortion
antibody

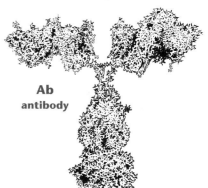

Ab

antibody

ABA   after born antibiotic
American Burn Association

aminobenzoic acid (topical sunscreen)

antibacterial agent

ABB acid-base balance (the net rate of the body's acid or alkali production is offset by the body's net rate of acid or alkali excretion)

air-blood barrier (the barrier separating the air from the blood in the alveoli of the lungs)

antibody-coated bacteria

abbr abbreviated

abbreviation

ABC abbreviated blood count

absolute band count

absolute basophil count

airway-breathing-circulation

alternative birthing center

aneurysmal bone cyst

antigen-binding capacity

antigen-binding cell

apnea, bradycardia and cyanosis

argon beam coagulator

aspiration biopsy cytology

ABD adrenergic blocking drugs

aged, blind, and disabled

abd abdomen

abdominal

abduct

abduction

ABDCT atrial bolus dynamic computer tomography

Abd Gth abdominal girth

abd poll abductor pollicis (muscle)

ABE acute bacterial endocarditis (infectious endocarditis caused by bacteria such as streptococci, staphylococci, and gram-negative bacilli)

American Board of Examiners

amobarbital elixir

aprobarbital elixir

ABEA American Broncho-Esophagological Association

ABEM American Board of Emergency Medicine

ABEP auditory brainstem-evoked potential

ABF androgen-binding fraction

aortobifemoral (bypass)

ABFP American Board of Forensic Psychiatry

ABGs arterial blood gases

ABI anterobasal infarct (heart infarct due to occlusion of the circumflex branch of the left coronary artery)

atherothrombotic brain infarction

ABIM American Board of Internal Medicine

ABJ anastomosis between bile duct and jejunum

ABK aphakic bullous keratopathy

ABL abeta-lipoproteinemia

ammonia blood level

angioblastic lymphadenopathy

antigen-binding lymphocyte

ABLB alternate binaural loudness balance

ABM acute bacterial meningitis

ABMT autologous bone marrow transplantation

ABMS Advisory Board for Medical Specialties

autologous bone marrow specialties

ABMT allogenic bone marrow transplant

autologous bone marrow transplantation

ABN aseptic bone necrosis

abn abnormal

abnormality

ABNM American Board of Nuclear Medicine

ABO   absent bed occupancy
absent bed occupant
American Board of
Orthodontists
antibiotic ointment
blood groups A, B, AB,
and O

ABOG   American Board of
Obstetrics and
Gynecology

ABOS   American Board of
Orthopaedic Surgery

ABP   actin-binding protein
acute bacterial prostatitis
acute biliary pancreatitis
American Board of
Pediatrics
American Board of
Periodontology
androgen-binding protein
antigen-binding protein
arterial blood pressure

ABPA   allergic
bronchopulmonary
aspergillosis

ABPC   antibody-producing cell

ABPM   ambulatory blood pressure
monitoring

ABPN   American Board of
Psychiatry and Neurology

ABR   absolute bed rest
auditory brainstem evoked
response
auditory brainstem
response

ABRCA   anterior branch of right
coronary artery
atrial branch of right
coronary artery

ABS   acrylonitrile-butadiene-
styrene
acute brain syndrome
admitting blood sugar
aging brain syndrome
American Board of
Surgery
anorexia-bulimia syndrome
arterial blood sample
aspiration biopsy syringe

at bedside

abs   absent
absolute
absorption

absc   abscess
abscissa

abs.feb.   *absente febre* [Latin] while
fever is absent

abstr   abstract

ABT   Allen blue test
aminopyrine breath test
autologous blood
transfusion
(autotransfusion)

abt   about

ABU   American Board of
Urology

ABUTO   acute bilateral upper tract
obstruction

ABV   acid-base values
Adriamycin (doxorubicin)
+ bleomycin + vinblastine
(combination chemo-
therapy)

ABVD   Adriamycin (doxorubicin)
+ bleomycin + vinblastine
+ dacarbazine
(combination
chemotherapy)

ABW   actual body weight

ABx   antibiotics

ABY   acid bismuth yeast

AC   abdominal cavity
abdominal circumference
abdominal compression
acarbose (precose; for
treating diabetes by
blocking the absorption
of glucose and
carbohydrates in the
intestine)
acromioclavicular (joint)
activated charcoal
acupuncture clinic
acute
acute cholecystitis
adenylate cyclase (adenyl
cyclase)
adrenal cortex

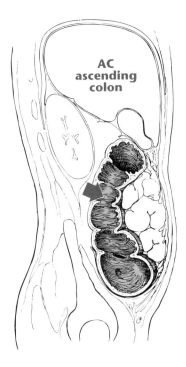

AC
ascending
colon

adrenocorticoid
Adriamycin (doxorubicin)
  + cyclophosphamide
  (combination chemo-
  therapy)
aftercare (services after
  discharge from hospital)
airborne contaminants
air conduction
alcoholic cirrhosis
  (Laennec's cirrhosis)
alternating current
alveolar cancer
  (adenocarcinoma)
alveolar crest
ambulatory care
amniocentesis
amniotic cavity
anal canal
anchored catheter
anodal closure
ansa cervicalis (a nerve
  loop in the cervical
  plexus consisting of fibers

from the first three
  cervical nerves)
antecubital
anterior chamber (of eye)
anterior cruciate
  (ligament)
anticoagulant
anti-inflammatory
  corticosteroid
aortic coarctation (a
  localized constriction of
  the aorta characterized by
  severe narrowing of the
  lumen)
appendiceal carcinoids
articular capsule
articular cartilage
ascending colon
auricular chondritis
axillary crutches

A/C   anterior chamber of eye

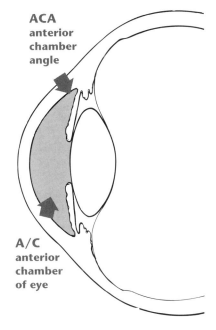

ACA
anterior
chamber
angle

A/C
anterior
chamber
of eye

A & C   ascites and cirrhosis
Ac   actinium (a rare metallic
              element)
aC   arabinosylcytosine
              (cytarabine)

ac   acute
air conduction
alternating current
anaerobic culture
anchored catheter
anterior commissure

a.c.   *ante cibum* [Latin] before meals

ACA   acquired chromosomal abnormalities
acute care (short-term health care, usually less than one month)
acute cerebellar ataxia
acyclovir (a synthetic nucleoside with antiviral activity against the herpes virus)
adenocarcinoma (malignant adenoma)
adult child of an alcoholic
air contrast arthrogram
American Chiropractic Association
American College of Angiology
aminocaproic acid (inhibits dissolution of fibrin in the blood; used to prevent bleeding)
Amplicor chlamydia assay
anterior cerebral artery
anterior chamber angle (of eye)
anterior choroidal artery
anterior communicating artery
anticardiolipin antibody
auditory canal atresia

AC/A   accommodative convergence-accommodation (ratio)

ACAD   asymptomatic carotid artery disease
asymptomatic coronary artery disease

ACAH   autoimmune chronic active hepatitis

ACAI   American College of Allergy and Immunology

ACAO   acyl coenzyme A oxidase

ACA ratio   accommodative convergence and accommodation ratio

ACAT   acyl cholesterol acyl transferase

ACATI   acyl cholesterol acyl transferase inhibitor
automated computerized axial tomography

ACB   antibody-coated bacteria
aortocoronary bypass
asymptomatic carotid bruit

AcB   assist with bath

ACBE   air contrast barium enema

ACBG   aortocoronary bypass graft

ACBYS   aortocoronary bypass surgery

ACC   acalculous cholecystitis
accelerin-convertin (factor)
accommodation
acentric chromosome (chromosome with no centromere)
acrocentric chromosome (chromosome with the centromere near one end)

ACC
acrocentric
chromosome

actinic cell carcinoma
acute cholecystitis
adenoid cystic carcinoma
alveolar cell carcinoma
ambulatory care center

American College of
  Cardiology
anodal closure contraction
aplasia cutis congenita
arm cylinder cast
articular chondrocalcinosis
  (pseudogout)

acc   acceleration
accident
accommodation

ACCBG   adenoid cystic carcinoma
of Bartholin gland

ACCESS   Ambulatory Care Clinic
Effectiveness Systems
Study

ACCH   Association for the Care of
Children's Health

AcCh   acetylcholine (a neuro-
transmitter)

AcChR   acetylcholine receptor
accid   accident
AcCoA   acetylcoenzyme A
accom   accommodation
ACCP   American College of Chest
Physicians
American College of
Clinical Pharmacology

ACCS   anterior cervical cord
syndrome

ACCSG   adenoid cystic carcinoma
of salivary glands

ACCU   acute coronary care unit
adenylate cyclase catalytic
unit

ACD   absolute cardiac dullness
acid citrate dextrose
actinomysin D
  (dactinomycin)
adult celiac disease
air conditioner disease
allergic contact dermatitis
anterior cervical
  diskectomy
anticonvulsant drug
area of cardiac dullness
Arnold-Chiari deformity
  (the medulla oblongata
  and part of the
  cerebellum protrude

through the foramen
  magnum)
augmentative communi-
  cation device (alternative
  communication device)

ACDCPR   active compression-
decompression
cardiopulmonary
resuscitation

ACDE   American Council for
Drug Education

ACD (F)   anterior cervical
decompression (fusion)

ACD & F   anterior cervical
diskectomy and fusion

ACDK   acquired cystic disease of
the kidney

ACDS   American Contact
Dermatitis Society
Association for Children
with Down Syndrome

ACE   acute coronary event
adrenocortical extract
alcohol, chloroform, and
  ether (anesthetic
  mixture)
American Council on
  Exercise

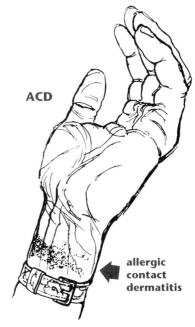

ACD

allergic
contact
dermatitis

angiotensin I-converting enzyme (its gene is located at 17q23)

anterior chamber of eye

ace acetone (dimethyl ketone)

ACED anhidrotic congenital ectodermal dysplasia

ACEHL American Council on Exercise Hot Line (1-800 529-8227)

ACEI angiotensin-converting enzyme inhibitor (its gene is located at 1q 42–q43)

A-cells alpha cells (of the adenopituitary)

alpha cells (of the pancreatic islets of Langerhans)

ACEP American College of Emergency Physicians

Acet acetone (dimethyl ketone)

acetab acetabulum (large cup-shaped cavity on the lateral side of the hipbone that accommodates the head of the femur)

a.c.& h.s. *ante cibum et hora somni* [Latin] before meals and at bedtime

acetyl CoA

acetyl-coenzyme A

ACF acute care facility

acute circulatory failure

ambulatory care facility

anterior cervical fusion

anterior cranial fossa (the front subdivision of the floor of the cranial cavity)

ACF

anterior cranial fossa

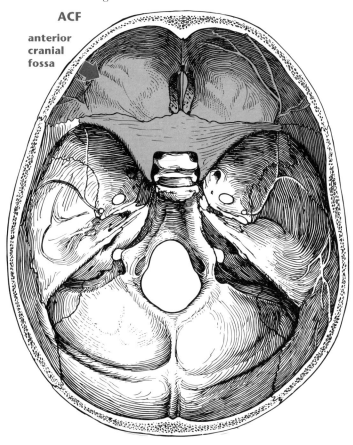

ACFS American College of Foot Surgeons

ACG active chronic gastritis (principally caused by *H. pylori*)
acycloguanosine
American College of Gastroenterology
angiocardiogram
angiocardiography
apexcardiography

AcG accelerator globulin

ac-g accelerator globulin

ACGIH American Conference of Governmental Industrial Hygienists

ACGME Accreditation Council for Graduate Medical Education

ACH acetylcholine (a neuro-transmitter)
active chronic hepatitis
acute care hospital
adrenal cortical hormone
air exchange per hour

ACh acetylcholine (a neuro-transmitter)

ACHD atherosclerotic coronary heart disease

AChE acetylcholinesterase (it deactivates the neuro-transmitter acetylcholine, released at neurohumoral junctions, thereby permitting transmission of new impulses)

AChR acetylcholine receptor

AChRAb acetylcholine receptor antibody

AChRP acetylcholine receptor protein

a.c. & h.s.
ante cibum et hora somni [Latin] before meals and at bedtime

ACI acoustic comfort index
acute cardiac ischemia
acute coronary infarction
acute coronary

insufficiency
adrenocortical insufficiency
autologous chondrocyte implantation (to repair damaged cartilage)

acid p'tase
acid phosphatase

ACIF anti-complement immunofluorescence

ACILI anterior chamber intraocular lens implantation

AC-IOL anterior chamber intraocular lens

ACIP Advisory Committee on Immunization Practices (part of CDC)

ACJ acromioclavicular joint
acute cholestatic jaundice

ACJD acromioclavicular joint dislocation

AC joint acromioclavicular joint

ACL anococcygeal ligament
anterior cruciate ligament (of knee joint)

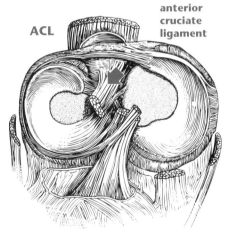

ACL — anterior cruciate ligament

aCL antibodies to cardiolipin

ACLA American Clinical Laboratory Association
anticardiolipid antibody

ACLD Association for Children with Learning Disabilities

ACLM	American College of Legal Medicine
ACLR	anterior cruciate ligament repair (of knee joint)
ACLS	advanced cardiac life support
ACM	acute cerebrospinal meningitis
	Adriamycin (doxorubicin) + cyclophosphamide + methotrexate (combination chemotherapy)
	air contrast myelography
	alveolar capillary membrane
	anterior chamber maintainer
	anticonvulsant medication
	Arnold-Chiari malformation
ACMC	Association of Canadian Medical Colleges
ACMV	assist-control mechanical ventilation
	assist-control mode ventilation
ACN	acute conditioned neurosis
	American College of Neuropsychiatrists
	American College of Nutrition
	anococcygeal nerve
ACNM	American College of Nuclear Medicine
	American College of Nurse-Midwives
ACO	acute coronary occlusion
	acyl coenzyme A oxidase
	Adriamycin (doxorubicin) + cyclophosphamide + Oncovin (vincristine) (combination chemo-therapy)
	alert, cooperative, and oriented
	American College of Otolaryngologists
ACoA	adult children of alcoholics

	anterior communicating artery
ACoA	acetyl coenzyme A
ACOE	anterior chamber of eye
ACOEM	American College of Occupational and Environmental Medicine
ACOG	American College of Obstetricians and Gynecologists
ACOM	American College of Occupational Medicine
ACOS	American College of Osteopathic Surgeons
ACOV	aortocranial occlusive vascular disease
ACP	achondroplasia
	acid phosphatase
	acute cor pulmonale
	acyl-carrier protein
	ambulatory care program
	American College of Pathologists
	American College of Pharmacists
	American College of Physicians
	amorphous calcium phosphate
	anterior cervical plate (internal fixation system)
	aortic counterpulsation
	aspirin-caffeine-phenacetin
	Association of Clinical Pathologists
ACPA	American Cleft Palate Association
	anticytoplasmic antibodies
ACPC	aminocyclopentane carboxylic (acid)
ACPCA	American Cleft Palate-Craniofacial Association
ACPD	absolute cephalopelvic disproportion
ACPE	American Council on Pharmaceutical Education
AcPh	acid phosphatase
ACPM	American College of

Preventive Medicine

ACPO acute colonic pseudo-
obstruction
ACPP adrenocorticopolypeptide
ACPS acrocephalopolysyndactyly
(Carpenter's syndrome)
acq acquired
ACR acetylcholine receptor
adenomatosis of colon and
rectum
American College of
Radiology
American College of
Rheumatology
anterior cruciate
(ligament) rupture (of
knee joint)
anticonstipation regimen
ACRM American Congress of
Rehabilitation Medicine
ACS acrocephalosyndactyly

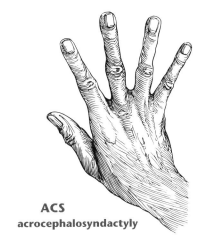

ACS
acrocephalosyndactyly

(craniostenosis marked
by acrocephaly and
syndactyly)
acute chest syndrome
acute confusional state
(delirium)
adhesive capsulitis of
shoulder (frozen
shoulder)
adnexal carcinoma of skin
adolescent coercive sex

American Cancer Society
American Chemical Society
American College of
Surgeons
anodal closing sound
anterior crus (limb) of
stapes (shorter and less
curved than the posterior
crus)
aortocoronary shunt
Association of Clinical
Scientists
asymptomatic carrier state
automated catheterization
system
ACSA aminocephalosporanic
acid
ACSD acrocephalosyndactyly
(type I Apert syndrome
and type II Apert-
Crouzon syndrome)
ACSL automatic computerized
solvent litholysis
ACSM American College of
Sports Medicine
ACSP adenylate cyclase-
stimulating protein
ACT activated clotting time
activated coagulation time
adjuvant chemotherapy
alternate cover test
androgen-control therapy
ankle clonus test
antichymotrypsin
anticoagulant therapy
axial compression test
Act-D actinomycin D
(dactinomycin)
ACTe anodal closure tetanus
Act Ex active exercise
ACTG AIDS clinical trials group
ACTH adrenocorticotropic
hormone (corticotropin)
ACTH RF
adrenocorticotropic
hormone releasing factor
ACTH ST
adrenocorticotropic
hormone (ACTH)

stimulation test

ACTP adrenocorticotropic
polypeptide

ACTS acute cervical traumatic
sprain

ACU ambulatory care unit

ACV acyclovir (exhibits selective
antiviral activity against
herpes simplex)

ACVD acute cardiovascular
disease
atherosclerotic
cardiovascular disease

ACVL aberrant congenital venous
loop

Acyl-CoA

organic compound –
coenzyme A ester

AD abdominal distention
active disease
acute diarrhea
addict
Addison's disease (adrenal
gland disorder marked by
reduced production of
adrenal steroids)
adductor
adenoid
adenovirus
adiposis dolorosa
(Dercum's disease)
admitting diagnosis
adrenal dysfunction
advanced directive (health
care decisions when
incapacitated)
affective disorder
after discharge
alcohol dehydrogenase
alcohol dependence
Alzheimer's dementia
Alzheimer's disease
amebic dysentery (amebic
colitis; intestinal
amebiasis)
analgesic dose
ankle drop
anodal duration
antidepressant

antigenic determinant
aortic dissection
Apert's disease
(acrocephalosyndactyly)
appropriate disability
arginase deficiency
Armstrong's disease
(lymphocytic chorio-
meningitis)
articular disk
atopic dermatitis
Aujeszky's disease
(pseudorabies)
autonomic dysreflexia
autosomal dominant
average dose

A & D admission and discharge
antiperspirants and
deodorants
antiseptics and
disinfectants
anxiety and dyspnea
asthma and dyspnea

a.d. *alternis diebus* [Latin] every
other day
aqua destillata [Latin]
distilled water
auris dextra [Latin]
right ear

ADA adenosine deaminase (a
deficiency of this enzyme
is evident in patients with
severe combined
immunodeficiency
syndrome)
American Dental
Association
American Diabetes
Association
American Dietetic
Association
Americans with Disabilities
Act
amnesic-dysnomic aphasia
anterior descending
(coronary) artery

ADAA Anxiety Disorders
Association of America

ADAM adjustment disorder with

anxious mood

ADAMHA
Alcohol, Drug Abuse, and Mental Health Administration

ADAP Alzheimer's disease associated protein

ADAS Alzheimer's disease assessment scale

ADATC Alcoholism and Drug Addiction Treatment Center

ADB accidental death benefit

ADBLCA anterior descending branch of left coronary artery

ADC affective disorders clinic
AIDS-dementia complex
average daily consumption

AdC adrenal cortex

ADCC adult day-care center
antibody-dependent cell cytotoxicity
antibody-dependent cell-mediated cytotoxicity
antibody-dependent cellular cytotoxicity

ADD adenosine deaminase deficiency
ampulla of deferent duct
attention deficit disorder
autosomal dominant disease
autosomal dominant disorder
average daily dose

A&DD alcohol and drug dependence

add adduction

add. *adde* [Latin] add

ADDH attention deficit disorder with hyperactivity

addict addiction

ADDM adjustment disorder with depressed mood

add poll adductor pollicis (muscle)

ADDS American Digestive Disease Society

ADDU alcohol and drug dependency unit

ADE absorption, distribution, and elimination
acute disseminated encephalitis
adrenalectomized
adverse drug event
audible Doppler enhancer

A-delta small-diameter myelinated axons

ADEM acute disseminating encephalomyelitis

adeno CA
adenocarcinoma (carcinoma derived from glandular tissue)

adeq adequate

ADG atrial diastolic gallop

ADGP albumin-dextrose-gelatin phosphate

ADH alcohol dehydrogenase (acetaldehyde reductase)
antidiuretic hormone (vasopressin)
arterial diastolic hypertension

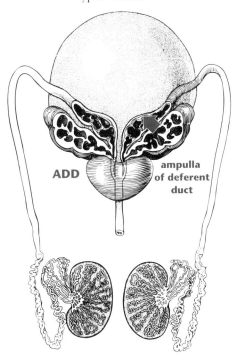

ADD   **ampulla of deferent duct**

atypical ductal hyperplasia
ADHD attention deficit
   hyperactivity disorder
ADI acceptable daily intake
   acetabular depth index
   allowable daily intake
   American Drug Index
   atlantodental interval
      (space between the back
      surface of the anterior
      arch of the 1st cervical
      vertebra and the front
      surface of the odontoid
      process of the 2nd
      cervical vertebra)
adj adjoining
ADL activities of daily living
ad. lib. *ad libitum* [Latin]
   as desired
ADM Adriamycin (doxorubicin)
   admission
AdM adrenal medulla
adm admission
ADMA aldehyde dimethyl acetate
adm Dr admitting doctor
ADME absorption, distribution,
   metabolism, and
   excretion (of a
   substance)
Admin administration
adm MD admitting physician
ADN autonomous diabetic
   nephropathy
ADN-Aase B
   antideoxyribonuclease B
ad naus. *ad nauseam* [Latin] to the
   level of producing nausea
ADO apnoic diffusion
   oxygenation
Ado adenosine (a nucleoside)
AdOAP Adriamycin (doxorubicin)
   + Oncovin (vincristine) +
   ARA-C (cytarabine) +
   prednisone (combination
   chemotherapy)
ADOD arthrodentosteodysplasia
ADODM adult-onset diabetes
   mellitus
adol adolescent

ADP acute demyelinating
   polyneuropathy
   adenosine diphosphate (a
   nucleotide)
   approved drug product
   automatic data processing
ad part. dolent.
   ad partes dolentes [Latin] to
   the painful area
ADPase adenosine diphosphatase
ADPG adenosine diphosphate
   glucose
ADPKD autosomal dominant
   polycystic kidney disease
ADPL average daily patient load
ADPR adenosine diphosphate
   ribose
ADPRT ADP-ribosyl transferase
ADQ abductor digiti quinti
   (abductor digiti minimi)
   (muscle)
adq adequate
ADR acquired drug resistance
   acute dystonic reaction
   Adriamycin (doxorubicin;
   antineoplastic agent)
   adverse drug reaction
   allergic drug reaction
   ataxia-deafness-retardation
   (syndrome)
adr adrenalin (epinephrine)
ADRDA Alzheimer's Disease and
   Related Disorders
   Association
   (800) 621-0379
ADRRS adverse drug reaction
   reporting system
ADS acute death syndrome
   acute diarrheal syndrome
   alcohol dependence scale
   alpha-delta sleep
   alternate delivery system
   anonymous donor's sperm
   antibody deficiency
   syndrome
   antidiuretic substance
   apnea during sleep
ad sat. *ad saturandum* [Latin]
   to saturation

ADSD alcohol-dependent sleep
disorder
arthritis-dermatitis
syndrome
ADST alternate-day steroid
therapy
adst. feb.
adstante febre [Latin] when
fever is present
ADT adenosine triphosphate
admission-discharge-
transfer
agar-gel diffusion test
alternate-day treatment
American dog tick
(*Dermacentor variabilis*)
anterior drawer test
anticipate discharge
tomorrow
any darn thing (a placebo
used during a random
controlled trial)
auditory discrimination
test
A. duodenale
Ancylostoma duodenale
(hookworm that attaches
to small bowel mucosa)

A.duodenale

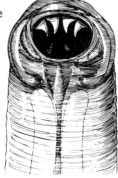

*Ancylostoma
duodenale*

ad us. *ad usum* [Latin] according
to custom
ad us. ext.
ad usum externum [Latin]
for external use
ADV adenovirus (worldwide
virus causing disease,
especially of the upper
respiratory tract)
adventitia (loose,
outermost layer of an
organ; tunica adventitia)
ADW assault with a deadly
weapon
A5D5W water solution with 5%
alcohol + 5% dextrose
ADWD Adams de Weese device
ADX acetyldigoxin
adrenalectomized
audiological diagnosis
AE above elbow (said of
amputations and
prostheses)
active euthanasia
active exercise
acute exacerbation
adverse effects
adverse event
agar-gel electrophoresis
air embolism
antiembolitic
antiepileptic
asteatotic eczema
atheroembolism
AEA above elbow amputation
alcohol, ether, and acetone
anti-endomysium antibody
anti-estrogenic agent (e.g.,
Tamoxifen)
AEB acute erythroblastopenia
as evidenced by
atrial ectopic beat
AEC at earliest convenience
Atomic Energy
Commission
AECB acute exacerbations of
chronic bronchitis
AECD allergic eczematous contact
dermatitis
AECG ambulatory
electrocardiography
AED antiepileptic drug
automated external
defibrillator
AEDH acute epidural hematoma
AEDP automated external

defibrillator pacemaker

AEE acute allergic encephalitis

AEF allogenic effector factor

amyloid enhancing factor

aortoenteric fistula

AEG air encephalogram

air encephalography

AEH adynamic episodica
hereditaria

AEL acute erythroblastic
leukemia

AELs attached ear lobes

AEMIS Aerospace and
Environmental Medical
Information System

AEN aseptic epiphyseal necrosis

AEP acute edematous
pancreatitis

auditory evoked potential

autonomous erythroid
proliferation

AEq age equivalent

aeq. *aequales* [Latin] equal

AER albumin excretion rate

aldosterone excretion rate

auditory evoked response

average evoked response

Aer M aerosol mask

AERP atrial excitation
repolarization phase

AERT auditory evoked response
test

Aer T aerosol tent

AES American
Electroencephalographic
Society

American Endocrine
Society

American Epilepsy Society

American Equilibration
Society

antiembolic stockings

aortic ejection sound

auger electron
spectroscopy

autoerythrocyte sensitivity
(Gardner-Diamond
syndrome)

AET antiestrogen therapy

atrial ectopic tachycardia

AEV avian erythroblastosis virus

AEW African eye worm

AF abnormal frequency

acanthosis factor

acetabular fossa

acid-fast

adult female

afebrile

age factor

amniotic fluid

anal fissure

angiogenesis factor

annulus fibrosus

anterior fontanel

antifibrinogen

aortic flow

Arthritis Foundation

Asian female

athlete's foot (tinea pedis)

atrial fibrillation

atrial flutter

AF

**atrial
flutter**

attributable fraction

attributable fraction for
covariates

audio frequency

avulsion fracture

axillary fossa (axilla;
armpit)

AFA American Fracture
Association

antifungal agent

AFAFP amniotic fluid alpha-
fetoprotein

AFB acid-fast bacilli

acid-fast bacteria

air fluidized bed

American Foundation for
the Blind (800) 232-5463

aortofemoral bypass (in
treatment of aortoiliac
occlusive disease)

	aspirated foreign body
AFBG	aortofemoral bypass graft
AFC	Adriamycin (doxorubicin) + 5-fluorouracil + cyclophosphamide (combination chemotherapy)
	air-filled cystogram
	antibody forming cells
AFCI	acute focal cerebral ischemia
AFCR	American Federation for Clinical Research
AFCs	antibody-forming cells (functionally same as plasma cells)
AFDC	Aid to Families with Dependent Children
AFE	amniotic fluid embolism
afeb	afebrile (without fever)
AFF	Aerobics and Fitness Foundation
aff	afferent (conveying a fluid or a nerve impluse toward a center)
AFG	amniotic fluid glucose
AFI	acute febrile illness
	amaurotic familial idiocy
	amniotic fluid index
	atrial filling index
AFIB	atrial fibrillation
AFib	atrial fibrillation
AFIBF	atrial fibrillation and flutter
AFIP	Armed Forces Institute of Pathology
AFIS	amniotic fluid infection syndrome
AFKO	ankle-foot-knee orthosis
AFL	acute fatty liver
	air-fluid level
	antifibrinolysin
	artificial limb
	atrial flutter
AFLNH	angiofollicular lymph node hyperplasia
AFLP	acute fatty liver of pregnancy
AFM	Academy of Family

AG

adrenal gland

	Mediators
	aerosol face mask
	atomic force microscope
	Austin Flint murmur
AFND	acute febril neutrophilic dermatosis (Sweet's syndrome)
AFO	ankle-foot orthosis
AFOU	anteflexion of uterus
AFP	acute febrile polyneuritis
	acute flaccid paralysis
	alpha-fetoprotein
	atypical facial pain
AfP	affiliate physician
AFP-MS	alpha fetoprotein maternal serum
AFPP	acute fibropurulent pneumonia
AFP-T	alpha fetoprotein tumor
AFRD	acute febrile respiratory disease
AFRI	acute febrile respiratory illness
AFS	American Fertility Society
	atomic fluorescence spectroscopy
AFSP	acute fibrinoserous pneumonia
AFT	antigen fixation test
AFTA	American Family Therapy Association
AFV	amniotic fluid volume
AFVSS	afebrile, vital signs stable
AFX	atypical fibroxanthoma

AG abdominal girth
acute gastritis
adrenal gland
(suprarenal gland)
antiglobulin
antigravity
apocrine glands (glands
producing secretions that
contain part of the
secreting cells)
atrial gallop

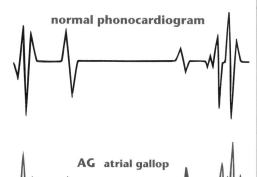

normal phonocardiogram

AG atrial gallop

audiogram
A/G albumin/globulin ratio
Ag antigen (a foreign
substance that stimulates
an immune response)
silver (metallic element)
AGA accelerated growth area
acute gonococcal arthritis
acute gouty arthritis
afferent glomerular
arteriole
American Geriatrics
Association
appropriate for gestational
age
AGAB aminoglycoside antibiotics
AGAG acidic glycosaminoglycans
AGBAD Alexander Graham Bell
Association for the Deaf
AGC absolute granulocyte count

adherence glycoprotein
complex
anatomic graduated
components
automatic gain control
AGCSP anterior gray column of
spinal cord
AGD adiposogenital dystrophy
agar gel diffusion
antigenic determinants
(epitopes)
AGE acute gastroenteritis
advanced glycation end
(product)
angle of greatest extension
AGEPC acetly glyceryl ether
phosphoryl choline
AGEs advanced glycation
endproducts
advanced glycosylation
endproducts
AGF adrenal growth factor
angle of greatest flexion
anti-gammaglobulin factor
AGG agammaglobulinemia (lack
of all classes of immuno-
globulins in the blood)
anti-gammaglobulin
AGGS anti-gas gangrene serum
AGI alpha-glucosidase inhibitor
agit. ante sum.
agita ante sumendum [Latin]
shake before taking
agit. bene
agita bene [Latin]
shake well
AGL acute granulocytic
leukemia
AGM antigenic modulation
AGN acute glomerulonephritis
AGNB anaerobic gram-negative
bacilli
AgNO$_3$ silver nitrate (a caustic
applied topically after
dipping in water)
AGP alkaline granulocyte
phosphatase
AGPA American Group Practice
Association

A/G R	albumin-globulin ratio
A/G ratio	albumin-globulin ratio
AGS	absorbable gelatin sponge (Gelfoam)
	adiposogenital syndrome
	adrenogenital syndrome (appearance of secondary male sex characteristics in the female resulting from adrenal hyperfunction)
	aminoglycoside (an antibiotic that inhibits protein synthesis)
AGT	abnormal glucose tolerance
	antiglobulin test (Coombs)
agt	agent
AGTH	adrenoglomerulotrophic hormone
AGTT	abnormal glucose tolerance test
AGU	aspartylglucosaminuria
AGV	aniline gentian violet
AGVHD	acute graft-versus-host disease (wasting disease)
AH	abdominal herniorrhaphy
	abdominal hysterectomy
	abductor hallucis (muscle)
	absolute humidity
	Access for the Handicapped
	accidental hemorrhage
	acetylhydrolase
	Aeromonas hydrophila
	alcoholic hepatitis
	alveolar hemorrhage
	aminohippurate
	antihyaluronidase
	anxiety hysteria
	aqueous humor (the watery fluid occupying the anterior and posterior chambers of the eye)
	arterial hypertension
	artificial heart
	autonomic hyperreflexia
	axillary hair
A & H	amenorrhea and hirsutism

ah	hyperopic astigmatism
AHA	acetohydroxamic acid (Lithostat; a bacterial enzyme blocker)
	acquired hemolytic anemia
	acute hemolytic anemia
	American Heart Association
	American Hospital Association
	arthritis, hives, and angioedema (syndrome)
	aspartyl-hydroxamic acid
	autoimmune hemolytic anemia
AHAb	alcoholic hyalin antibody
	antihemagglutinin antibody
AHAg	alcoholic hyalin antigen
AHARD	acute hantavirus-associated respiratory disease
AHB	alpha-hydroxybutyric acid
AHBc	hepatitis B core antibody
AHC	academic health center
	acute hemorrhagic conjunctivitis
	acute hemorrhagic cystitis
	anterior horn cell
	antihemophilic factor C
AHCDs	alpha heavy chain diseases

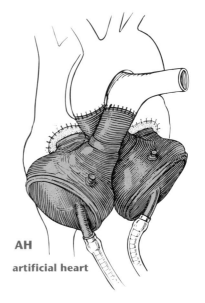

AH

artificial heart

23

AHCPR   Agency for Health Care
Policy and Research

AHD   acquired heart disease
acute heart disease
adrenocorticotropic
hormone deficiency
antihyaluronidase
antihypertensive drug
arteriosclerotic heart
disease
autoimmune hemolytic
disease

AHE   acute hypertensive
encephalopathy

AHF   acute heart failure
American Hepatic
Foundation
antihemophilic factor
Argentine hemorrhagic
fever

AHFS   American Hospital
Formulary Service

AHG   aggregated human
globulin
aluminum hydroxide gel
antihemophilic globulin
antihuman globulin
ataxia-hypogonadism
syndrome

AHGS   acute herpetic gingival
stomatitis
antihuman globulin serum

AHH   adenohypophyseal
hormone
anosmia and
hypogonadotropic
hypogonadism
(syndrome)
aryl-hydrocarbon
hydroxylase

AHHD   arteriosclerotic hypertensive heart disease

AHI   apnea-hypopnea index

AHJ   artificial hip joint

AHL   acute hemorrhagic
leukoencephalitis
apparent half-life
Asbestos Hotline
(800) 334-8571

AHLD   aspergillus hypersensitivity
lung disease

AHLE   acute hemorrhagic
leukoencephalitis

AHLG   antihuman lymphocyte
globulin

AHM   adductor hallucis muscle

AHMA   American Holistic Medical
Association

AHN   adenomatous hyperplastic
nodule

AHO   Albright's hereditary
osteodystrophy

AHOM   acute hematogenousosteo-
myelitis

AHP   acute hallucinatory
paranoia
acute hemorrhagic
pancreatitis

AHR   antihyaluronidase reaction
Association for Health
Records

AHRF   American Hearing
Research Foundation

AHS   American Hearing Society

AHSC   anterior horn of spinal
cord

AHT   antihyaluronidase test/titer

AHTG   antihuman thymocyte
globulin

AHU   arginine, hypoxanthine
and uracil

AI   abdominal irradiation
accidental injury
adhesion index
adrenal insufficiency
alcoholic intoxication
allergy index
alternating isometrics
anaphylatoxin inhibitor
anterior-inferior
aortic incompetence
aortic insufficiency
arbovirus infection
articulation index
artificial insemination
artificial intelligence
autoinfection (infection by
a pathogen already

present in the body)

A & I allergy and immunology

AIA allergen-induced asthma
allyl-isopropyl acetamide
anti-insulin antibody
aspirin-induced asthma

AIBA aminoisobutyric acid

AIBS American Institute of
Biologic Sciences

AIC aminoimidazole-
carboxamide
antigen-
immunosuppressive
conjugate
Arthritis Information
Clearinghouse
(703) 558-8250
autologous immune
complex

AICA anterior inferior cerebellar
artery
anterior inferior
communicating artery

AICAR aminoimidazole
carboxamide
ribonucleotide

AICD acute irritant contact
dermatitis
autologous immune
complex disease
automatic implantable
cardioverter defibrillator

AICF auto-immune complement
fixation

AICR American Institute for
Cancer Research

AID acute infantile diarrhea
acute infectious disease
Agency for International
Development
antigen-independent
determinants
anti-inflammatory drug
artificial insemination by
donor
autoimmune deficiency
autoimmune disease (a
disease resulting from an
immune response

directed against self
antigens)
automatic implantable
defibrillator

AIDH artificial insemination,
donor husband

AI(DO) artificial insemination
(with donated oocyte)

AIDP acute inflammatory
demyelinating
polyneuritis

AIDS acquired immune
deficiency syndrome

AIDS IH AIDS Information Hotline
(800) 342-AIDS

AIDSKS AIDS with Kaposi's
sarcoma

AIDSLINE
acquired
immunodeficiency
syndrome, information
online

AIE acute infectious
encephalitis
acute infective endocarditis

AIF anti-inflammatory

AIFD acute intrapartum fetal
distress

AIG anti-immunoglobulin

AIH alcohol-induced
hypoglycemia
artificial insemination by
husband (homologous
insemination)
autoimmune hemolytic
anemia

AIHA American Industrial
Hygiene Association
autoimmune hemolytic
anemia

AIHD acquired immune
hemolytic disease

AII acute intestinal infection

AIIS anterior inferior iliac spine

AIL acute infectious
lymphocytosis
angio-immunoblastic
lymphadenopathy

AILD alveolar interstitial

lung disease
angioimmunoblastic
lymphadenopathy with
dysproteinemia

AIM *Abridged Index Medicus*
Annals of Internal Medicine
Archives of Internal Medicine
artificial intelligence in
medicine

AIMs abnormal involuntary
movements

AIMS abnormal involuntary
movement scale

AIN acute interstitial nephritis

AINS anti-inflammatory nonsteroidal

AINT anterior internodal tract
(between S-A node and
A-V node)

AIO abdominal incontinence
operation

AIOD aortoiliac occlusive disease

AION anterior ischemic optic
neuropathy

AIP acute inflammatory
polyneuropathy
acute intermittent
porphyria
acute interstitial
pneumonia

AIPO acute intestinal
pseudoobstruction
(Ogilvie's syndrome)

AIR amino-imidazole
ribonucleotide

AIS abbreviated injury scale
abbreviated injury severity
(score)
adenocarcinoma *in situ*
adolescent idiopathic
scoliosis
androgen insensitivity
syndrome

AIS-C androgen insensitivity
syndrome, complete

AIS-I androgen insensitivity
syndrome, incomplete

AISM artificial insemination of
surrogate mother

AIT acute intensive treatment
allergy immunotherapy

AITN acute interstitial tubular
nephritis

AITP acute idiopathic
thrombocytopenic
purpura

AIU absolute iodine uptake

AIUM American Institute of
Ultrasound in Medicine

AIVDB anterior interventricular
descending branch (of
coronary artery)

AIVR accelerated idioventricular
rhythm

AJ ankle jerk (Achilles jerk;
reflex test)

AJAO American Juvenile Arthritis
Organization

AJC acrylic jacket crown

AJCC American Joint Committee
on Cancer

AJCCS American Joint Committee
for Cancer Staging

AJMC *American Journal of*
Managed Care

AJPH *American Journal of Public*
Health

AJR abdomino–jugular reflex
abnormal jugular reflex

AK above knee (said of
amputations or
prostheses)
acetate kinase
actinic keratosis (senile
keratosis)
Addison keloid
adenylate kinase
angiokeratoma
arsenical keratosis
(keratosis resulting from
prolonged arsenic
poisoning)
artificial kidney
astigmatic keratotomy
(corneal surgery for
vision correction)

AKA above-the-knee amputation
alcoholic ketoacidosis

aka	also known as
AKF	American Kidney Fund
AKPS	anterior knee pain syndrome
AKS	alcoholic Korsakoff syndrome
	arthroscopic knee surgery
AL	abdominal laparotomy
	acute laryngitis
	acute leukemia
	argon laser (used for photocoagulation)
	arrested labor
	immunologic amyloid
Al	aluminum
ALA	aerobic lung abscess
	amebic liver abscess
	American Laryngological Association
	American Lung Association
	aminolevulinic acid
	anti-lymphocyte antibody
Ala	alanine (amino acid)
AL-Anon	Alcoholic Anonymous
ALARA	as low as reasonably achievable
ALAT	AlaSTAT latex allergy test
alb	albumin
ALC	alcoholic liver cirrhosis

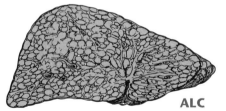

ALC
alcoholic liver cirrhosis

	alternative lifestyle checklist
	approximate lethal concentration
alc	alcohol
	alcoholic
AlcR	alcohol rub
ALD	adrenoleukodystrophy
	alcoholic liver disease

	aldolase (an enzyme)
	assistive listening device
ALDF	American Lyme Disease Foundation
ALDH	aldehyde dehydrogenase
ALD-L	liver aldolase
ALD-M	muscle aldolase
ALDOST	aldosterone (a potent electrolyte-regulating hormone)
ALE	active life expectancy
	allowable limits of error
ALEC	artificial lung expanding compound
ALF	American Liver Foundation
ALFs	assisted living facilities
ALG	antilymphocyte globulin
ALH	angiolymphoid hyperplasia
	anterior lobe of hypophysis

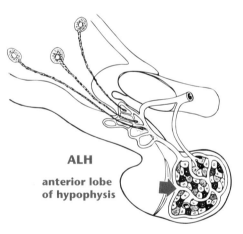

ALH

anterior lobe of hypophysis

A-line	arterial line
ALI	acute lung injury
	anterolateral infarct (heart infarction due to occlusion of the anterior interventricular branch of the left coronary artery)
	argon laser iridotomy
ALK	alkaline
	avian leukosis virus keratomileusis

alk alkaline
alk p'tase alkaline phosphatase
ALL acute lymphatic leukemia
acute lymphoblastic
leukemia
acute lymphocytic
leukemia
allorhythmia (recurring
irregularity in the heart
rhythm)
anterior longitudinal
ligament

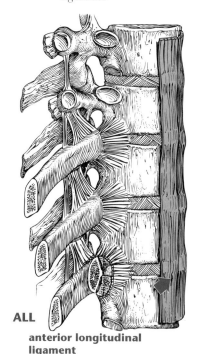

ALL
**anterior longitudinal
ligament**

ALLA acute lymphocytic
leukemia antigen
ALM acral lentiginous
melanoma
acrolentiginous melanoma
adductor longus muscle
ALMI anterior lateral myocardial
infarct
ALN aortic lymph node
axillary lymph node
ALNC axillary lymph node
carcinoma

ALND axillary lymph node
dissection
Al(OH)$_3$ aluminum hydroxide
ALOS average length of stay
ALP acute lupus pericarditis
alkaline leukocyte
phosphatase
allopurinol (reduces
urinary excretion of uric
acid)
alveolar lung proteinosis
anterior lobe of pituitary
apolipoproteins
argon laser
photocoagulation
ALPC argon laser
photocoagulation
ALPE apolipoprotein E
ALPS angiolymphoproliferative
syndrome
anterior locking plate
system
Aphasia Language
Performance Scale
ALPSA anterior labrum
periosteum shoulder
arthroscopic (lesion)
ALR agglutination lysis reaction
annular ligament of radius
arterial light reflex
ALRI acute lower-respiratory-
tract infection
anterolateral rotatory
instability
ALROS American Laryngological,
Rhinological, and
Otological Society
ALS acute lateral sclerosis
advanced life support
afferent loop syndrome
amyotrophic lateral
sclerosis (Lou
Gehrig's disease)
angiotensin-like substance
anticipated life span
antilymphocytic serum
ALSA Amyotrophic Lateral
Sclerosis Association
ALSCD ampulla of lateral

semicircular duct

ALSD adult lipid storage disease

Alzheimer-like senile dementia

ALT acid-loading test

alanine aminotransferase (alanine transaminase; formerly GPT)

argon laser trabeculoplasty

ALTB acute laryngotracheobronchitis

alt.dieb. *alternis diebus* [Latin] every other day

ALTE apparent life-threatening event

alt.hor. *alternis horis* [Latin] every other hour

alt.noct. *alternis noctis* [Latin] every other night

ALTP argon laser trabeculoplasty

ALTS acute lumbar traumatic sprain

A. lumbricoides

Ascaris lumbricoides (largest intestinal nematode parasite)

ALV adeno-like virus

ALZ Alzheimer's disease

AM achievement motivation

actinomycosis

actomyosin

adolescent medicine

adult male

alcoholic myopathy

alternative medicine

alveolar macrophage

amalgam (an alloy of mercury and other metals)

ammoniated mercury

anovular menstruation

apomorphine

arterial mean

Asian male

atrial myxoma

augmentation mammaplasty

aviation medicine

myopic astigmatism

Am americium (artificial trans-uranic clement)

aM atypical mycobacteriosis

am myopic astigmatism

ametropia

a.m. *ante meridiem* [Latin] before noon; morning

ante mortem [Latin] prior to death

AMA acute metabolic acidosis

against medical advice (usually, self-discharge from hospital without physician's approval)

American Medical Association

antibasement membrane antibody

antimalarial agent

antimitochondrial antibodies

AMA-DE *American Medical Association Drug Evaluation*

amal amalgam (filling)

AMAP as much as possible

AMAs antimicrobial agents

AMAT antimalignant antibody test

AMB as manifested by

amb ambulatory

AMBA antimycobacterial agent

ambig ambiguous

AMBL acute megakaryoblastic leukemia

ambul ambulatory

AMC academic medical center

acute myocardial (infarction)

antibody-mediated cytotoxicity

arthrogryposis multiplex congenita

AMCI acute meningococcal infection

acute myocardial infarction

AMD acid maltase disorder (type II glycogenosis)

age-related macular degeneration

alpha methyldopa

American Medical Directory

arthroscopic micro-
diskectomy
Association for Macular
Diseases

AMDGF alveolar macrophage-
derived growth factor

amDNA antimessenger DNA

AME amebic
meningoencephalitis
amphotericin methyl ester
aseptic
meningoencephalitis

AMEA American Medical
Electroencephalographic
Association

AMegL acute megokaryoblastic
leukemia

Amer J Med
American Journal of Medicine

Amer J Radiol
*American Journal of
Radiology*

AMESLAN
American sign language

AMF acute mallet finger
Asian, middle-aged female

AmFAR American Foundation for
AIDS research
aminoglycoside (an
antibiotic that inhibits
protein synthesis)

A2MG alpha-2-macroglobulin

AMH acute migraine headache
anti-mullerian hormone
(prevents uterine
development in
the male)

AMHF American Mental Health
Fund

AMI acquired monosaccharide
intolerance
acute myocardial infarction
Advancement of Medical
Instrumentation
amitriptyline
(antidepressant)
anterior myocardial
infarction

AMIA American Medical

Informatics Association

AMJA American Medical Joggers
Association

AMKL acute megakaryoblastic
leukemia

AML acute monocytic leukemia
acute myeloblastic
leukemia
acute myelocytic leukemia
acute myelogenous
leukemia
acute myeloid leukemia
angiomyolipoma (a
hamartoma containing
vascular, adipose, and
muscle elements)
anterior mitral leaflet

AMM adductor magnus muscle
agnogenic myeloid
metaplasia
Asian, middle-aged male

AMMBL acute myelomonoblastic
leukemia

AMML acute myelomonocytic
leukemia

AMMMF agnogenic myeloid
metaplasia with
myelofibrosis

AMN adrenomyeloneuropathy

AMN FS amniotic fluid scan

amnio amniocentesis

AMO ammoniated mercury
ointment

AMOL acute monoblastic
leukemia
acute monocytic leukemia

AMP ACV (acyclovir)-5-
monophosphate
acid mucopolysaccharide
adenosine monophosphate
amniotic membrane
perforator
amphetamine
amputation
Austin-Moore prosthesis
average mean pressure

3'5'-AMP cyclic adenosine
monophosphate
cyclic AMP

Amp ampicillin

amp   ampere (A is preferred)
ampule (ampul; small glass
   container sealed to
   preserve the sterile
   condition of its contents)
amputation
AMP-c   cyclic adenosine
   monophosphate
amphet   amphetamine (speed; any
   of a group of synthetic
   chemicals that stimulate
   the central nervous
   system)
AMPRA   American Medical Peer
   Review Association
AMPS   acid mucopolysaccharide
AMPT   alphamethylpara tyrosine
   (metyrosine; an
   antihypertensive agent)
ampul   ampule (ampul; small glass
   container sealed to
   preserve the sterile
   condition of its contents)
AMRA   American Medical Records
   Association
AMRL   Aerospace Medical
   Research Laboratories
AMRN   American Medical Radio
   News
AMRS   automated medical record
   system
AMS   acute mountain sickness
antimacrophage serum
aseptic meningitis
   syndrome
atypical measles syndrome
auditory memory span
AMSA   American Medical
   Students Association
AMSIT   part of the mental status
   examination (A = appearance; M = mood; S = sen-
   sorium; I = intelligence;
   T = thought process)
AMSSO   anterior mandibular
   subapical segmental
   osteotomy
AMST   antimicrobial susceptibility
   test

AMT   alpha-methyltyrosine
American Medical
   Technologists
antimicrobial therapy
amt   amount
amu   atomic mass unit
AMV   assisted mechanical
   ventilation
assisted mechanical
   ventilator
AMVI   acute mesenteric vascular
   insufficiency
AMVL   anterior mitral (right
   atrioventricular) valve
   leaflet
AMWA   American Medical
   Women's Association
American Medical Writers
   Association
AMWS   American Men and
   Women of Science
AMX   amoxicillin (a
   semisynthetic derivative
   of ampicillin)
AMY   amylase (an enzyme of the
   hydrolase class secreted
   by the salivary glands and
   pancreas)
AMZ   astemizole (second-
   generation
   antihistamine)
AN   abducent nerve (6th
   cranial nerve)
acanthosis nigricans
   (diffuse thickening of the
   prickle-cell layer of the
   skin with brownish-black
   pigmentation, generally
   seen in the axillae)
accessory nerve (11th
   cranial nerve)
acne neonatorum
   (infantile acne)
acoustic neuroma (acoustic
   neurilemoma)
acute nephritis
afferent nerve
alkaptonuria
   (homogentisuria)

amyl nitrite (inhaled to relieve pain in angina pectoris)
anesthesia
aneurysm
anode
anorexia nervosa
anxiety neurosis
aseptic necrosis
ataxic nystagmus
attributable number
autonomic neuropathy
avascular necrosis
axillary node
axonal neuropathy

An actinon
(old name for radon-219)
anodal
anode (positive electrode)

ANA absolute neutrophil count
acetylneuraminic acid
alanine beta-naphthylamide
American Narcolepsy Association
American Neurological Association
American Nurses' Association
antineoplastic agent
antineutrophil cytoplasmic antibody
antinuclear antibody

ANAD anorexia nervosa and associated disorders

ANADase antinicotinyl adenine dinucleotidase

ANAG acute narrow angle glaucoma

anal analgesia
analgesic
analysis

ANB avascular necrosis of bone

ANC absolute neutrophil count
acid-neutralizing capacity
antigen-neutralizing capacity

ANCA antineutrophil cytoplasmic antibody

ANCOVA (one-way) analysis of covariance

AND anterior nasal discharge
axillary node dissection

ANDA abbreviated new drug application

Andro androsterone (a male sex hormone derived from testosterone metabolism)

ANE angioneurotic edema (acute, transient edema of skin or mucous membranes, especially of the throat)

Anes anesthesia

ANF antinuclear factor (factor directed against nuclear antigens)
atrial natriuretic factor

ANFF antinuclear fluorescent factor

ANG acute necrotizing gingivitis
angiogram (an x-ray film of blood vessels containing contrast medium)

Angio angiogram (an x-ray film of blood vessels containing contrast medium)

ang pect angina pectoris

ANHE acute necrotizing hemorrhagic encephalopathy

ANI acute nerve irritation
axillary nodal irradiation

ANIS Anorexia Nervosa Inventory (self-rating)

ank ankle

ANL all-or-none law

ANLL acute nonlymphoblastic leukemia
acute nonlymphoid leukemia
acute nonlymphocytic leukemia

ann fib annulus fibrosus (anulus fibrosus; the ringlike portion of the intervertebral disk)

ANOV	analysis of variance
ANOVA	analysis of variance
ANP	acute necrotzing pancreatitis
	A-norprogesterone
	atrial natriuretic peptide
ANS	acute nephritic syndrome
	American Nutrition Society
	answer
	anterior nasal spine

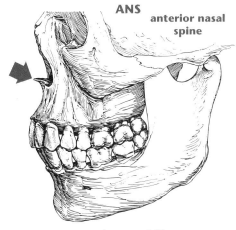

ANS **anterior nasal spine**

antineutrophilic serum
arteriolar nephrosclerosis
asymptomatic

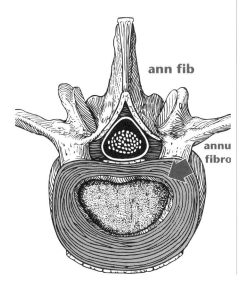

ann fib

annu fibro

neurosyphilis

autonomic nervous system

ANSCII	American National Standard Code for Information Interchange
ANSD	autonomic nervous system disorder
	autonomic nervous system dysfunction
ANSI	American National Standards Institute
ANT	acoustic noise test
ant	anterior
antag	antagonist
ante	*ante* [Latin] before
anti-ChE	anticholinesterase
anti-GBM	antiglomerular basement membrane (disease)
anti-HAV	antibody to hepatitis A virus
anti-HBcAg	antibody to hepatitis B core antigen
anti-HBeAg	antibody to hepatitis B e antigen
anti-HBsAg	antibody to hepatitis B surface antigen
anti-P Ab	anti-P antibody (important antibody in reproductive failure)
anti-TPO	antithyroid peroxidase
ant.jentac.	*ante jentaculum* [Latin] before breakfast
ANTR	apparent net transfer rate
ANTU	alpha-naphthylthiourea
ANuA	antinuclear antibody
ANUG	acute necrotizing ulcerative gingivitis (trench mouth)
ANUM	acute necrotizing ulacerative mucositi
anx	anxiety
AO	abdominal aorta
	Agent Orange (herbicide)
	airway obstruction

	ankle orthosis
	anodal opening
	anovulation (cessation of ovulation)
	antioxidants (a substance that interferes with or prevents oxidation)
	aorta
	aortic opening
Ao	aorta
A & O	alert and oriented
A & O x3	alert and oriented to person, place and time
Ao	aorta
AOA	Administration on Aging
	American Optometric Association
	American Orthopaedic Association
	American Osteopathic Association
	anterior osseous ampulla
	arch of aorta
AOAA	amino-oxyacetic acid
AOAC	arthroper oblong acetabular cup
AOAP	as often as possible
AOB	alcohol on breath
AoBC	aortic blood pressure
AOBS	acute organic brain syndrome
AOC	American Orthoptic Council
	anodal opening contraction
	area of concern
AOCA	American Osteopathic College of Anesthesiologists
AOCD	American Osteopathic College of Dermatology
	anemia of chronic disease
AOCPA	American Osteopathic College of Pathologists
AOCR	American Osteopathic College of Radiology
AOD	adult-onset diabetes
	alcohol and other drug

	alleged onset date (for Social Security disability claim)
	anti-obesity drug
	arterial occlusive disease
	arteriosclerotic occlusive disease
	auriculo-osteodysplasia
AODA	alcohol and other drug abuse
AODM	adult onset diabetes mellitus
AoE	aortic enlargement
AOF	American Optometric Foundation
AOFP	atypical orofacial pain (oral complaint syndrome)
AoG	aortography
AOHS	angio-osteohypertrophy syndrome
AOI	apnea of infancy
AOL	acro-osteolysis
	angle of Lewis (at manubriosternal junction)
	atlanto-occipital ligament
AOM	acute osteomyelitis
	acute otitis media
AOMA	American Occupational Medical Association
AoMP	aortic mean pressure
AON	acute optic neuritis
	all-or-none (law)
AOO	acute outflow obstruction
	age of onset
AOP	adiposity-oligomenorrhea-parotid swelling (syndrome)
	apnea of prematurity
AoP	aortic pressure
AOPA	American Orthotics and Prosthetics Association
AOR	at own risk
	auditory oculogyric reflex
AORN	Association of Operating Room Nurses
AOS	acridine orange stain
	ambulatory

outpatient surgery

American Ophthalmological Society

American Otological Society (Inc)

anodal opening sound

AOSC acute obstructive suppurative cholangitis

AOSD adult-onset Still's disease

AOSSM American Orthopedic Society for Sports Medicine

AoSt aortic stenosis

AOT Association of Ocupational Therapists

AOTA Amerian Occupational Therapy Association

analysis of variance

AOV ampulla of Vater (greater papilla; short dilated tube formed by the union of the pancreatic and bile ducts just before they empty into the duodenum)

AoV aortic valve

AOVM angiography occult vascular malformation

AOW admitted from other ward

AP abdominal pregnancy

abruptio placentae (premature detachment of a normally affixed placenta)

acid phosphatase

action potential

acute pain

acute pancreatitis

acute panniculitis (nodular fat nccrosis)

acute peritonitis

acute parotitis

acute pneumonia

adenomatous polyp

adenomatous polyposis

adolescent pregnancy

air pollution

alkaline phosphatase

Alliston procedure (to correct gastroesophageal reflux)

Altemeier's procedure (to correct rectal prolapse)

Amanita phalloides

amylopectinosis

anaphylactic purpura

angina pectoris (suppressive chest pain resulting from inadequate blood supply to the heart muscle)

antepartum

anterior pituitary

anterior-posterior

anteroposterior (view)

anterior pituitary

antiperspirant (aluminum chlorohydrate)

appendectomy

appendicitis

appendix

arterial pressure

artificial pneumothorax

Arum pin (to treat Colles' fracture)

aspiration pneumonia

atherosclerotic plaque

auditory performance

auditory prosthesis

Auerbach's plexus

A.P. *accouchement premature* [French] premature birth

A & P adoption and parenting

anxiety and palpitation

atelectasia and pneumonia

auscultation and palpation

auscultation and percussion

A-P antero-posterior (x-ray)

A-5-P adenosine-5-phosphate

Ap angina pectoris

a.p. *ante partum* [Latin] before delivery

ante prandium [Latin] before dinner

APA acute parenteral alimentation

aldosterone-producing

adenoma

American Pancreatic
Association

American Paralysis
Association

American Pharmaceutical
Association

American Podiatric
Association

American Psychiatric
Association

American Psychoanalytic
Association

American Psychological
Association

antipernicious anemia
(factor)

antiphospholipid antibody

antipyretic-analgesics

ascending pharyngeal
artery

APAA aldosterone-producing
adrenal adenoma

APAb antiplatelet antibody

antithyroid peroxidase
antibody

APACHE Acute Physiology and
Chronic Health
Evaluation (scoring
system)

APAD acetylpyridine-adenine
dinucleotide

APAF antipernicious anemia
factor

APAP acetaminophen (acetyl-
para-aminophenol;
paractamol)

APB abductor pollicis brevis
(muscle)

atrial premature beat

APC abdominal paracentesis

absolute phagocyte count

acetylsalicylic acid
(aspirin), phenacetin,
and caffeine (analgesic
preparation)

activated protein C

acute pericarditis

acute

pharyngoconjunctival
fever

adenomatous polyposis of
colon

airplane cast (shoulder
spica)

anterior polar cataract

antigen-presenting cell
(carries antigen in a form
that can stimulate
lymphocytes)

aspirin, phenacetin and
caffeine

atrial premature complex

atrial premature
contraction

autologous packed cells

APCA Air Pollution Control Act

APC-C acetylsalicylic acid +
phenacetin + caffeine,
with codeine

APCD adult polycystic disease

APCKD adult-type polycystic kidney
disease

APCv adeno-pharyngeal-
conjunctival virus

A-P-C virus

adeno-pharyngeal-
conjunctival virus

APD accessory pancreatic duct

action potential duration

acute polycystic disease

afferent pupillary defect

antiplatelet drug

antisocial personality
disorder

aorto-pulmonary defect

atrial premature
depolarization

autoimmune progesterone
dermatitis

automated peritoneal
dialysis

avoidant personality
disorder

APDC ammonium-pyrrolidone
dithiocarbamate

Anxiety and Panic Disorder
Clinic

APDT	antiplatelet drug therapy
APE	acute polioencephalitis
	acute psychotic episode
	acute pulmonary edema
	aminophylline + phenobarbital + ephedrine
	anteior pituitary extract
APECED	autoimmune polyendocrinopathy-candidiasis-ectodermal dystrophy
APF	anabolism promoting factor
	anterior pillar of fauces
	antiperinuclear factor
APFA	Adult Personality Functioning Assessment (interview)
APG	acute proliferative glomerulonephritis
	aluminum phosphate gel
	anterior pituitary gonadotrophin
	Apgar (score)
APGAR	American Pediatric Gross Assessment Record
APH	antepartum hemorrhage
	anterior pituitary hormone
APh	alkaline phosphatase
Aph	aphasia (language disorder due to brain dysfunction)
APHA	American Public Health Association
APhA	American Pharmaceutical Association
	American Pharmacists Association
API	alkaline protease inhibitor
	arterial pressure index
	Asian/Pacific Islander
	Association for Practitioners of Infection Control
APIE	assessment + plan + implementation + evaluation
APIP	acute postinfectious polyneuropathy

APKD	adult-onset polycystic kidney disease
	adult polycystic kidney disease
APL	abductor pollicis longus (muscle)
	acute promyelocytic leukemia
	anaphylaxis (an immediate, severe hypersensitivity reaction induced by second exposure to a specific antigen)
	anterior pituitary-like (hormone)
APLA	antiphospholipid antibody
APLC	anterior-posterior lower cervical (x-ray view)
APLD	automated percutaneous lumbar diskectomy
APLN	anterior pectoral lymph node
APM	Academy of Physical Medicine
	Academy of Psychosomatic Medicine
	adductor pollicis muscle
	anterior papillary muscle
	Apophysomyces
	aspartame (a nutritive sweetner approximately 180 times sweeter than table sugar)
APm	mean arterial pressure
APMA	American Podiatric Medical Society
APMI	abrupt pacemaker inhibition
APN	acute painful neuropathy
	acute pyelonephritis
	average peak noise
APO	Adriamycin (doxorubicin) + prednisone + Oncovin (vincristine) (combination chemotherapy)
	apomorphine
Apo	apolipoprotein

apoprotein

Apo A-1 apolipoprotein A-1 (a protein constituent of HDL)

Apo A-1 Milano

genetic variation of apolipoprotein A-1

ApoB apolipoprotein B

ApoC apolipoprotein C

ApoD apolipoprotein D

ApoE apolipoprotein E

ApoE2 apolipoprotein E2

ApoE3 apolipoprotein E3

Apo E4 apolipoprotein E4

Apo-Lp apolipoproteins

APORF acute postoperative renal failure

APOs apolipoproteins

APP acute-phase protein

acute purulent pericarditis

Alzheimer precursor protein

amyloid precursor protein

arginine-enriched polypeptide

antiplatelet plasma

arterial pressure pulse

avian pancreatic polypeptide

app apparent

appendix

appr approximate

approx approximate

APPs acute-phase proteins

appt appointment

appx appendix

appy appendectomy

APRD adult polycystic renal disease

AProL acute promyelocytic leukemia

APRT adenine phosphoribosyl-transferase

APRTD adenine phosphoribosyl-transferase deficiency

APS adenosine-phosphosulfate

airplane splint

American Pediatric Society

American Physiological

Society

aminopolystyrene

antiphospholipid syndrome

aortopulmonary shunt

apple peel syndrome

APSA American Pediatric Surgical Association

APSAC anisoylated plasminogen streptokinase activator complex

APSCD ampulla of posterior semicircular duct

APSD Alzheimer's presenile dementia

aorto-pulmonary septal defect

APSGN acute poststreptococcal glomerulonephritis

APSS Association for the Psychophysiological Study of Sleep

APT acid perfusion test

acid phosphatase test

alum-precipitated toxoid

antiplatelet therapy

antipyrine test

APTA American Physical Therapy Association

APS

airplane splint

APTP	angina pectoris-type pain
APTS	acid phosphatase test for semen
aPTT	activated partial thromboplastin time
APU	ambulatory procedure unit
APUD	amine precursor uptake and decarboxylation (by chromaffin cells of the gatrointestinal tract)
APUD cells	amine precursor uptake and decarboxylation cells (secrete hormones)
APVD	acropectorovertebral dysplasia (F syndrome)
APW	alkaline peptone water
AQ	achievement quotient
	any quantity
aq	aqueous
aq.	*aqua* [Latin] water
AQA	Air Quality Act
aq. ad	*aqua ad* [Latin] add water
aq. bull.	*aqua bulliens* [Latin] boiling water
aq. cal.	*aqua calida* [Latin] hot water
AQCESS	automated quality of care evaluation support system
aq. dest.	*aqua destillata* [Latin] distilled water
aq. ferv.	*aqua fervens* [Latin] hot water
aq. frig.	*aqua frigida* [Latin] cold water
AQI	air quality index
aq. tep.	*aqua tepida* [Latin] tepid water
aqu	aqueous
AR	absorption rate
	accelerated reaction
	acne rosacea (chronic inflammatory disorder characterized by papules, pustules, and dilation of capillaries on the middle third of the face)
	active resistive (exercise)
	admitting room

	age regression
	airway resistance
	alarm reaction
	alcohol related
	allergic rhinitis
	anger rape
	antigen receptor
	aortic regurgitation
	artificial respiration
	assisted respiration
	at risk
	atrophic rhinitis
	attributable risk
	autosomal recessive
A & R	advised and released
Ar	argon
ARA	Academy of Rehabilitative Audiometry
	acute respiratory acidosis
	acute respiratory akalosis
	adenosne regulating agent
	American Rehabilitation Association
	American Rheumatism Association
	antiribosomal antibody
	awaiting receipt of application
ARA-A	vidarabine (Vira-A) (adenine arabinoside)
ARA-AC	fazarabine
ARA-C	cytarabine (cytosine arabinoside)
ARA-Hx	arabinosyl hypoxanthine
ARAS	ascending reticular activating system
ARB	adrenergic receptor binder
	antibiotic-resistant bacteria
	anticoagulant-related bleeding
	any reliable brand
ARBA	adrenergic receptor blocking agent
ARBD	alcohol-related birth defects
ARBOR	arthropod-borne (viruses)
ARBOW	artificial rupture of bag of water
ARC	acute rheumatic carditis

age-related cataract
AIDS-related complex
American Red Cross
anomalous retinal
  correspondence
Association for Retarded
  Children

ARCA   acquired red cell anemia
ARD   acute radiation disease
acute renal dysfunction
acute respiratory disease
acute respiratory distress
allergic respiratory disease
altitude-related disorder
anorectal disorders
anti-rejection drug
autosomal recessive disease
autosomal recessive
  disorder

ARDS   acute respiratory distress
  syndrome (shock lung)
adult respiratory distress
  syndrome

ARDs   anti-reflux drugs
ARE   active resistive exercises
amount (of substance) to
  be excreted

ARF   acute renal failure (most
  serious renal disorder)
acute respiratory failure
acute rheumatic fever
Addiction Research
  Foundation

ARG   activin receptor gene
alkaline reflux gastritis
aortorenography
autoradiography

Arg   arginine (amino acid)
ArgP   arginine phosphate
ARI   acute renal insufficiency
acute respiratory infection
acute respiratory
  insufficiency

ARID   AIDS-related immune
  dysfunction

ARIF   arthroscopically-assisted
  reduction and internal
  fixation

Ar ion laser
argon ion laser

ARK   adrenergic receptor kinase
ARL   anorectal line
average remaining lifetime
ARLD   alcohol-related liver
  disease
ARM   anxiety reaction, mild
artificial rupture of (fetal)
  membranes
ARMD   age-related macular
  degeneration
ARMS   adverse reaction
  monitoring system
ARN   acute radiation nephritis
acute retinal necrosis
A RNA S   alternate RNA splicing
ARNS   acute retinal necrosis
  syndrome
AROM   active range of motion
artificial rupture of
  membranes
A(ROM)   active range of motion
ARP   aggressive risk profile
alcohol rehabilitation
  program
Argyll Robertson pupil
assimilation regulatory
  protein
at-risk period
ARPE   acute reactive psychotic
  episode
ARPP   age-related pain
  perception
ARPT   American Registry of
  Physical Therapists
ARR   adverse reaction report
assessment of risk for
  release
ARRD   asymptomatic
  rhegmatogenous retinal
  detachments
ARRE-1   antigen receptor response
  element 1
ARRE-2   antigen receptor response
  element 2
ARRHTH   arrhythmia
ARRS   American Roentgen Ray
  Society
ARRT   adenine phosphoribosyl-
  transferase

American Registry of
Radiologic Technologists

Arry arrhythmia (a variation
from the normal rhythm
of the heart beat)

ARS activating reticular system
acute radiation syndrome
acute repetitive seizure
akinetic-rigid syndromes
American Radium Society
anorectal sphincters
antirabies serum

ARSD acute repetitive seizure
disorder

ART accredited record
technician
acid reflux test
acoustic reflex test
active resistance training
adjuvant radiation therapy
alcohol-related treatment
antibiotic-resistant
tuberculosis
arterial
assessment, review, and
treatment
assisted reproductive
technology
automated reagin test

art artery

ARTFs alcohol-related traffic
fatalities

ARTS assisted reproductive
technology services

ARV AIDS-associated retrovirus
AIDS-related virus

ARVD arrhythmogenic right
ventricular dysplasia

ARVDs antiretroviral drugs

ARVO Association for Research in
Vision and
Ophthalmology

ARVS acute retroviral syndrome

ARVT antiretroviral therapy

AS Aarskog syndrome
(faciogenital dysplasia)
abdominal striae
absence seizure (petit mal)
absolute scotoma

active sleep
acute sinusitis
Adams-Stokes (disease)
Albright's syndrome
(polyostotic fibrous
dysplasia)
Alport's syndrome
(hereditary nephritis
associated with deafness)
alveolar sac
ampere second
anabolic steroid
anal sphincter
anal stenosis
anaphylactic shock
anatomic snuffbox
angioid streaks
angiosarcoma
ankylosing spondylitis
(Marie-Strumpell disease)
annular scotoma
antiserum
antisocial
anxiety syndrome (feeling
of panic accompanied by
palpitation of the heart,
sweating, pallor, and
shallow respiration)
aortic sinuses (of Valsalva)
aortic sound
aortic stenosis

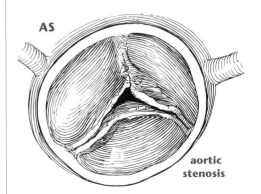

AS

aortic
stenosis

Apert syndrome
(acrocephalosyndactyly)
aqueous solution
arcuate scotoma

arteriosclerosis

artificial sweetner

Asherson's syndrome (cricopharyngeal achalasia syndrome)

asplenia syndrome (Ivemark's syndrome)

assessment

assisted suicide

atherosclerosis

atonic seizure

atrial septum

atropine sulfate

attempted suicide

As arsenic

astigmatism

a.s. *auris sinistra* [Latin] left ear

ASA acetylsalicylic acid (aspirin)

Adam-Stokes attack

Acoustical Society of America

American Schizophrenia Association

American Society of Anesthesiologists

American Surgical Association

antisperm antibody

argininosuccinic acid

arylsulfatase A

aspirin (acetylsalicylic acid)

aspirin-sensitive asthma

5-ASA 5-aminosalicylate

ASAA acquired severe aplastic anemia

ASAHP American Society of Allied Health Professionals

ASAIO American Society for Artificial Internal Organs

ASAL arginine succinate lyase

ASAM American Society of Addiction Medicine

ASAP American Society for Adolescent Psychiatry

American Society for Adolescent Psychology

as soon as possible

ASAS American Society of Abdominal Surgeons

arginine succinate synthetase

ASAT aspartate aminotransferase (formerly SGOT)

ASB anesthesia standby

assisted spontaneous breathing

asymptomatic bacteriuria

ASC Aarskog-Scott syndrome (faciodigitogenital syndrome)

acetylsulphanilyl chloride

acute suppurative cholangitis

adenosquamous carcinoma

altered state of consciousness

ambulatory surgical center

American Society of Cytology

anterior subcapsular cataract

antigen-sensitive cell

arousal-sleep cycle

arylsulfatase C

ascorbic acid (vitamin C)

automatic sensitivity control

asc ascending

ASCAD arteriosclerotic coronary artery disease

A scan amplitude scan (ultrasonography)

ASCB American Society for Cell Biology

ASCC American Society for the Control of Cancer

anterior (superior) semicircular canal

ASCI American Society for Clinical Investigation

ASCII American Standard Code for Information Interchange

ASCLD American Society of Crime Laboratory Directors

ASCLT American Society of Clinical Laboratory Technicians

ASCN American Society of Clinical Nutrition

ASCO American Society of Clinical Oncology

ASCP American Society of Clinical Pathologists
American Society of Cytopathology

ASCRS American Society of Colon and Rectal Surgeons

ASCUS Atypical squamous cells of undetermined significance

ASCVD arteriosclerotic cardiovascular disease
atherosclerotic cardiovascular disease

ASD acrosyndactyly (fusion of the ends of two or more digits)
adjustment sleep disorder
Albers-Schönberg's disease (osteopetrosis)
Alzheimer senile dementia
arteriosclerotic dementia
atrial septal defect

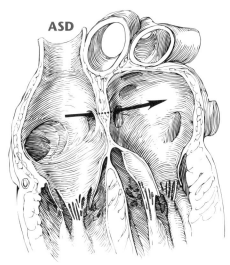

atrial septal defect

ASDA American Sleep Disorders Association

ASDC Association of Sleep Disorders Centers
automated source data collection

ASDH acute subdural hematoma

ASDP American Society of Dermatopathology

ASE acute stress erosion

ASECS antigen-specific electrophoretic cell separation

ASFR age-specific fertility rate

ASG American Society for Genetics
aortic valved graft
apocrine sweat gland

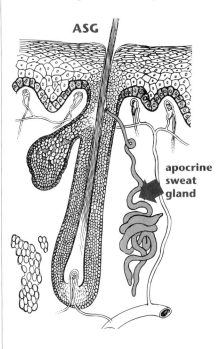

ASG

apocrine sweat gland

ASGE American Society for Gastrointestinal Endoscopy

ASGs apocrine sweat glands

ASH aldosterone-stimulating hormone
alkylosing spinal hyperostosis
American Society of Hematology

antistreptococcal
hyaluronidase

appetite-suppressing
hormone

asymmetrical septal
hypertrophy

As H hypermetropic astigatism

ASHD arteriosclerotic heart
disease

atherosclerotic heart
disease

atrial septal heart defect

ASHG American Society for
Human Genetics

ASHI Association for the Study of
Human Infertility

ASHN acute sclerosing hyaline
necrosis

ASI acromial spur index

addiction severity index

American Statistics Index

anteroseptal infarct (heart
infarct usually due to
occlusion of the anterior
intraventricular branch of
the left coronary artery)

ASIA American Spinal Injury
Association

ASIF Association for the Study of
Internal Fixation

ASII American Science
Information Institute

ASIM American Society of
Internal Medicine

ASIP American Society for
Investigative Pathology

ASIS anterior superior
iliac spine

ASK acyl-streptokinase

antistreptokinase

ASL American sign language

antistreptolysin (titer)

ASLHA American Speech-
Language Hearing
Association

ASLMS American Society for Laser
Medicine and Surgery

ASLO antistreptolysin-O

ASLT antistreptolysin test

ASM anal sphincter muscle

anterior scalene muscle

AsM myopic astigmatism

ASMC arterial smooth muscle cell

ASMD atonic sclerotic muscular
dystrophy

ASMI anteroseptal myocardial
infarction

ASMT American Society for
Medical Technology

ASN American Society of
Nephrology

American Society of
Neurochemistry

arteriosclerotic nephritis

Asn asparagine (nonessential
amino acid)

ASNE annulospiral nerve ending

ASO alleles-specific
oligonucleotides

antistreptolysin-O (titer)

arteriosclerosis obliterans
(obliterating
arteriosclerosis)

automatic stop order

ASOS American Society of Oral
Surgeons

ASOT antistreptolysin-O titer

ASO titer antistreptolysin-O titer

ASP abnormal spinal posture

ASIS

anterior
superior
iliac
spine

acute suppurative parotitis

acute symmetric
polyarthritis

American Society of
Parasitology

ankylosing spondylitis

antisocial personality

aortic systolic pressure

asparaginase (enzyme used
in the treatment of
childhood leukemia)

aspiration

atherosclerotic plaque

Asp aspartate (salt of
aspartic acid)

aspartic acid (nonessential
amino acid)

ASPAT aspartate aminotransferase
A-streptococci
polysaccharide
antibody titer

ASPD antisocial personality
disorder

ASPEN American Society of
Parenteral and Enteral
Nutrition

ASPM American Society of
Paramedics

ASPO American Society for
Psychoprophylaxis in
Obstetrics

ASPRS American Society of Plastic
and Reconstructive
Surgeons

ASPS advanced sleep
phase syndrome

ASPVD atherosclerotic peripheral
vascular disease

ASR aldosterone secretion rate
automatic speech
recognition

ASPVD atherosclerotic peripheral
vascular disease

ASQ anxiety scale questionnaire

ASR aldosterone secretion rate
antistreptolysin reaction

ASRA American Society of
Regional Anesthesia

ASS acute schistosomiasis

(Katayama fever)

acute serum sickness
(hypersensitivity reaction
to the infusion of
foreign serum)

acute spinal stenosis

Adams-Stokes syndrome
(heart block disorder
marked by sudden loss of
consciousness)

African sleeping sickness

anterior superior
(iliac) spine

ASSC antigen-specific suppressor
cells

ASSE American Society of Safety
Engineers

ASSH American Society for
Surgery of the Hand

Assn association

ASSO American Society for the
Study of Orthodontics
anterior subapical sliding
osteotomy

Assoc association

ASST antegrade scrotal
sclerotherapy

asst assistant

AST abduction stress test
adduction stress test
alcohol screening test
angiotensin sensitivity test
anterior spinothalamic
tract
antibiotic sensitivity test
antishock therapy
antistreptolysin test
audiometry sweep test

ASt antistaphylolysin

Ast astigmatism

Asth asthenopia

ASTI acute soft tissue injury
antispasticity index

Astigm astigmatism (unequal
curvature of the
refractive surfaces of
the eye)

ASTM American Society of
Testing and Materials
(standards)

ASTMH American Society of
Tropical Medicine and
Hygiene
ASTO antistreptolysin O
as tol as tolerated
ASTRO American Society for
Therapeutic Radiology
and Oncology
Astro astrocytoma (tumor
composed of astrocytes)
ASTS American Society of
Transplant Surgeons
ASTZ antistreptozyme (test)
ASU acute stroke unit
ASV antisnake venom
assisted spontaneous
ventilation
ASX asymptomatic
ASW artificial sweetener
asym asymmetric
AT abdominal toxoplasmosis
achievement test
Achilles tendinitis
Achilles tendon
Adam's test (for scoliosis)
adipose tissue
adjuvant therapy
agglutination titer
air temperature
alpha-tocopherol
(vitamin E)
aminotransferase
(transaminase)
3-amino-1,2,4-triazole
anaphylatoxin
angiotensin (a polypeptide
present in the blood
plasma and formed by
the action of the enzyme
renin on a globulin)
antithrombin
antitrypsin
applanation tonometry
Aschoff-Tawara (node)
ataxia-telangiectasia
(syndrome)
atraumatic
atrial tachycardia
atropine (an alkaloid with

antimuscarinic actions)
atypical teratomas
(germinomas)
auditory tube (eustachian
tube)
autologous transfusion
(patient's own blood)
axial tomography
axonal terminal
A-T adenine-thymine
ataxia telangiectasia
AT-I angiotensin I
AT-II angiotensin II
AT-III angiotensin III
A.T. 10 dihydrotachysterol (oral
antihypocalcemic agent)
At astatine (a radioactive
element)
atom
atrium
ATA alcohol-tobacco amblyopia
alimentary toxic aleukia
American Thyroid
Association
anterior tubercle of atlas
antithrombin activity
antithrombocyte antibody
antithyroglobulin antibody
A tape adhesive tape
Atax ataxia (lack of muscle
coordination)
ATB alpha-tocopherol,
beta carotene
antibiotic
at the bedside
atrial tachycardia
with block
ATBI acute traumatic
brain injury
ATC activated thymus cell
anterior tibial
compartment
(syndrome)
around-the-clock
AT-II C alveolar type II cell
(unique to lung)
AT-IIIC antithrombin-III
concentrate
ATCC American Type

Culture Collection

ATCS anterior tibial compartment syndrome

ATD Alzheimer's type dementia
anticipated time of discharge
antitrypsin deficiency
articulotrochanteric distance
asphyxiating thoracic dystrophy (Jeune syndrome)

AT-IIID antithrombin-III deficiency

ATE acute thromboembolism
acute toxic encephalopathy
adenotonsillectomy
adipose tissue extraction (liposuction)

ATF Bureau of Alcohol, Tobacco, and Firearms

At Fib atrial fibrillation

At Fib

atrial fibrillation

ATFL anterior talofibular ligament

ATG adenine-thymidine-guanine
antithrombocyte globulin
antithymocyte globulin

ATGAM antithymocyte gammaglobulin

AT/GC adenine-thymine/guanine-cytosine (ratio)

ATH anthropometric total hip

ATHC allotetrahydrocortisol

ATHS astringedent topical hemostatic solution

ATI abdominal trauma index
Achilles tendon inflammation

ATIN acute tubulointerstitial nephritis

ATL Achilles tendon lengthening

adult T cell leukemia
adult T cell lymphoma
atypical lymphocyte

ATLAS Training and Learning to Avoid Steroids (program)

ATLL adult T cell leukemia/lymphoma

ATLPL adipose tissue lipoprotein lipase

ATLS acute tumor lysis syndrome
advanced trauma life support

ATLV adult T-cell leukemia virus
aortic trileaflet valve

ATM acute transverse myelopathy

atm atmosphere (1 atm = mean atmospheric pressure at sea level)

ATMA antithyroid-plasma membrane antibody

at mass atomic mass (ma)

ATMI acute transmural myocardial infarction

ATN acute tubular necrosis
auriculotemporal nerve

at no atomic number

ATOD alcohol, tobacco, and other drugs

ATP adenosine triphosphate (cell's major energy currency)
autoimmune thrombocytopenic purpura
azathioprine (an immunosuppressive agent for prevention of transplant rejection)

AtP attending physician

ATPase adenosine triphosphatase

ATPC angioplasty, transluminal, percutaneous coronary

ATP-2Na adenosine triphosphate disodium

ATPR average threshold of pain reaction

ATPS ambient temperature, pressure and saturation

ATR Achilles tendon reflex
atrial
atropine (anticholinergic alkaloid)
ATr antitrypsin (a substance that inhibits the action of the proteolytic enzyme trypsin)
atr atrial
atrophy
Atre atresia (absence of a normal body opening)
Atro atrophy (wasting away)
atropine (anticholinergic alkaloid)
ATS absent testes syndrome (anorchia)
acid test solution
American Thoracic Society
American Trauma Society (800) 556-7890
antitetanic serum
antitetanus serum
antithymocyte serum
anxiety tension state
atherosclerosis
atropine sulfate
ATSD Alzheimer type senile dementia
ATSDR Agency for Toxic Substances and Disease Registry
ATT antitetanus therapy
antitetanus toxoid
antitoxin titer
aspirin tolerance time
atty attorney
ATU alcoholism treatment unit
ATVL anterior tricuspid (right atrioventricular) valve leaflet
at vol atomic volume
at wt atomic weight (former name for relative atomic mass)
atyp atypical
ATZ anal transitional zone
AUs allergenic units
Angstrom units
antitoxin units
aphthous ulcers
arbitrary units
Au gold (aurum)
Au 198 radioactive gold
a.u. *auris uterque* [Latin] each ear
AUA American Urological Association
asymptomatic urinary abnormalities
AuAg Australian antigen
AuAg P Australian antigen protein
AUAN acute uric acid nephropathy
AUB abnormal uterine bleeding
AuBMT autologous bone marrow transplant
AUBP acute uncomplicated back pain
AUC area under the curve
aud auditory
AUDI International Society of Audiology
AUE acute uremic encephalopathy
AUG acute ulcerative gingivitis
adenine-uridine-guanine
AUGIB acute upper gastrointestinal bleeding
AUGH acute upper gastrointestinal hemorrhage
AuHAA Australian hepatitis-associated antigen
AUL acute undifferentiated leukemia
AUO amyloid of unknown origin
AUR Association of University Radiologists
acute urinary retention
AUS acute urethral syndrome
ausc auscultation
AuSH Australia serum hepatitis
AuSH-Ag Australia serum hepatitis antigen
AUTI acute urinary tract infection
asymptomatic urinary

	tract infection
aux	auxiliary
AV	acne vulgaris (chronic acne, occurring commonly on the face, chest and back of adolescents and young adults)
	adenovirus
	allergic vasculitis
	anteversion
	anticipatory vomiting
	aortic valve

AV

aortic valve

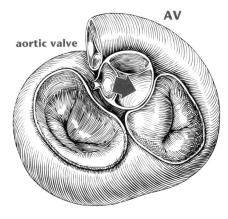

	arteriovenous
	artificial ventilation (artificial respiration)
	assisted ventilation
	atrioventricular
	azygos vein
A-V	arteriovenous
	atrioventricular
aV	abvolt
Av	arteriovenous
	average
AVA	antiviral antibody
	aortic-valve atresia
	arrhythmogenic ventricular activity
	arteriovenous angioma
AVB	atrioventricular block
	atrial premature beat
AVC	aberrant ventricular conduction
	acrylic veneer crown

	acute vertebral collapse
	allantoid vaginal cream
	anovulatory cycle
	atrioventricular conduction
	atrioventricular cushions (swellings)
AVCMF	Adriamycin (doxorubicin) + vincristin (Oncovin) + cyclophosphamide + methotrexate + 5-fluorouracil (combination chemotherapy)
AVCS	atrioventricular conduction system
AVCs	aortic-valve cusps
AVCT	antiviral chemotherapy
AVD	aoritic valve defect
	aortic valve disease
	arbovirus disease
	atrioventricular dissociation
avD	arteriovenous difference
avD-O$_2$	arteriovenous oxygen saturation difference
AVDP	average diastolic pressure
	avoirdupois
AVE	amniotic-fluid embolism
	antral vascular ectasia (watermelon stomach)
	aortic valve echocardiogram
AVF	antiviral factor
	aortic-valve fistula
	arteriovenous fistula (abnormal communication between an artery and a vein)
aVF	augmented unipolar foot (limb lead in which the positive terminal is secured to the left foot during electrocardiography)
AVG	aortovenography
Avg	average
AVGP	aortic valved graft prosthesis

AVH	acute viral hepatitis
AVHD	acquired valvular heart disease
AVI	adenovirus infection
	aortic-valve incompetence
	aortic-valve insufficiency
	arbovirus infection
AVJ	atrioventricular junction
AVJA	atrioventricular junctional arrhythmia
AVJT	atrioventricular junctional tachycardia
AVL	avian leukosis virus
aVL	augmented unipolar left (limb lead in which the positive terminal is secured to the left arm during electrocardiography)
AVLINE	audiovisual online
AVM	arteriovenous malformation
AVMA	American Veterinary Medical Association
AVMF	arteriovenous malformation
AVN	acute vasomotor nephropathy

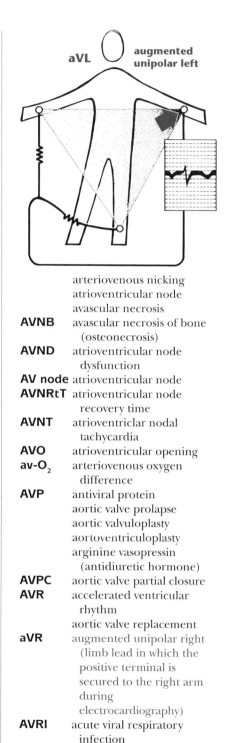

	arteriovenous nicking
	atrioventricular node
	avascular necrosis
AVNB	avascular necrosis of bone (osteonecrosis)
AVND	atrioventricular node dysfunction
AV node	atrioventricular node
AVNRtT	atrioventricular node recovery time
AVNT	atrioventriclar nodal tachycardia
AVO	atrioventricular opening
av-O$_2$	arteriovenous oxygen difference
AVP	antiviral protein
	aortic valve prolapse
	aortic valvuloplasty
	aortoventriculoplasty
	arginine vasopressin (antidiuretic hormone)
AVPC	aortic valve partial closure
AVR	accelerated ventricular rhythm
	aortic valve replacement
aVR	augmented unipolar right (limb lead in which the positive terminal is secured to the right arm during electrocardiography)
AVRI	acute viral respiratory infection

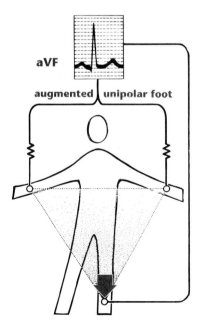

AVRT	atrioventricular reciprocating tachycardia
	atrioventricular reentrant tachycardia
AVS	aortic valve stenosis
	arteriovenous shunt
	auditory vocal sequencing
AVSD	atrioventricular septal defect
AVSP	atrioventricular sequential pacing
AVSS	afebrile, vital signs stable
AVT	antiviral therapy
	arginine vasotonin
AVV	atrioventricular valve
AVVCs	atrioventricular-valve cusps
AVVI	atrioventricular-valve insufficiency
AVZ	avascular zone
AW	abdominal wall
	able to work
	above waist
	abrupt withdrawal
	airway
	alcohol withdrawal
	atomic weight (former name for relative atomic mass)
A & W	alive and well
AWA	as well as
AWB	autologous whole blood
AWD	alcohol withdrawal

	delirium
AWI	anterior wall infarction
AWMI	anterior wall myocardial infarction
AWO	airway obstruction
AWOL	absent without leave
AWP	airway pressure
AWR	airway resistance
AWS	alcohol withdrawal syndrome
	Ayre wooden spatula
AWU	alcohol withdrawal unit
Ax	axillary
	axis (of cylindric lens)
ax	axis (of cylindric lens)
AXG	adult xanthogranuloma
AXL	axillary lymphoscintigraphy
AXM	acetoxycyclohexamine
AXR	abdominal x-ray
Ax-Ro joint	
	axial rotation joint
AYF	anti-yeast factor
AYV	aster yellow virus
AZ	autonomous zone (isolated zone)
	azathioprine (Imuran; immunosuppressive agent for prevention of transplant rejection)
AZA	azathioprine (Imuran; immunosuppressive agent for prevention of transplant rejection)
AzC	azacytosine
AzG	azaguanine (blocks nucleic acid synthesis)
AZT	Ascheim-Zondek test (pregnancy test)
	zidovudine (azidothymidine; Retrovir)
A-Z test	Ascheim-Zondek test (pregnancy test)
AZU	azauracil
AzUMP	6-azauridylic acid monophosphate
AzUR	azauridine (used in the treatment of acute leukemia)

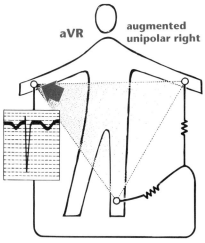

aVR **augmented unipolar right**

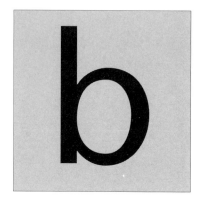

B   bacillus
base (of prism)
basophil
bath
bel
bicuspid
black
blastocyst
blood type B+, B–
boil (furuncle)
bolus

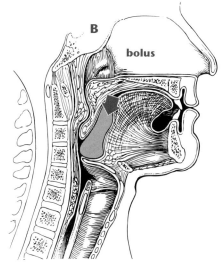

boron
brachial
bregma (skull landmark
where the sagittal and
coronal sutures meet)

bronchus
bruit (abnormal sound
heard during
auscultation)
bubo (inflammatory
swelling of a lymphatic
gland, usually in the
groin or axilla)
buccal
bulimia
bunion
bursa

B I   Billroth I (operation;
partial resection of
stomach with anastomosis
to the duodenum)

B II   Billroth II (operation;
partial resection of
stomach with anastomosis
to the jejunum)

B1   vitamin B1 (thiamine)
B2   vitamin B2 (riboflavin)
B4   before
B6   vitamin B6 (pyridoxine)
B7   vitamin B7 (biotin)
B8   vitamin B8 (adenosine
phosphate)
B9   benign
B12   vitamin B12
(cyanocobalamin)
b   base (nucleic acids)
bel
blood (as a subscript)
born
b.   *bis* [Latin] twice
BA   bacillary angiomatosis
Bacillus anthracis
backache
bacterial agglutination
balloon angioplasty
basilar artery
basion
benzanthracene
benzyladenine
benzyl alcohol
bile acid
biliary atresia
blocking antibody
blood alcohol

bone age
boric acid
brachial artery
breast augmentation
Broca's area
bronchial adenoma
bronchial asthma
bronchial atresia
buffered acetone

Ba barium
basion (craniometric landmark located on the midpoint of the anterior margin of the foramen magnum)

BAA bacterial antigen assay
benzoyl arginine amide
beta-adrenergic agonist
branched amino acid

BAAF Bensley's acid aniline fuchsin

BAB blood agar base
blood-air barrier
blood-aqueous barrier
bronchoarterial bundle

BABA beta-adrenergic blocking agent

BABT bile acid breath test

BAC bacterial antigen complex
blood alcohol concentration
bronchoalveolar carcinoma
bronchoalveolar cells

BACM benign acute childhood myositis

BACON bleomycin + Adriamycin (doxorubicin) + CCNU (lomustine) + Oncovin (vincristine) + nitrogen mustard (mechlorethamine) (combination chemotherapy)

BACOP bleomycin + Adriamycin (doxorubicin) + cyclophosphamide + Oncovin (vincristine) + prednisone (combination chemotherapy)

bact bacteria

BAD bipolar affective disorder

BAE bronchial arterial embolization

BaE barium enema

BAEE benzoyl L-arginine ethyl ester

BaEn barium enema

BAEP brainstem auditory evoked potential

BAER brainstem auditory evoked response

BAF B cell-activating factor
bimalleolar ankle fracture

BAGG buffered azide glucose glycerol (broth)

BAH biatrial hypertrophy
bilateral adrenal hyperplasia

BAI basilar artery insufficiency
Broca's area infarction
building-associated illness

BAIB beta-aminoisobutyric (acid)

BAL blood alcohol level
British antilewisite
bronchoalveolar lavage
dimercaprol (an antidote to poisoning by mercury and arsenic)
2,3-dimercaptopropanol

BALF bronchoalveolar lavage fluid

BALT bronchus-associated lymphoid tissue

BAM bacillary angiomatosis
brachial artery mean (pressure)

BaM barium meal (light meal which contains barium opaque to Roentgen rays)

BAME benzoylarginine methyl ester

BAN benign acute nephritis
British Adopted Name

B. anthracis
Bacillus anthracis

BAO basal acid output

	basal gastric acid output
	bilateral arterial occlusion
BAP	bacillary angiomatosis-bacillary peliosis
	bacterial alkaline phosphatase
	beta-amyloid peptide
	brachial artery pulse
BAPA	benzoylarginyl-*p*-nitroanilide
BAQ	brain-age quotient
BAR	beta-adrenergic receptor
barb	barbiturate (sedative-hypnotic agent)
BARI	Bypass Angioplasty Revascularization Investigation
BARVT	bilateral acute renal vein thrombosis
BAS	beta-adrenergic stimulation
	boric acid solution
	Butler-Albright syndrome
BASA	baby aspirin (acetylsalicylic acid)
	beta-adrenergic stimulating agent
BASH	Bulimia Anorexia Self-Help (800) 227-4785
Baso	basophil
BAST	beta-adrenergic stimulant therapy
BAT	blunt abdominal trauma
	breathalyzer test
BAV	balloon aortic valvuloplasty
BAVP	balloon aortic valvuloplasty
BAW	bronchoalveolar washing
BB	bad breath
	Barr's body (can be used to determine genotypic sex of an individual)
	bed bath
	bed board
	belly button
	benzyl bromide (war gas)
	beriberi (form of polyneuritis due to deficiency of thiamine)
	beta blocker

	Bier block
	blood bank
	Blount brace
	blue baby (an infant with a congenital heart defect in which the ductus arteriosus or foramen ovale of the heart fails to close)
	bone bank
	bone biopsy
	breast biopsy
	breech birth
	bronchial block
	brush biopsy
	brush border
	bundle branch (fasciculi atrioventricularis)
BBA	born before arrival (of physician or midwife)
	butyl benzoic acid
BBB	blood-brain barrier (blood-cerebral barrier)
	bundle-branch block
BBBB	bilateral bundle branch block
BBD	benign breast disease
	brittle bone disease
BBE	baseball elbow (arthritic changes in elbow of veteran pitchers)
BBF	baseball finger (mallet finger) (avulsion of the common extensor tendon)
	basketball foot (medial subtalar dislocation)
BBL	bird breeder's lung
BBM	brush border membrane
BBOW	bulging bag of water
BBPs	blood borne pathogens
BBS	benign breast syndrome
	bilateral breath sounds
	broad Brucher shoe
	brown bowel syndrome
	buried bumper syndrome
BBSD	Besnier-Boeck-Schaumann disease (sarcoidosis)
BBT	basal body temperature

B. burgdorferi
　Borrelia burgdorferi (the
　　causative agent of Lyme
　　borreliosis)
B Bx　breast biopsy
BC　Baker's cyst (popliteal cyst)
　　balloon catheter
　　beta-carotene
　　biliary cirrhosis
　　biliary colic
　　bipolar cell
　　birth canal
　　birth certificate
　　birth control
　　birthing center
　　birthing chair
　　black cancer (malignant
　　　melanoma)
　　Blalock clamp
　　blepharoconjunctivitis
　　　(inflammation of the
　　　eyelids and conjunctiva)
　　blind spot
　　blood count
　　blood culture
　　bone cement
　　　(polymethylmethacrylate)
　　bone conduction
　　brachiocephalic
　　breast cancer
　　bronchial carcinoma
B₁C　beta-1 component
　　of complement
B & C　biopsy and curettage
　　board and care
b/c　benefit/cost
BCA　balloon catheter
　　　angioplasty
　　basal cell atypia
　　breast cancer antigen
BCAA　branch chain amino acids
　　Brandt cytology balloon
B-CAV　bleomycin + CCNU
　　　(lomustine) + Adriamycin
　　　(doxorubicin) +
　　　vinblastine (combination
　　　chemotherapy)
BCB　blood - CSF barrier
BC-BS　Blue Cross-Blue Shield

　　(insurance plan)
BCC　basal cell carcinoma
　　　(the most common
　　　human cancer)

BCC basal cell
carcinoma

BCD　basal cell dysplasia
　　bleomycin +
　　　cyclophosphamide +
　　　dactinomycin
　　　(combination
　　　chemotherapy)
　　blood coagulation disorder
BCDDP　Breast Cancer Detection
　　　Demonstration Project
BCDF　B cell differentiation
　　　factors
BCDM　biocompatible dialysis
　　　membrane
BCE　basal cell epithelioma
　　benign childhood epilepsy
B cell　bone marrow derived
　　　lymphocyte (lymphocyte
　　　produced in the bone
　　　marrow)
BCF　basophil chemotactic
　　　factor
BCG　bacille Calmette-Guerin
　　　(attenuated form of
　　　TB vaccine)
　　ballistocardiogram
　　bronchocentric
　　　granulomatosis

BCGF B cell growth factor
BCH basal cell hyperplasia
BCIS Bowen's carcinoma *in situ*
BCKA branched-chain keto acid
BCL B cell lymphoma
bcl-2 active version of a proto-oncogene
BCLL B cell chronic lymphocytic leukemia
BCLSS Basic Cardiac Life Support System
BCM below costal margin
BCME bis(chloromethyl) ether
BCN basal cell nevus
BCNS basal cell nevus syndrome
BCNU bischloroethylnitrosourea (carmustine, an antineoplastic agent)
BCOC bowel cathartic of choice
BCP basal cell papilloma (seborrheic keratosis)
BCNU (carmustine) + cyclophosphamide + prednisone (combination chemotherapy)
birth control pill
Blue Cross Plan
BCR birth control regimen
blunt cardiac rupture
BCS battered child syndrome (must be reported to authorities for investigation)
Budd-Chiari syndrome (endophlebitis hepatica obliterans)
BCSI breast cancer screening indicator
BCSU Bard Clamshell septal umbrella (to close ventricular septal defects)
BCT Barany's caloric test
benign cystic teratoma
brachiocephalic trunk
BCU burn care unit
BCV brachiocephalic vein
BCVS bicaval venous cannulation
BCYE buffered charcoal yeast extract (agar)

BD Baastrup disease (kissing osteophytes; kissing spine)
bacillary dysentery
balance disorder
Bannister's disease (angioedema)
barbiturate dependent
Barlow's disease (infantile scurvy)
Basedow's disease (partial lipodystrophy)
behavioral disorder
Bekhterev's disease (rheumatoid spondylitis)
belladonna
below diaphragm
Benson's disease (asteroid hyalosis)
Bennett dislocation
Best's disease (congenital macular degeneration)
Biermer's disease (pernicious anemia)
bile duct
bipolar disorder
birth date
birth defect

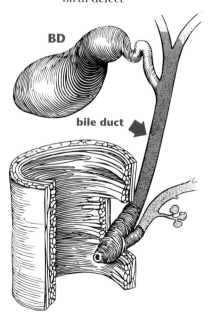

blood donor

Bloodgood's disease
(cystic disease of breast)

bloody diarrhea

Blount's disease
(tibia vara)

Boeck's disease
(sarcoidosis)

bone densitometry

bone dysplasia

Bornholm disease
(epidemic pleurodynia)

Bouillaud's disease
(rheumatic endocarditis)

Bourneville's disease
(tuberous sclerosis)

Boutonniere deformity
(buttonhole deformity)

Bowen's disease
(intraepidermal
squamous cell
carcinoma)

Bradley's disease
(epidemic nausea
and vomiting)

brain damage

brain dead

breech delivery

Bright's disease
(glomerulonephritis)

bronchodilator

Buchanan disease

Buerger disease
(thromboangiitis
obliterans)

Bureau of Drugs

Burns disease

Buschke's disease
(cryptococcosis)

B & D   bloating and diarrhea

bronchiectasis and dyspnea

b.d.   *bis die* [Latin] twice a day

BDA   balloon dilation
angioplasty

bile duct atresia

bromocriptine-dopamine
agonist

BDC   blood donor center

bulldog clamp

burn-dressing change

BDD   bronchodilator drug

BD-DT   biliary duct-dwelling
trematodes

BDH   black dot heel

bdh   bubble-diffusion
humidifier

BDI   bacterial disk infection

Beck Depression Inventory

BDL   below detectable limits

bone density loss

BDM   Becker's muscular
dystrophy

bDNA   bacterial DNA

BDNF   brain-derived neurotrophic factor

BDO   bile duct obstruction

B-DOPA   bleomycin + dacarbazine +
Oncovin (vincristine) +
prednisone + Adriamycin
(doxorubicin)
(combination
chemotherapy)

BDP   benzodiazepine

bronchopulmonary
dysplasia

BDR   background diabetic
retinopathy

bedbug rash

BDRW   black-dot ringworm

BDS   blue-diaper syndrome

b.d.s.   *bis in die summendus* [Latin]
to be taken twice a day

BDT   bronchodilator therapy

BDUR   bromodeoxyuridine

BDZ   benzodiazepines

BE   bacterial endocarditis

barium enema

baseball elbow

below elbow (said of
amputations or
prostheses)

binge eating

biologically equivalent

Bohr effect

boxer's elbow

brain edema

bread equivalent

breast examination

bronchitis-emphysema
bronchoesophagology
bullous emphysema

Be beryllium (metallic element)

be bacterial endocarditis
barium enema

BEA bacillary epithelioid angiomatosis
below-the-elbow amputation
bioelectric activity
brain electric activity

BEAM brain electric activity mapping
brain electric activity monitoring

BEAP bronchiectasis, eosinophilia, asthma and pneumonia

BEC bacterial endocarditis

BED branching enzyme deficiency (type IV glycogenosis)

BEE basal energy expenditure

BEF bronchoesophageal fistula

BEH benign essential hypertension
benign exertional headache

BEI backscattered electron imaging
biological exposure indices
butanol-extractable iodine; also called butanol-extractable radioactive iodine

BEIP Biomedical Engineering and Instrumentation Program

BEIR biological effects of ionizing radiation

BEN Balkan endemic nephropathy

benz benzene (volatile carcinogenic liquid hydrocarbon)

BEP bleomycin + etoposide +

Platinol (cisplatin) (combination chemotherapy)
brain evoked potential
brainstem evoked potential

B-EP beta-endorphin

BER basic electrical rhythm

BERS benign epilepsy with rolandic (or midtemporal) spikes

BES balanced electrolyte solution
Bongiovanni-Eberlein syndrome

BEST bicycle exercise stress test

BET Buck's extension traction

Beth unit Bethesda unit (a measure of the level of inhibitor to factor VIII)

BEV bleeding esophageal varices (bleeding of the branches of the azygos vein that anastomose with tributaries of the portal vein in the distal esophagus)

bev beverage

BEXR barium enema x-ray

BF bacterial flora
Barton fracture
baseball finger
Bennett fracture
biofeedback
black female
blastogenic factor
blister fluid
blood fluke (*Schistosoma mansoni*)
body fat
body fluids
bone fragment
Bosworth fracture
boxer's fracture
breast fed
breastfeeding
bumper fracture
burst fracture

BFB	biofeedback
	bronchial foreign body
BFC	benign febrile convulsion
BFD	black-fly disease
BFF	backfire fracture
	(chauffeur's fracture)
bFGF	basic fibroblast growth
	factor
BFH	benign familial hematuria
BFHC	biofilter hemoconcentrator
BFL	bird fancier's lung
BFM	biceps femoris muscle
	blood flow monitoring
BFO	balanced forearm orthosis
	blood-forming organ
BFP	beta fetoprotein
	biologic false-positive
	bleomycin + etoposide +
	cisplatin (combination
	chemotherapy)
BFPR	biologic false-positive
	reaction
BFR	blood flow rate
B. fragilis	
	B. fragilis
BFS	Babinski-Frohlich
	syndrome
	blood fasting sugar
	burning feet syndrome
	(Gopalan's syndrome)
BFT	biofeedback technique
BFU	burst-forming unit
BG	basal ganglia
	Bender Gestalt (test)
	beta-galactosidase
	beta-glucuronidase
	blood glucose
	blood group
	bone graft
BGA	biogenic amines
	blood gas analysis
	Brunner's gland adenoma
BGAg	blood group antigen
BGC	Bartholin gland carcinoma
	bronchogenic carcinoma
	bronchogenic cyst
BGCa	bronchogenic carcinoma
BGCT	benign glandular cell
	tumor

bGH	bovine growth hormone
BGL	blood gas level
	blood glucose level
BGlu	blood glucose
BGM	blood glucose monitoring
BGN	background noise
BGP	beta-glycerophosphatase
	bone Gla protein (test)
BGR	background radiation
BGT	Bender gestalt test
BGTT	borderline glucose
	tolerance test
BGU	benign gastric ulcer
BH	bill of health
	blackhead (comedone)
	Board of Health
	borderline hypertensive
	bowel habits
	brain hemorrhage
	bronchial hyper-reactivity
	bundle of His
BH2	dihydrobiopterin
BH4	tetrahydrobiopterin
BHA	bilateral hilar adenopathy
	butylated hydroxyanisole
BHB	beta-hydroxybutyrate
BHBA	beta-hydroxybutyric acid
BHC	benzene hexachloride
	(hexachlorocyclohexane)
	Braxton Hicks contraction
	Bremer halo crown
	(for cervical traction)
bHCG	beta human chorionic
	gonadotropin
BHD	buttonhole deformity
	(buttonhole mitral
	stenosis)
BHE	benign
	hemangioendothelioma
	(benign neoplasm of
	blood-vessel
	endothelium)
BHF	Bolivian hemorrhagic fever
BHI	Better Hearing Institute
	biosynthetic human insulin
BHL	biological half-life
BHM	Bureau of Health
	Manpower
BHN	Brinell hardness number

BHP   basic health profile
       benign hypertrophy of
          prostate
BHPr   Bureau of Health
          Professions
       benign hypertrophic
          prostatitis
BHR   Boerema hernia repair
       bronchial
          hyperresponsiveness
BHS   benign hypermobility
          syndrome
       beta-hemolytic streptococci
       black heel syndrome
       breathholding spell
BHT   black hairy tongue
       breath hydrogen test (used
          in acute gastroenteritis
          and fat absorption tests)
       bucket handle tear
          (longitudinal tear of
          knee's meniscus)

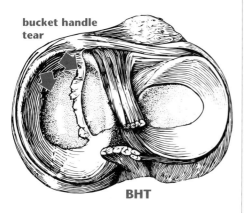

bucket handle tear

BHT

       butylated hydroxytoluene
          (food additive)
BI   behavioral intervention
       birth injury
       blunt injury
       bodily injury
       bowel impaction
       bowel incontinence (fecal
          incontinence)
       bowel injury
       brain injury
       breast implant

       burn index
       bullous impetigo
Bi   bismuth
BIA   bioimmunoassay
BIB   brought in by
bib.   *bibe* [Latin] drink
biblio bibliography
BICAP bipolar electrocoagulation
          therapy
Bicarb bicarbonate
BICU burn intensive care unit
BID   brought in dead
b.i.d. *bis in die* [Latin]
          twice a day
BIDS brittle hair, impaired
          intelligence, decreased
          fertility and short stature
          (syndrome)
BIF   beta interferon
       bifocal
BIH   benign intracranial
          hypertension
BIL   biceps interval lesion
bilat bilateral
bili   bilirubin (bile pigment)
bilirub bilirubin (bile pigment)
BIMC blessed-information-
          memory-concentration
          (test)
BIN   benign intradermal nevus
b.i.n. *bis in nocte* [Latin]
          twice a night
BIO   binocular indirect
          ophthalmoscopy
biochem biochemistry
BIOD bony intraorbital distance
BIOETHICSLINE
       bioethical information
          online
BioF   biofeedback
BIOI   BioResearch Index
BI or BO base in or base out (prism)
BIOSIS *Biological Abstracts List*
          of Serials
BIP   bacterial intravenous
          protein
       bismuth iodoform paraffin
BiPD biparietal diameter
          (distance between the

two fetal parietal
eminences)

BIUG benign intrauterine
growths

BJ Bence Jones (protein)
biceps jerk (biceps
reflex test)
bicondylar joint
bilocular joint

B & J bones and joints

BJM benign juvenile melanoma
bones, joints, and muscles

BJP Bence Jones protein

BK back
band keratopathy
below-the-knee (said of
amputations or
prostheses)

Bk berkelium (a synthetic,
transuranic radioactive
element)

bk back

BKA below-knee amputation

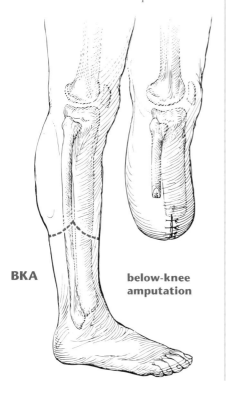

BKA   **below-knee
amputation**

BK-A basophil kallikrein of
anaphylaxis

bka below-knee amputation

BKC below-knee cast

bkf breakfast

bkg background

BKO below-knee orthosis

BKTT below knee to toes

BKV BK virus

BKWC below the knee
walking cast

BL basal lamina
black light
blind loop
blood loss
body lice
bronchial lavage
Burkitt lymphoma
bowleg

bl blood

blad bladder

BlBk blood bank

BLB m Boothby, Lovelace,
Bulbulian mask (oxygen
mask for use at high
altitudes)

BLCM below left costal margin

BLD benign lymphoepithelial
disease
black lung disease

Bld blood

Bld Bk blood bank

BLE basal layer of endometrium
blood levels of enzymes

BLEL benign lympho-epithelial
lesion

BLEO bleomycin (cytotoxic
glycopeptide)
bleomycin sulfate
(antineoplastic agent)

bleph blepharitis (inflammation
of an eyelid)

BLEs both lower extremities

BLG beta-lactoglobulin

BLI bombesin-like
immunoreactivity

blk black

BLL blood lead level

	bone lead level
	borderline leprosy
BLN	brachial lymph node
BLNs	bronchial lymph nodes
BLOBS	bladder obstruction
BLOC	brief loss of consciousness
BLP	beta-lipoprotein
BLPOs	beta-lactamase-producing organisms
BLQ	both lower quadrants
BLS	basic life support
	blind loop syndrome (syndrome which may occur following operations of the small intestine, that form a blind loop resulting in stagnation of intestinal contents)
	blood sugar
	Bureau of Labor Statistics
BIS	blood sugar
BLT	bilateral tubal ligation
	bleeding time
	blood clot lysis time
	blood type
BLU	broad ligament of uterus
BLV	blood volume
Blx	bleeding time
BM	bacterial meningitis
	basal metabolism
	basement membrane
	basilar membrane (of cochlear duct)
	behavioral medicine
	birthmark (nevus)
	birth membranes (amnion and chorion)
	body mass
	bone marrow
	bone mass
	bowel movement
	Bowman's membrane (thin layer of cornea)
	Boyden meal (meal consisting of flour, egg yolks, milk and port wine, used to test the evacuation time of

	the gallbladder)
	Bureau of Medicine
BMA	biceps muscle of arm
	bone marrow aspiration
BMB	bone marrow biopsy
BMBL	benign monoclonal B cell lymphocytosis
BMC	bacterial myocarditis
	bone marrow cell
BMCG	beta-methyl-crotonyl-glycinuria
BMD	Bamberger-Marie disease
	Becker's muscular dystrophy
	bone marrow depression
	Bureau of Medical Devices
BMDD	bipolar manic-depressive disorder
BME	bone marrow embolism
	bone marrow examination
	brief maximal effort
	brompheniramine maleate elixir
BMEON	borderline malignant epithelial ovarian neoplasm
BMF	black, middle-aged female
BMG	benign monoclonal gammopathy (presence of serum M component without indications of multiple myeloma)
BMI	body mass index (calculated from height and weight)
B.microti	*Babesia microti*
BML	benign metastasizing leiomyomas
BMJ	bones, muscles, and joints
	British Medical Journal
	breast milk jaundice
bmk	birthmark
BML	bone marrow lymphocytosis
BMM	black, middle-aged male
BMMRP	Biological Models and Materials Research Program
BMN	bone marrow necrosis

Bmod behavior modification
B-mode brightness modulation
BMP bimanual palpation
bone marrow pressure
BMPP benign mucous membrane
pemphigus
BMQA Board of Medical Quality
Assurance
BMR basal metabolic rate
BMS Bureau of Medicine and
Surgery
burning mouth syndrome
bleomycin sulfate
(antineoplastic agent)
BMT basement membrane
thickening
benign mesenchymal
tumor
bone marrow toxicity
bone marrow transplant
BMTU bone marrow
transplant unit
BN benign neoplasm
bladder neck
blue nevus (circumscribed
blackish-blue nodule
beneath the skin, chiefly
composed of dopa-
positive pigment-
producing cells)
Bouchard's node (a small,
hard nodule located in
the proximal
interphalangeal joint of a
finger in osteoarthritis)
brachial neuritis
bronchial node
bulimia nervosa
BNA Basle Nomina Anatomica
(official anatomical
nomenclature)
BNC benign neonatal
convulsions
bladder neck contracture
BND barely noticeable
difference
BNDD Bureau of Narcotics and
Dangerous Drugs
BNF bilateral neurofibromatosis

BNFE benign neonatal familial
epilepsy
BNO bladder-neck obstruction
BNOE benign necrotizing otitis
externa
BNS benign nephrosclerosis
(hyaline arteriolar
nephrosclerosis)
BO beeper obliterans
biliary obstruction
blackout
body odor
bowel obstruction
breath odor
B & O belladonna and opium
BOA benzoquinone-acetic acid
bifurcation of aorta
born out of asepsis
BOC butyloxycarbonyl
BOD biochemical oxygen
demand
borderline
breach of duty
BOH Board of Health
bundle of His
(atrioventricular bundle)
BOLD bleomycin + Oncovin
(vincristine) + lomustine
+ dacarbazine
(combination
chemotherapy)
blood oxygen level-
dependent
BoLV bovine leukemia virus
BOM bilateral otitis media
BOMC blessed-orientation-
memory-concentration
(test)
BOO bladder outlet obstruction
BOOP bronchiolitis obliterans
with organizing
pneumonia
BOS bacterial overgrowth
syndrome
bail-out stenting
BOT benign ovarian tumor
botulinum toxin
bowing of tibia
bot bottle

BOU   burning on urination
BOW   bag of waters (amniotic sac)
BOW-B   bag of waters broke
BP   bacillary peliosis
back pain
barbital poisoning
bathroom privileges
bedpan
Bell's palsy (facial paralysis with characteristic distortion)
beta-protein
biological parent
biphenyl
bipolar
bipolar prosthesis
bleach poisoning
blood pressure
boiling point
bone paste
bowenoid papulosis
brachial plexus
breech presentation

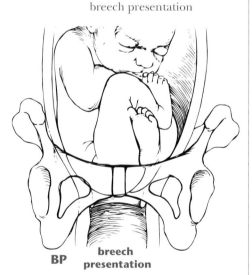

BP   **breech presentation**

bronchopneumonia (inflammation of the lungs, usually originating in the bronchioles)
bubonic plague (the most common form of plague, marked by inflammatory

enlargement of lymphatic glands)
bullous pemphigoid
bypass (a shunt; a diverted flow)
B/P   blood pressure
bp   base pair
bed pan
boiling point
bronchopulmonary aspergillosis
BPAD 1   bipolar affective disorder type 1
BPB   biliopancreatic bypass
black-pigmented bacteroides
brachial plexus block
bromophenol blue (indicator of hydrogen ion concentration)
BPC   bipolar cell (a neuron with afferent and efferent processes, as those in the retina)
blood pressure cuff
BPD   bipolar disorder (manic-depressive disorder)
borderline personality disorder
bronchopulmonary dysplasia
BPDAU   Bard patent ductus arteriosus umbrella (to close patent ductus arteriosus defects)
bronchopulmonary dysplasia (chronic lung disease of infants)
BPDscale   borderline personality disorder scale
BPEC   bipolar electrocardiogram
bipolar electrocautery
B.pertussis
Bordetella pertussis
BPF   Brazilian purpuric fever
bronchopleural fistula
buccopharyngeal fascia
BPG   baseline pinch gauge (determines

thumb-finger grasp)
blood pressure gauge
bypass graft
2,3-BPG 2,3-bisphosphoglycerate
BPH benign prostatic
hyperplasia

BPH
benign prostatic
hyperplasia

benign prostatic
hypertrophy
BPI bactericidal/permeability-
increasing protein
beef-pork insulin
BPIG bacterial polysaccharide
immune globulin
BPIP bactericidal permeability-
increasing protein
BPL benign proliferative lesion
beta-propiolactone
(disinfectant)
bronchopulmonary lavage
BPLNs bronchopulmonary lymph
nodes
BPM beats per minute
breaths per minute
brompheniramine maleate
bpm beats per minute
breaths per minute
BPMD benign pseudohypertropic
muscular dystrophy

BPN bacitracin, polymyxin B,
and neomycin
bacterial pyelonephritis
brachial plexus neuropathy
BPP backpack palsy
biophysical profile
bovine pancreatic
polypeptide
B protein precursor
brachial plexus palsy
brachial plexus paralysis
BP&P blood pressure and pulse
BPPD body-powered prosthetic
device
BPPN benign paroxysmal
positional nystagmus
BPPV benign paroxysmal
positional (postural)
vertigo (precipitated by
specific movements or
when the head is in a
certain position)
BPQA Board of Physician Quality
Assurance
BPS beats per second
binge-and-purge syndrome
breaths per second
bypass surgery
BPSD bronchopulmonary
segmental drainage
BPT bronchial provocative test
(to induce
bronchoconstriction)
BPTI brachial plexus
traction injury
BPV benign paroxysmal vertigo
benign positional vertigo
bilateral parietal vasectomy
BQ bentoquatum (Ivy Block;
protection against poison
ivy, poison oak and
poison sumac rash)
Bq becquerel (a unit of
radioactivity)
BR bathroom
bedrest
bedroom
biceps reflex (biceps jerk)
bilirubin (pigment formed

from hemoglobin during destruction of red blood cells by the reticuloendothelial system)
biologic response
biologic rhythms
birthing room
breathing rate
breech
butterfly rash

Br breast
breech
bregma
bromine
bronchitis
brucellosis

BRA brain
brain-reactive antibody

BRAC basic rest activity cycle

BRADY bradycardia (abnormal slowness of the heartbeat, a rate usually less than 60 beats per minute)

BRAO branch retinal artery occlusion

BrAP brachial artery pressure

BRAT Baylor rapid autologous transfusion

BRAT diet bananas, rice, applesauce, and toast diet

BRATT diet bananas, rice, applesauce, tea, and toast diet

BRBPR bright red blood per rectum

BrBx breast biopsy

BRCA1 breast cancer gene 1 (mutant human gene for breast cancer)

BRCA2 breast cancer gene 2 (mutant human gene for breast cancer)

BRcBRP bedrest with bathroom privileges

BRCM below right costal margin

BRF behavioral risk factor
bone-resorbing factor

BRFSS Behavioral Risk Factor Surveillance System

BRH benign recurrent hematuria
Bureau of Radiological Health

brkf breakfast

BRM biologic response modifier
biologic response modulator
brachioradialis muscle

BrM breast milk

BRNS Breathe Right nasal strips

Bron bronchial

Broncho bronchoscopy

Bronk bronchoscopy

BRP bathroom privileges
bilirubin production
brief reactive psychosis

BRPs biorational pesticides

BRR baroreceptor reflex
brachioradialis reflex
breathibg reserve ratio

BRS battered root syndrome

BrS breath sounds

BrU bromouracil (a pyrimidine analogue)

BRVO branch retinal vein occlusion

BS Babinski's sign

BS
Babinski's
sign

Bacillus subtilis
bacterial septicemia

Barlow's syndrome (mitral regurgitation)
Bartter's syndrome
Battle's sign (discoloration behind the ear, seen in fracture of the base of the skull)
bedsore
before sleep
Behcet's syndrome (mucocutaneous oral syndrome)
Bernheim's syndrome
Bethesda system
bile salts
bismuth subsalicylate (Pepto Bismol)
blind spot
blood sugar
Boeck sarcoid
bone scan
bone spur
border schizophrenia
Bouveret's syndrome (paroxysmal tachycardia)
bowel sounds
breath sounds
Brett's syndrome
Brudzinski's sign
Buckley's syndrome (hyperimmunoglobulinemia E syndrome)
buffered saline
Bunnel stitch
Bywaters' syndrome (crush syndrome)

bs   bedside
bowel sounds
breath sounds

BSA   benzenesulfonic acid
Biofeedback Society of America
body surface area
bovine serum albumin
bowel sounds audible (active)
brainstem audiometry
broad-spectrum antibiotic

BSAP   brief, short-action potential

BSB   body surface burned (%)
BSC   bedside commode
broomstick cast
burn scar contracture
BSCCs   bony semicircular canals
BSD   bedside drainage
BSE   bovine spongiform encephalopathy (mad cow disease) (human equivalent, Creutzfeldt-Jakob disease)
brainstem encephalitis
breast self-examination
BSEP   brainstem evoked potential
BSER   brainstem evoked response
BSF   busulfan (antineoplastic agent)
BSFs   B cell stimulating factors
BSGA   beta-streptococci group A
BSGS   branchio-skeleto-genital syndrome
BSH   Bassini-Shouldice hernioplasty
BSI   bicycle spoke injury
bound serum piron
brainstem injury
BSID   Bayley Scale of Infant Development
BSIP   Baer's sacroiliac point
BSJ   ball and socket joint (sphenoidal joint)

BSJ

ball and socket joint

BSK	breaststroker's knee
BSL	blood sugar level
BSN	bowel sounds normal
BSNA	bowel sounds normal and audible (active)
BSO	bilateral sagittal osteotomy
	bilateral salpingo-oophorectomy
	bilateral serous otitis (media)
BSP	sulfobromophthalein (Bromosulphalein)
BSp	bronchospasm
BSPD	burn stress pseudodiabetes
BSPT	Bromsulphalein test
BSR	blood sedimentation rate
	bowel sounds regular
BSS	balanced salt solution (balanced saline solution)
	basic salt solution
	Bernard-Soulier syndrome (Bernard-Soulier disease)
	bismuth subsalicylate (active ingredient of Pepto-Bismol; diarrhea prophylaxis)
	bowstring sign
	Brown-Sequard syndrome (ipsilateral paralysis with contralateral loss of pain and temperature sensation)
	buffered salt solution (buffered saline solution)
BSSC	bismuth subsalicylate (active ingredient of Pepto-Bismol; diarrhea prophylaxis)
BSSO	bilateral sagittal split osteotomy (of mandible)
BST	blood serologic test
	bowstring test
	buccal smear test
	bullet shot trauma
bST	bovine somatotropin
B. subtilis	*Bacillus subtilis*
BSUTD	baby shots (vaccinations) up-to-date

BT	balanced traction (balanced suspension traction)
	Barlow's test (maneuver test for dislocation)
	Bechterew's test (to detect sciatica)
	bedtime
	benign tumor
	benzidine test (for occult blood in feces or urine)
	biceps tendonitis
	bicipital tendonitis (bicipital tenosynovitis)
	biliary tract
	biologic therapy
	birth trauma
	biuret test
	bleeding time
	blind test
	blood test
	blood transfusion
	blood type (antigen phenotype)
	body temperature
	bowler's thumb (perineural fibrosis of the thumb's ulnar digital nerve)
	breast tumor
	breath test
BTA	bilateral tubal anastomosis
	bladder tumor assay
	Blood Transfusion Association
BTB	back to bed
	blood-testis barrier
	blood-thymus barrier
BTC	balloon-tipped catheter
	basal temperature charting
	bioavailable testosterone concentration
	body temperature charting by the clock
BTE	behind the ear (hearing aid placement)
	bladder training exercise
BTF	boot top fracture
BTFS	breast tumor

frozen section

BTH bitemporal hemianopia

BTHS broad thumb-hallux
syndrome

BTI biliary tract infection

BTL bilateral tubal ligation

BTLS basic trauma life support

BTO Blalock-Taussig operation
(the anastomosis of the
subclavian artery to the
pulmonary artery to
direct blood from the
systemic circulation to
the lungs)

BTP biliary tract pain

BTPS body temperature,
pressure and saturation

BTR biceps tendon reflex

BTRA Bolton tooth ratio analysis

BTS bleeding time test
blue toe syndrome
burning tongue syndrome

B-TS bradycardia-tachycardia
syndrome

BTT botulinum toxin therapy

BTU British thermal unit

BTV blue tongue virus

BTW beef tapeworm (*Taenia
saginata*)

BTX benzene, toluene, xylene

BU bacteriuria (bacteria in
the urine)
Behnken's unit
below umbilicus
Bethesda unit
blood urea
Bodansky unit
burn unit
busulfan (antineoplastic
agent)

Bu butyl (hydrocarbon
radical)

BU-CY busulfan +
cyclophosphamide
(combination
chemotherapy)

BUdR bromodeoxyuridine (it
causes breakage in
chromosomal regions)

BUDS bilateral upper dorsal
sympathectomy

BUE both upper extremities

BUG bulbourethral gland

BUI brain uptake index

BULIT bulimia test

BUN blood urea nitrogen
bundle

BUN/CR blood urea nitrogen-
creatine ratio

BUO bilateral ureteral
obstruction
bleeding of undetermined
origin
bleeding of
unknown origin
bruising of
undetermined origin
bruising of
unknown origin

BUQ both upper quadrants

BUS Bartholin, urethral, and
Skene's glands

BUSG biopsy with ultrasonic
guidance

BV bacterial vaginosis
black vomit
blood vessel
blood volume
bronchovesicular

BVAD biventricular assist device
blood vessel endothelium

BVE blood volume expander
(blood volume extender)

BVH biventricular hypertrophy

BVL bilateral vas ligation

BVMGT Bender Visual-Motor
Gestalt Test

BVP balloon valvuloplasty
blood vessel prosthesis

BVS blue velvet syndrome

BW battered woman
bed-wetting (enuresis)
below waist
birth weight
bladder washout
body weight
bullet wound
burn wound

bw   body weight
BWF   blackwater fever
bwf   bite wing film
BWR   baby with reflux
BWS   battered wife syndrome
        battered woman syndrome
        black widow spider
BWSBs   black widow spider bites
BWSV   black widow spider venom
BWt   birth weight
BWX   bite-wing x-ray
Bx   biopsy
BX BS   Blue Cross and Blue Shield
BXE   bedside x-ray examination
BXO   balanitis xerotica

        obliterans
BXRE   bedside x-ray examination
BYCPR   bystander-initiated
        cardiopulmonary
        resuscitation
BZ   benzodiazepine
        (minor tranquilizer)
BZC   benzocaine
        (local anesthetic)
BZD   benzodiazepine
        (minor tranquilizer)
        Brill-Zinsser disease
        (recrudescent
        typhus fever)
BZZI   Brunner zigzag incision

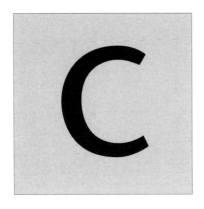

C

calcaneus
calculus
callus (new bone
 formation around
 fragments of a fracture)
Campylobacter
capacitation
capitulum
carbohydrate
carbon

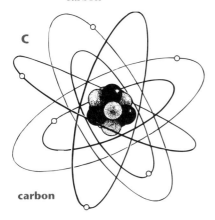

carbon

cardiac
carpus
carrier
cartilage
caruncle
cathode
Caucasian
cell
Celsius (a temperature

scale that indiates the
freezing point of water as
0°C and the boiling point
as 100°C under normal
atmospheric pressure)
centigrade (Celsius is
 preferred)
centriole
cerebellum
cerebrum
certified
cervical (vertebrae)
cesarean
cestodes (tapeworms,
 segmented worms)
chigger (agent of
 scrub typhus)
cholesterol (a fatlike
 steroid alcohol)
chorea (St. Vitus' dance)
chorion
chromosome
cilium
clavicle
cleavage
coccyx
cochlea
coefficient
collagen
colon

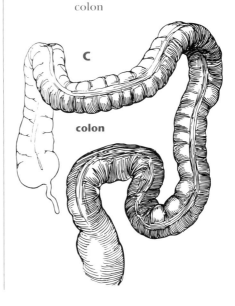

colon

comedo (blackhead)
complement (from C1 through C9)
concentration
constant
contraction
cornea
cortex
coryza (head cold)
coulomb
creatine (creatin; a nitrogenous compound found mainly in muscle tissue)
creatinine (a normal metabolic waste)
croup (acute respiratory illness characterized by resonant barking cough and hoarseness)
cuspid
cyanosis
cysteine (an amino acid present in most proteins)
cystine (a sulfur-containing amino acid present in many proteins)
cytidine (a nucleoside consisting of cytosine attached through a ß-glycosidic linkage to ribose)
cytosine (a decomposition product of nucleic acid)
large calorie

C   heat capacity

C'   complement (a multifactorial immune system consisting of nonspecific proteins present in normal serum that are essential for the destruction of cellular antigens in the presence of antibody)

C1   first cervical spinal nerve
first cervical vertebra
first component of complement

C2   second cervical spinal nerve
second cervical vertebra
second component of complement

C3   third cervical spinal nerve
third cervical vertebra
third component of complement

C4   fourth cervical spinal nerve
fourth cervical vertebra
fourth component of complement

C5   fifth cervical spinal nerve
fifth cervical vertebra
fifth component of complement

C6   sixth cervical spinal nerve
sixth cervical vertebra
sixth component of complement

C7   seventh cervical spinal nerve
seventh cervical vertebra

C7

seventh cervical vertebra

seventh component of complement

C8   eighth component of complement

C9   ninth component of complement

C3-4   space between third and fourth cervical vertebrae

C4-5 space between fourth and
fifth cervical vertebrae

C5-6 space between fifth and
sixth cervical vertebrae

C6-7 space between sixth and
seventh cervical vertebrae

C7-T1 space between seventh
cervical and first thoracic
vertebrae

c centi (prefix denoting
decimal factor 10^{-2})
cup
curie
cycle
cylinder
small calorie
with

c. *cum* [Latin] with

CA calcium antagonist
calcium oxalate
cancer
carbonic anhydrase
carcinoma
cardiac allograft
cardiac angiography
cardiac apnea
cardiac arrest
cardiac arrhythmia
cathode
Caucasian adult
cerebellar ataxia
cerebral aqueduct
Chemical Abstracts
chemotactic activity
child abuse
Chopart amputation
chromosome aberration
chronologic age
citric acid
coarctation of aorta
Cocaine Anonymous
congenital anosmia
conus arteriosus
coronary angioplasty
coronary artery
corpus albicans
crista ampullaris
croup-associated (virus)
cutaneous administration

(transdermal
administration)
cytotoxic antibody

C-A co-alcoholic

Ca calcium
cancer

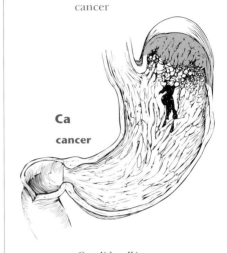

Ca

cancer

Candida albicans
carbolic anhydrase
cardiac arrest
carotid artery
cathode
cerebral aneurysm
cerebral angiography
cerebral aqueduct
cervicoaxial
Charcot arthropathy
chemical asphyxiants
child abuse
chromosomal aberration
chromosomal analysis
(chromatin)
chronological age
Cocaine Anonymous
conduction aphasia
cognitive avoidance
common antigen
condylomata acuminata
Cooley's anemia (beta-
thalassemia)
coronary angiography
coronary artery
corpus albicans
cortisone acetate

cystadenoma
cytosine arabinoside

C & A catabolism and anabolism
ca cancer
ca. *circa* [Latin] about
CAA carbamylaspartate
cerebral amyloid
angiopathy
cervical aortic arch
circulating anodic antigen
Clean Air Act
computer-assisted
assessment
coracoacromial arch
CA & A cardiac arrest and asystole
CAB captive air bubble
coronary artery bypass

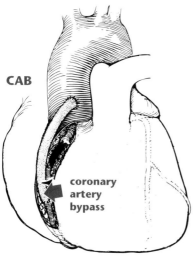

CAB

coronary
artery
bypass

CABG coronary artery bypass
graft(ing)
coronary artery bypass
graft (surgery)
CABI calcium bone index
CABPG coronary artery bypass
graft(ing)
CABS coronary artery bypass
surgery
CAC certified alcohol counselor
citric acid cycle
colon adenocarcinoma
coronary arterial calcinosis
cystadenocarcinoma
CA & CD cerebellar ataxia and
chorioretinal
degeneration
CACI computer-assisted
continuous infusion
CaCl$_2$ calcium chloride
CaCO$_3$ calcium carbonate
CACP cisplatin
(antineoplastic agent)
CaCX cancer of cervix
CAD chlamydia antigen
detection
computer-aided dispatch
computer-assisted
diagnosis
congenital abduction
deficiency
congenital articular
dysplasia

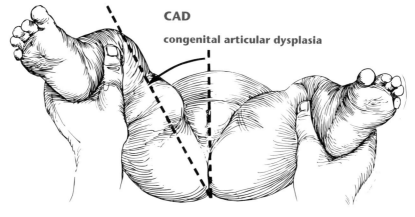

CAD

congenital articular dysplasia

coronary artery disease
Cad cadaver
CADD central axis depth dose
CAE centriacinar emphysema
cerebral artery embolism
childhood absence
  epilepsy (pyknolepsy)
coronary artery embolism
coronary artery
  endarterectomy
cyclophosphamide +
  Adriamycin
  (doxorubicin) +
  etoposide (combination
  chemotherapy)
CaE calcium excretion
CAF Children of Alcoholics
  Foundation
  (212) 949-1404
chronic atrial fibrillation
  (atrial arrhythmia)
cyclophosphamide +
  Adriamycin
  (doxorubicin)
  + 5-fluorouracil
  (combination
  chemotherpy)
cystadenofibroma
Caf caffeine
CAG chronic atrophic gastritis
closed angle glaucoma
congenital
  agammaglobulinemia
coronary angiogram
CaG calcium gluconate
  (calcium salt of
  gluconic acid)
CAGE cut down + annoyed by
  criticism + guilty about
  drinking + eye-opener
  drinks (alcoholism test)
CAH carbaminohemoglobin
chronic active hepatitis
  (chronic aggressive
  hepatitis)
congenital adrenal
  hyperplasia (most
  common adrenal
  disorder of childhood)

CAHD coronary artery heart
  disease
coronary atherosclerotic
  heart disease
coronary arteriosclerotic
  heart disease
CAHEA Committee on Allied
  Health Education and
  Accreditation
CAI carbonic anhydrase
  inhibitor
chronic adrenal
  insufficiency
chronic adrenocortical
  insufficiency
community-acquired
  infection
computer-assisted
  instruction
computer-aided instruction
CAJO cricoarytenoid joint
CAL café-au-lait (having the
  color of coffee with milk)
computer-assisted learning
coracoacromial ligament
Cal large calorie (kilocalorie,
  1000 calories)
cal small calorie
  (gram calorie)
Calb albumin clearance
C. albicans
  Candida albicans
CALD chronic active liver disease
calef. *calefac* [Latin] make warm
CALLA common acute
  lymphoblastic leukemia
  antigen
CALM café-au-lait macules
CALP café-au-lait pigment
CALS café-au-lait spots
  (pigmented macules with
  color resembling coffee
  with milk)
CAM child adult mist (tent)
chorioallantoic membranc
community-acquired
  meningitis
computer-assisted
  myelography

cyclic adenosine
monophosphate

cystic adenomatous
malformation

CAMF cyclophosphamide +
Adriamycin
(doxorubicin) +
methotrexate +5-
fluorouracil
(combination
chemotherapy)

CAMP cyclophosphamide +
Adriamycin
(doxorubicin) +
methotrexate +
procarbazine
(combination
chemotherapy)

cAMP cyclic adenosine
monophosphate

CAN child abuse and neglect
cord (umbilical)
around neck

CA/N child abuse and neglect

Canc cancelled

CANCER-LIT
cancer literature online

CANCER-PROJ
cancer research
projects online

CANS central auditory
nervous system

CANs cardioaccelerator nerves

CAO chronic airway obstruction
coronary artery
obstruction
cystadenoma of ovary

CaO₂ arterial oxygen
concentration

CAOD coronary artery
occlusive disease
coronary artery occlusion

CAOR central artery of retina

CaOx calcium oxalate

CaOxDD calcium oxalate
deposition disease

CAP cancer of prostate
capsule
carbamyl phosphate

catabolite activator protein

chloramphenicol (broad-
spectrum antibiotic)

chloroacetophenone
(tear gas)

chronic alcoholic
pancreatitis

chronic axonal poly-
neuropathy

College of American
Pathologists

colonic adenomatous
polyp

community-acquired
pneumonia

complement-activated
plasma

compound action potential

cyclophosphamide +
Adriamycin
(doxorubicin) +
prednisone (combination
chemotherapy)

cystine aminopeptidase

CaP cancer of prostate

cap capsule

cap. *capiat* [Latin] let him
(the patient) take
capacity
capsule

CAPA cancer-associated
polypeptide antigen

CaP CURE
Association for Cure of
Cancer of the Prostate

CAPD chronic ambulatory
peritoneal dialysis
continuous ambulatory
peritoneal dialysis

CAPER computer-assisted
pathology encoding and
reporting (system)

capiend. *capiendus* [Latin] to be
taken

CAPOC computer assisted practice
of cardiology

cap. quant. vult
capiat quantum vult [Latin]
take as much as desired

CAPS clinician administered posttraumatic stress (disorder)

CAPTA Child Abuse Prevention and Treatment Act

CAR cancer-associated retinopathy
chronic articular rheumatism
conditioned avoidance response
cutaneous axon reflex

CARB cilia-associated respiratory bacillus

CARBO Carbocaine (mepivacaine hydrochloride, an analogue of lidocaine)

carbo carbohydrate

CARE computerized audit and record evaluation (system)

CARES Cancer Rehabilitation Evaluation System

CARF Commission on Accreditation of Rehabilitation Facilities

CARM Children Against Rape and Molestation

CARN certified addiction registered nurse

cart cartilage

CAS calcific aortic stenosis
carotid artery stenosis
Center for Alcohol Studies
cerebral arteriosclerosis
chrome alum stain
cold agglutinin syndrome
congenital alcoholic syndrome
congenital aortic stenosis
coronary artery spasm
coronary atherosclerosis

cas castration

CASA computer-assisted self assessment
computer-assisted semen analysis
court appointed special advocate

CASH cancer and sex hormone
corticoadrenal stimulating hormone
cruciform anterior spinal hyperextension (orthosis)

CASHD coronary arteriosclerotic heart disease

CASMD congenital atonic sclerotic muscular dystrophy

CASOD chronic arteriosclerotic occlusive disease

CAST cardiac arrhythmia suppression trial
children of alcoholics screening test

CAT cataract
catecholamine (a group of compounds having a sympathomimetic action, such as epinephrine, norepinephrine, and dopamine)
children's apperception test
choline acetyltransferase
cognitive abilities test
combination antibiotic therapy
computed-aided transcription
computerized axial tomography (CAT scan)

CATCAM contour- adducted trochanteric controlled alignment method

cath cathartic (purgative; a substance that promotes evacuation of intestinal contents in a more or less fluid state)
catheter
catheterize

cath'd catheterized

CAT-LINE Catalogue OnLINE

CATS carotid artery territory stroke

CAT scan computed axial tomography scan
computer-assisted

tomography scanner

CaTT   calcium tolerance test

Cau   Caucasian

Cauc   Caucasian

caut   cauterization

CAUTI   catheter-associated urinary tract infection

CAV   computed-aided ventilation
congenital adrenal virilism
croup-associated virus
cyclophosphamide + Adriamycin (doxorubicin) + vincristine (combination chemotherapy)

CAVB   common atrioventricular bundle (bundle of His)
complete atrioventricular block
coronary arteriovenous fistula

CAVE   cyclophosphamide + Adriamycin (doxorubicin) + vincristine + etoposide (combination chemotherapy)

CAVH   continuous arteriovenous hemofiltration

CAVHD   continuous arteriovenous hemodialysis

CAVP-16   cyclophosphamide + Adriamycin (doxorubicin) + vincristine + etoposide + cisplatin (combination chemotherapy)

CAVS   calcified aortic valve stenosis

CAWO   closing abductory wedge osteotomy

CB   campylobacteriosis
capillary bed
carotid body
catheterized bladder
cell body (of neuron)
cesarean birth
chalk bone
chemical burns

childbearing
childbirth
chromatin body
chronic bronchitis
Clensicair bed (dignity bed)
code blue (designation for the hospital resuscitation team or for the resuscitation procedure)
color blindness
compact bone
cone biopsy
contrast baths
cost-benefit

C & B   crown and bridge (collar crown)

Cb   columbium (former name for the element niobium)

CBA   childbearing age
cholinergic blocking agent
chronic bronchitis-asthma
collar button abscess
cost-benefit analysis
coronary balloon angioplasty

CBAb   complement-binding antibody

CBB   chronic bad breath

CBBB   complete bundle branch block

CBC   complete blood (cell) count
child behavior checklist

CBD   closed bladder drainage

CBE   candle-blowing excrcise
clinical breast examination

CBF   cerebral bloodflow
collarbone fracture
coronary blood flow

CBG   cancellous bone graft
capillary blood gases
capillary blood glucose
coronary bypass graft
cortical-binding globulin (transcortin)
cortical bone graft
corticosteroid-binding globulin
corticosterone-binding

globulin

cortisol-binding globulin (transcortin)

CBH cutaneous basophil hypersensitivity

CBI *Campylobacter* infection

continuous bladder irrigation

CBL circulating blood lymphocytes

cord (umbilical) blood leukocytes

CbI cobalamin (vitamin B12)

CBLCA circumflex branch of left coronary artery

CBM capillary basement membrane

cognitive behavior modification

Cruveilheir-Baumgarten murmur

CBN chronic benign neutropenia

C. botulinum
Clostridium botulinum

CBP calcium-binding protein

Campylobacter pylori

carbohydrate-binding protein

chronic bacterial prostatitis

complete breech presentation

condylar blade plate

C4-bp C4 binding protein

CBPG coronary bypass grafting

CBPS coronary bypass surgery

CBR carotid-body reflex

complete bed rest

CBS cervicobrachial syndrome

chronic brain syndrome

closed building syndrome

conjugated bile salts

constriction band syndrome

Cruveilhier-Baumgarten syndrome

cystathionine beta-synthase

CBT carotid-body tumor

cognitive-behavioral

therapy

Coleman block test

cord (umbilical) blood transplantation (effective alternative to conventional bone marrow transplants; it is a rich source of stem and progenitor cells needed to reconsititute the blood-forming tissues)

cytokine-base therapy

C. burnetii
Coxiella burnetii (causative agent of Q fever)

CBV catheter-balloon valvuloplasty

circulating blood volume

Coxsackie B virus

CBVD cerebrovascular disease

CBW childbearing woman

CBZ carbamazepine (anticonvulsant and analgesic)

CC cardiac catheterization

cardiac contusion

cardiac cycle (a complete heart beat)

CC

cardiac cycle

cell count
cell cycles (the cycles
  occurring in a
  reproducing cell
  population)
cerebellar cortex
cerebral cortex
cervical cancer
cervical cap
cervical collar
chief complaint
cholecalciferol
chronic cholecystitis
chronic complainer
chronic constipation
cisterna chyli
clean catch
  (of urine specimen)
closing capacity
collateral circulation
colon carcinoma
colorectal cancer
common cold
common complaint
complex carbohydrate
congenital cataracts
congenital cholesteatoma
  (keratoma)
contrast cystogram
(umbilical) cord
  compression
corpora cavernosa
corpus callosotomy
corpus callosum
correlation coefficient
cortical cataract
costal cartilage
costochondritis
Couinaud classification
  (grading liver disease)
crack cocaine
creatinine concentration
cricoid cartilage
critical care
critical condition
Crohn's colitis
croupy cough
cryocautery
current complaint

cystocele
C & C cold and clammy
C-C convexo-concave
Cc concave
Cc creatinine clearance
cc cubic centimeter(s)
with correction

CCA calcium channel antagonist
Child's class A
  (classification of
  esophageal varices)
choriocarcinoma
  (carcinoma developed
  from chorionic
  epithelium)
cine coronary
  arteriography
circumflex coronary artery
clear cell adenocarcinoma
common carotid artery

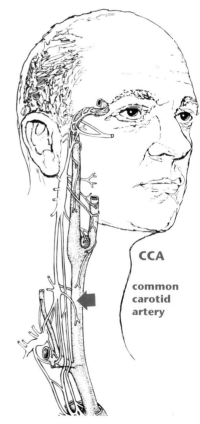

CCA

**common
carotid
artery**

congenital contractual
arachnodactyly

cupula of crista ampullaris

CCAC clear cell adenocarcinoma

C. canis *Ctenocephalides canis*

CCB calcium channel blocker
(nifedipine, verapamil; it
inhibits the entry of
calcium into cells)

carbon-carbon bond

Child's class B
(classification of
esophageal varices)

cold cup biopsy

CCC central corneal clouding

Child's class C
(classification of
esophageal varices)

chronic calculus
cholecystitis

chronic catarrhal colitis

chronic cigarette cough

clear cell carcinoma

comprehensive care clinic

CC&C colony count and culture

C/cc colonies per cubic
centimeter

CCCG cavum conchal
cartilage graft

CCCR closed-chest cardiac
resuscitation

CCCS condom-catheter
collecting system

CCD central core disease

cerebellar cortical
degeneration

cerebral cortical
degeneration

Chagas-Cruz disease (form
of trypanosomiasis)

charged-coupled device
(electronic device)

cleidocranial dysostosis
(cleidocranial dysplasia)

colony count for diarrhea

cortical collecting duct (of
kidney)

contract completion date

CCDC Canadian Communicable

Disease Center

CCE cardiogenic cerebral
embolism

clear-cell endothelioma

countercurrent
electrophoresis

CCEB Culture Collection of
Entomogenous Bacteria

C-cells calcitonin-producing cells
(of thyroid gland)

CCF cancer coagulation factor

carotid-cavernous fistula

compound comminuted
fracture

congestive cardiac failure

CCFE cyclophosphamide +
cisplatin + 5-fluorouracil
+ extramustine (combi-
nation chemotherapy)

CCG cholecystogram

chronic cystic gastritis

conchal cartilage graft

CCH chronic cholestatic
hepatitis

CCHD cyanotic congenital heart
disease

CCHF chronic congestive heart
failure

Crimean-Congo
hemorrhagic fever

CCHS congenital central
hypoventilation syndrome

CCI candidate for cochlear
implant

cardiocirculatory
insufficiency

chronic coronary
insufficiency

colocolic intussusception

CCID congenital cytomegalic
inclusion disease

CCJ calcaneocuboid joint

costochondral junction

CCK cholecystokinin
(pancreozymin)

CCL chronic catarrhal laryngitis

coracoclavicular ligament

costoclavicular ligament

costocoracoid ligament

critical condition list
CCl₄ carbon tetrachloride
CCLs craniocervical ligaments
CCM calcium citrate malate
closed chest massage
congestive cardiomyopathy
costoclavicular maneuver
critical care medicine
cyclophosphamide +
   CCNU (lomustine) +
   methotrexate
   (combination
   chemotherapy)
cysteine codon mutation
CCMS cerebro-costo-mandibular
   syndrome
clean catch midstream
   (urine specimen)
CCMSU clean catch midstream
   urine
CCMT cathechol-O-
   methyltransferase
CCN Computer Communication
   Network
condylocephalic nail
coronary care nursing
critical care nursing
curved Calapinto needle
CC NIH Clinical Center at NIH
Consensus Conference
   at NIH
CCNU chloroethyl-cyclohexyl-
   nitrosourea (lomustine)
CCO chronic contiguous
   osteomyelitis
C. coli *Campylobacter coli*
C-collar cervical collar
CCOS congenital corneal
   opacity syndrome
CCP chronic calcifying
   pancreatitis
chronic constrictive
   pericarditis
complement control
   protein (repeat)
complete cleft palate
cryptococcal pneumonitis
cytidine cyclic phosphate
CCPD chronic cyclic

peritoneal dialysis
continuous cycling
   peritoneal dialysis
Ccr creatinine clearance
CCR carotid chemoreflex
continuous complete
   remission
CCRC continuing care retirement
   community
CCRIS Chemical Carcinogenesis
   Research Information
   System (data bank)
CCRN critical care
   registered nurse
CCRPAT Critical Care Response
   Pattern Assessment Tool
CCRU critical care recovery unit
CCS celiac compression
   syndrome
central cord syndrome
cerebral calcification
   syndrome
cervical cell sample
cholecystosonography
chronic compartment
   syndrome
chronic congestive
   splenomegaly
coated compressed tablet
computerized cranial
   tomography
coronary care team
costoclavicular syndrome
critical care services
Cronkhite-Canada
   syndrome
CCSE cognitive capacity
   screening examination
CCT cancer chemotherapy
central conduction time
certified cardiographic
   technician
chronic catarrhal tonsillitis
closed cerebral trauma
combination
   chemotherapy
coronary care team
craniocerebral trauma
cuneocerebellar tract

cyclocryotherapy

CCTD craniocarpotarsal
dystrophy (whistling face
syndrome)

CCTV closed-circuit television

CCU cardiac care unit
critical care unit

CCUA clean catch urinalysis

CCUP culpocystourethropexy

CCV critical care ventilator

CCVM congenital cardiovascular
malformation

CCW counterclockwise

CD cadaver donor
Caffey disease
caisson disease
campomelic dysplasia
capillary drainage
cardiac disease
cardiac dysrhythmia
cardiovascular disease
carnitine deficiency
Carrion's disease
(bartonellosis)
celiac disease
(childhood sprue)
cerebellar degeneration
cervical dysplasia
cesarean delivery
Chagas' disease
(causative agent
Trypanosoma cruzi)
Charcot's disease
(neuropathic joint
disease)
chemical dependency
chondrodysplasia (results
in dwarfism)
Chopart dislocation
chromosomal disorder
chronic dialysis
chronic diarrhea
clinical death
closed drainage (airtight
drainage)
cluster designation
(of antigens)
cluster determinant
cluster of differentiation

(classification of
leukocyte antigens)
cochlear duct
cognition disorder
combination drug
communicable disease
communication disorder
complicated delivery
conductive deafness
congenital deafness
congenital defect
consanguineous donor
contact dermatitis

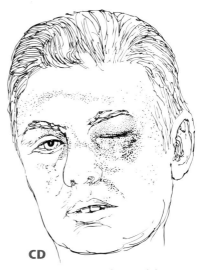

CD

contact dermatitis

contagious disease
corneal dystrophy
cranial dysraphism
Crohn's disease
cross dresser (transvestite)
cross dressing
(transvestism)
Crouzon's disease
cumulative dose
curative dose
cystine deficiency
cystic duct

CD3 antigenic marker on T cell
associated with
T cell receptor

CD4 antigenic marker of

helper/inducer T cells
(lymphocytes)

CD4 cc CD4 cell counts

CD8 antigenic marker of
suppressor/cytotoxic
T cells (lymphocytes)

CD$_{50}$ median curative dose

C/D cigarettes (cigars) per day

C & D curettage and desiccation
cytoscopy and dilatation

Cd cadmium (a metallic
element found in nature
associated chiefly with
zinc; excessive absorption
may produce interstitial
nephritis; inhalation may
produce pulmonary
edema)
caudal

cd candela

c/d cigarettes (cigars) per day

c.d. *conjugata diagonalis*
[Latin] diagonal
conjugate

CDA chlorodeoxy adenosine
(antiviral agent)
complement-dependent
antibody
congenital
dyserythropoietic anemia

2CDA 2-chlorodeoxy adenosine

CD18A CD18 antibodies

CDAD *Clostridium difficile-*
associated diarrhea

CDAP continuous distending
airway pressure

CDAPCA Comprehensive Drug
Abuse Prevention and
Control Act

CDB Center for Drugs and
Biologics

CDC capillary diffusion capacity
cell division cycle
Centers for Disease
Control and Prevention
(404) 329-3534 (formerly
called Communicable
Disease Center)
certified drug counselor

chronic disseminated
candidiasis
congenital dacryocystocele
Consensus Development
Conference (NIH
sponsored)
coronary dilatation
catheter

CDCA chenodeoxycholic acid
(chenic acid, an
abundant acid of human
bile with gallstone-
dissolving properties)
Consensus Development
Conference (NIH
sponsored)

CDCP Centers for Disease
Control and Prevention

CDCS cri-du-chat syndrome
(partial deletion of short
arm of chromosome 5)

CDD cervical disk disease
chronic degenerative
disease
chronic disabling
dermatosis
clot dissolving drug

CDDD cervical degenerative
disk disease

CDDP cisplatin (an antineoplastic
agent)

CDE certified diabetes educator

CDF chondrodystrophia fetalis

CDG chronic desquamative
gingivitis
cine-defecography

CDH congenital diaphragmatic
hernia
congenital dislocation
of hip (developmental
dysplasia of hip)
congenital dysplastic hip

CDI children's depression
inventory
color Doppler imaging

CD-I compact disk – interactive

C. difficile *Clostridium difficile*

CDILD chronic diffuse interstitial
lung disease

C. diphtheriae
Corynebacterium diphtheriae

CDJ choledochoduodenal junction

CDK congenital dislocation of knee

CDL carbon dioxide laser

CDLE chronic discoid lupus erythematosus

CDLT carbon dioxide laser therapy

CDM chondrodystrophic myotonia
clinical decision making

CDMAS computerized database management and analysis systems

CDML carbon dioxide membrane lung

cDNA complementary deoxyribonucleic acid (DNA)
copy of deoxyribonucleic acid (DNA)

CDP chemical dependence profile
chondrodysplasia punctata (stippled epiphysis disease)
chronic destructive periodontitis
cytidine diphosphate (a nucleotide that is a carrier for choline and ethanolamine in phospholipid synthesis)

CDPC cytidine diphosphate choline

CDR calcium-dependent regulator
complementarity determining regions of immunoglobulin
continuing disability review

CDRH Center for Devices and Radiological Health

CDROM compact disk-read-only memory

CDRs complementarity-determining regions (of immunoglobulin)

CDS caudal dysplasia syndrome
cervical disk syndrome
chronic dislocating shoulder (Bankart lesion)
closed drainage system
cul de sac

CDSC Communicable Disease Surveillance Center

CDSS cystic duct stump syndrome

CDT carbon dioxide therapy
combination drug therapy
combined diphtheria and tetanus

CDUS carotid Doppler ultrasonography
carotid duplex ultrasonography

CDX chlordiazepoxide (a benzo-diazepine tranquilizer)

CE California encephalitis
cardiac embolism
cardiac emergency
carotid endarterectomy
cauda equina (the sacral and coccygeal bundle of nerves in which the spinal cord ends; its appearance resembles the tail of a horse)
central episiotomy
cerebral edema
cerebral embolism
chorio-epithelioma
ciliated epithelium
columnar epithelium
conjugated estrogen
continuing education
converting enzyme

C/E angle center – edge angle

C & E cough and expectoration

Ce cerium (metallic element)

CEA carcinoembryonic antigen
carotid endarterectomy (most common operation in vascular surgery)
cholesterol-esterifying activity

cost-effectiveness analysis

cranial epidural abscess

CEBV chronic Epstein-Barr virus (infection)

CEC ciliated epithelial cell

CECT contrast-enhanced computed tomography

CED capacitance electronic disk

chondroectodermal dysplasia (Ellis-van Crevald syndrome)

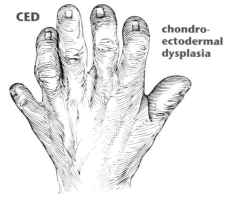

CED chondro-ectodermal dysplasia

chronic erosive gastritis

CEE childhood epileptic encephalopathy

conjugated equine estrogen

CEEG computer-analyzed electroencephalogram

CEFTAZ ceftazidime (cephalosporin derivative)

CEH chronic essential hypertension

CEI clinical ecological illness

coexisting illness

converting enzyme inhibitor

CEJ cemento-enamel junction

C. elegans

Caenorhabditis elegans

Cels Celsius (a temperature scale that indicates the freezing point of water as 0°C and the boiling point as 100°C under normal atmospheric pressure)

CEN certified emergency nurse

cent centigrade (Celsius is preferred)

CEO₂ cerebral extraction of oxygen

CEP chronic eosinophilic pneumonia

congenital erythropoietic porphyria

counter electrophoresis (counterimmuno-electrophoresis)

CEPH cephalosporin

CEp-S chromosome eighteen p-syndrome

CEq-S chromosome eighteen q-syndrome

chromosome eleven q-syndrome

CER cholesterol ester ratio

conditioned emotional response

cortical evoked response

cost-effectiveness ratio

CE & R central episiotomy and repair

CERCLA Comprehensive Environmental Response Compensation and Liability Act (superfund)

CERD chronic end-stage renal disease

Cert certified

CERULO ceruloplasmin (ferroxidase, an enzyme that oxidizes iron for transport in the blood)

cerv cervical

cervix

CES cauda equina syndrome

central excitatory state

cerebral edema syndrome

conditioned escape response

conjugated estrogen substance

cranial electrical stimulation

CEs conjugated estrogens

CESARS Chemical Evaluation Search and Retrieval System

CESC chorda equina of spinal cord

CESD cholesterol ester storage disease (mild lysosomal storage disease)

CETS chromosome eighteen trisomy syndrome
chromosome eight trisomy syndrome

CEUS cerebral embolism of unknown source

CEV California encephalitis virus
cyclophosphamide + etoposide + vincristine (combination chemotherapy)

CEX clinical evaluation exercise

CEx consultative examination

CF calcaneus fracture
calcarine fissure
cancer-free
cardiac failure
Caucasian female
cavus foot (talipes cavus)
centrifugal force
cerebral fissure
Chance fracture
chemotactic factor
Chiari-Frommel (syndrome)
chip fracture
chloroform
citrovorum factor
clavicle fracture
cleft foot (foot deformity in which the division between the third and fourth toes extends deep into the metatarsal area)
clotting factor
clubfoot (talipes equinovarus; one of the most common congenital deformities of the foot)
coccyx fracture

Colles' fracture (a fracture of the lower end of the radius bone)
complement fixation (test)
complement-fixing (antibody)
compound fracture
compression fracture

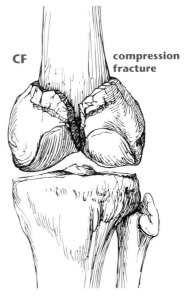

CF compression fracture

condylar fracture
constant frequency
conversion factor
coronary force
Cotton fracture
cough frequency
counting fingers (used in ophthalmology)
coupling factor
crush syndrome
cubital fossa
cystic fibrosis
Cystinosis Foundation

C & F chills and fever

Cf californium (radioactive element with a half life of 45 minutes)
complement fixation (test)

cf. *confer* [Latin] compare

CFA call for action

cervicofacial actinomycosis
colonization factor
  antigens
colony-forming assay
complement-fixing
  antibody (test)
Cystic Fibrosis Association

CFB Center for Bioethics
CFC capillary filtration
  coefficient
chlorinated fluorocarbon
chlorofluorocarbon
colony-forming cell
CFCP cystic fibrosis chest pain
CFD central fracture dislocation
chronic foot dermatitis
congenital facial diplegia
  (Mobius syndrome)
craniofacial dysostosis
craniofacial dyssynostosis
C. felis *Ctenocephalides felis*
C. fettus *Campylobacter fettus*
CFF critical fusion frequency
cystic fibrosis factor
Cystic Fibrosis Foundation
CFG chronic follicular gastritis
CFGH chorionic thyrotropin
  follicle-stimulating
  hormone
CFI complement fixation
  inhibition
C fiber unmyelinated axons
CFIDS chronic fatigue and
  immune dysfunction
  syndrome
CFL calcaneofibular ligament
  (of the ankle joint)
CFM craniofacial microsomia
CFND craniofrontonasal
  dysostosis
CFP cerebrospinal fluid protein
congenital facial palsy
cyclophosphamide +
  fluorouracil + prednisone
  (combination chemo-
  therapy)
cystic fibrosis of pancreas
cystic fibrosis protein
CFp-S chromosome five

p-syndrome
CFPT cyclophosphamide +
  5-fluorouracil
  +prednisone + tamoxifen
  (combination
  chemotherapy)
chromosome four p-
  syndrome
CFR Code of Federal
  Regulations
CFRs cumulative fertility rates
CFS Chiari-Frommel syndrome
  (galactorrhea-
  amenorrhea syndrome
  seen after pregnancy)
childhood febrile seizure
  (convulsions associated
  with high fever)
chronic fatigue syndrome
continuous filtration
  system
craniofacial stenosis
crush fracture syndrome
Cystic Fibrosis Society
CFs clotting factors
coagulation factors
CFSV cerebrospinal fluid shunt
  valve
CFT capillary filling time
capillary fragility test
  (Rumpel-Leede
  tourniquet test)
chronic fibrous thyroiditis
complement-fixation test
conjoint family therapy
CFTR cystic fibrosis
  transmembrane regulator
CFU close follow-up
colony-forming unit
CFU-C colony-forming unit,
  colony stimulating activity
  (granulopoietic
  progenitor)
CFU-E colony-forming unit,
  erythroid
CFU-L colony-forming unit,
  lymphoid
CFU-M colony-forming unit,
  macrophage

CFU-S colony-forming unit, spleen
CFV continuous-flow ventilation
CFX circumflex coronary artery
CG cerebral gigantism
cholecystogram
chorionic gonadotropin
chronic gastritis
chronic glomerulonephritis
congenital glaucoma
control group (subjects not exposed to special conditions)
corneal grafting
crista galli (a perpendicular bony ridge on the upper surface of the ethmoid bone in the anterior cranial fossa)
cryoglobulin
cystine guanine
cg centigram
CGA chlamydia group antibody
clonogenic assay
CGB chronic gastrointestinal bleeding
CGC Caenorhabditis Genetics Center
CGCE chronic glucocorticoid excess (hyperadrenalism)
CGD chronic granulomatous disease (immunodeficiency of X-linked or autosomal recessive inheritance)
CGE capillary gel electrophoresis
CGFs corticogeniculate fiber
CGH chorionic gonadotropic hormone
CGHP chorionic growth hormone-prolactin
CGI chronic granulomatous inflammation
CGKD complex glycerol kinase deficiency
CGL chronic granulocytic leukemia (chronic myelocytic leukemia)
correction with glasses
cgm centigram
cGMP cyclic guanosine monophosphate
CGN chronic glomerulonephritis

CGN chronic glomerulonephritis

CG/OQ cerebral glucose-oxygen quotient
CGP circulating granulocyte pool
CGRP calcitonin-gene-related peptide
CGS cardiogenic shock
caregiver stress
catgut suture (absorbable collagen from healthy animals)
centimeter-gram-second (system)
cryogenic surgery
CGT chorionic gonadotropin
CGTT cortisol-glucose tolerance test
CGVHD chronic graft-versus-host disease
cGy centigray (unit of absorbed radiation dose equal to 1 rad)
CH capillary hemorrhage
cardiac hypertrophy
case history
cerebral hemisphere

cerebral hemorrhage

charley-horse (muscle spasm, soreness and stiffness resulting from a direct injury)

chemical hazard

child

cholesterol (a fatlike steroid alcohol)

chronic halitosis

chronic hepatitis

chronic hypertension

chronic thyroiditis (Hashimoto's disease)

cluster headache

completely healed

corpus hemorrhagicum

cystic hygroma (lymphangioma cavernosum)

C-H crown–heel (applied to the length of a fetus)

C & H cocaine and heroin

Ch chest

choline (a precursor of acetylcholine)

chronic

CHA calcium hydroxyapatite

chronic hemolytic anemia

compound hypermetropic astigmatism (all meridians are hyperopic)

congenital hemolytic anemia

congenital hypoplastic anemia

cyclohexylamine

ChAC choline acetyltransferase

CHAD cyclophosphamide + hexamethylmelamine + Adriamycin (doxorubicin) + DDP (cisplatin) (combination chemotherapy)

CHAMPUS Civilian Health and Medical Program of the Uniformed Services

CHAP cyclophosphamide +

hexamethylmelamine + Adriamycin (doxorubicin) + cisplatin (combination chemotherapy)

ChAT choline acetyltransferase

CHB carbon-hydrogen bond

chronic hepatitis B

complete heart block

CHC community health center

Comprehensive Health Care

consumer health care

CHCC Comprehensive Healthcare Clinic

CHCl cocaine hydrochloride

CHD cartilage hair dysplasia

Chediak-Higashi disease (Chediak-Higashi syndrome)

childhood disease

chronic hemodialysis

claw hand deformity

common hepatic duct

congenital hip dislocation

congenital heart disease

congestive heart disease

coronary heart disease

CHE chronic hepatic encephalopathy (acquired cerebral degeneration)

chronic hypertrophic emphysema

ChE cholinesterase (an enzyme that removes acetylcholine discharged at the neuromuscular junction and prevents it from re-exciting the muscle)

CHEMLINE chemical dictionary online

chemical information online

Chemo chemotherapy

chemo chemotherapy

CHES Certified Health Education Specialist

CHF	chronic heart failure
	congenital hepatic fibrosis
	congestive heart failure
CHFV	combined high-frequency ventilation
CHH	cartilage-hair hypoplasia
CHI	closed head injury
CHINS	children in need of supervision
CHIP	catastrophic health insurance plan
	comprehensive health insurance plan
CHL	chloramphenicol (broad-spectrum antibiotic)
	conductive hearing loss
	coracohumeral ligament
chlor	chloride (any compound of chlorine)
CHM	congestive hepatomegaly
CHN	carbon + hydrogen + nitrogen
	certified hemodialysis nurse
	congenital hairy nevus
CHO	carbohydrate
C_{H_2O}	water clearance
Cho	choline (a precursor of acetylcholine)
CH₃OH	methyl alcohol
CHOL	cholesterol (a fatlike steroid alcohol)
Chol	cholesterol (a fatlike steroid alcohol)
c hold	withhold
Chole	cholecystectomy
CHOP	cyclophosphamide + hydroxydaunorubicin (Adriamycin) + Oncovin (vincristine) + prednisone (combination chemotherapy)
CHP	charcoal hemoperfusion
	Comprehensive Health Planning (and Public Health Services Amendments)
	cutaneous hepatic porphyria

chpx	chickenpox
CHR	cerebrohepatorenal (syndrome)
chr	chromosome
	chronic
CHRS	cerebro-hepato-renal syndrome (Zellweger syndrome)
	congenital hereditary retinoschisis (splitting of the retina)
CHS	Chediak-Higashi syndrome
	Composite Healthcare System
	compression hip screw
	congenital hip subluxation
	congenital hypoventilation syndrome
CHT	chemohormonal therapy
	closed head trauma
	combined hormonal therapy
CI	calcaneal index
	cardiac index
	cardiac insufficiency
	cartilage implantation
	cell immunity
	cephalic index
	cerebral infarction
	cerebral insufficiency
	cervical incompetence
	chronic impotence
	chronic infection
	chronic inflammation
	clinical investigator
	Coccidioides immitis
	cochlear implant
	coitus interruptus
	color index
	colostomy irrigation
	confidence interval
	contamination index
	coronary insufficiency
	counterincision
	counterirritant
	cross-infection
	cutaneous ileostomy
C & I	cataract and ichthyosis

Ci	curie(s)
CIA	chemiluminescent immunoassay
	chronic idiopathic anhidrosis (deficiency of sweating)
	colony-inhibiting activity
	common iliac artery
	congenial intestinal aganglionosis
CIB	crying-induced bronchspasm (spasmodic contraction of the smooth muscles of the bronchi)
cib.	*cibus* [Latin] food
CIBD	chronic inflammatory bowel disease
CIBP	chronic intractable benign pain
CIBPS	chronic intractable benign pain syndrome
CIC	calcium ion concentration
	cardioinhibitory center
	chronic inflammatory cell
	circulating immune complex
	clean intermittent catheterization
	common iliac catheter
	completely in canal (hearing aid)
	crisis intervention center
CICD	chronic irritant contact dermatitis
	circulating immune-complex disease
CICU	cardiac intensive care unit
	coronary intensive care unit
CID	cellular immunodeficiency
	central inspiratory drive
	chronic irritant dermatitis
	cytomegalic inclusion disease
	cytomegalovirus inclusion disease
CIDP	chronic idiopathic polyradiculopathy
	chronic inflammatory demyelinating polyneuritis
	chronic inflammatory demyelinating polyneuropathy
	chronic inflammatory demyelinating polyradiculoneuropathy
CIDS	cellular immunity deficiency syndrome
	continuous insulin delivery system
CIE	countercurrent immuno-electrophoresis
	counter-immunoelectrophoresis (technique in which antibody and antigen are placed in separate wells in an agar plate and attracted toward each other by an electric field)
CIEN	cervical intraepithelial neoplasia
	conjunctival intraepithelial neoplasia
CIEP	counterimmuno-electrophoresis
CIF	clipping injury fracture
	clonal inhibitory factor
	cyclooxygenase (COX) inhibition factor
Cig	cytoplasmic immunoglobulin
CIH	carbohydrate-induced hyperlipemia (hyperlipoproteinemia, type IV)
	chronic interstitial hepatitis (cirrhosis of the liver)
CIHD	chronic ischemic heart disease
CII	catheter-induced infection
	chronic intestinal ischemia
	continuous insulin infusion (with the insulin pump)

CILN	common iliac lymph node
CIM	chronic idiopathic megacolon
	Cumulated Index Medicus
CIMP	closed intramedullary pinning
CIN	central inhibition (inhibitory state)
	cervical intraepithelial neoplasia
	chronic interstitial nephritis (disease that destroys nephrons)
CIN I	cervical intraepithelial neoplasia (with mild dysplasia)
CIN II	cervical intraepithelial neoplasia (with modeate dysplasia)
CIN III	cervical intraepithelial neoplasia (with severe dysplasia)
C_{in}	insulin clearance
CINE	chemotherapy-induced nausea and emesis (vomiting)
	cineangiography
	cinematography
	cineradiography
CIP	chronic intestinal pseudoobstruction
CIPD	chronic intermittent peritoneal dialysis
CIPN	chronic inflammatory polyneuropathy
Circ	circular
	circulation
	circumcision
CIRF	cocaine-induced respiratory failure
CIS	Cancer Information Service (800) 4-CANCER
	carcinoma *in situ*
	catheter-induced spasm
CIs	counterirritants
CISC	carcinoma *in situ* of cervix
CISCA	cisplatin + cyclophosphamide + Adriamycin

	(doxorubicin) (combination chemotherapy)
CISP	chronic intractable shoulder pain
CISV	carcinoma *in situ* of vagina
CIT	Casoni intradermal test
	conventional insulin therapy
cit. disp.	*cito dispensetur* [Latin] dispense immediately
CITH	cytomegalovirus-induced thrombocytopenia and hemolysis
CITP	chronic idiopathic thrombocytopenic purpura
CIU	chronic idiopathic urticaria
CIVII	continuous intravenous insulin infusion
CJ	Charcot joint (neuropathic joint)
	Chopart joint (talonavicular and calcaneocuboid joints)
	conjunctivitis
CJD	Creutzfeldt-Jakob disease
C. jejuni	*Campylobacter jejuni*
CJR	centric jaw relation
CJS	Creutzfeldt-Jakob syndrome
CK	check
	choline kinase
	congenital kyphosis
	creatine kinase
	creatinine kinase
	crush kidney (lower nephron nephrosis)
	cytokinin
CK-BB	creatine kinase-BB isoenzyme (found primarily in brain)
CKC	cold knife conization
CK-MB	creatine kinase-MB isoenzyme (found primarily in heart muscle)
CK-MM	creatine kinase-MM

isoenzyme (found primarily in skeletal muscle)

CKP compartmental knee prosthesis

CL capillary lumen
cardiac lipomas
cholelithiasis
chronic leukemia
cirrhosis of liver
clavicle
clear liquid
cleft lip
coin lesion
confidence level
contact lens
corpus luteum

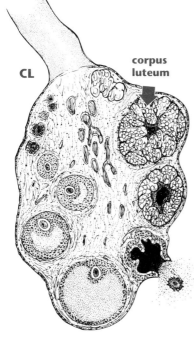

CL   **corpus luteum**

crab lice
critical list
cruciate ligament
cruciform ligament
cutis laxa (loose skin)
cytotoxic lymphocyte

Cl chlorine (a gaseous element used as a disinfectant and bleaching agent)

cl centiliter

CLA certified laboratory assistant
conjugated linoleic acid
contralateral local anesthesia
cutaneous lichen amyloidosis

Class classification

Class I congestive heart failure (no restrictons on ordinary activities)

Class II congestive heart failure (with some restrictions on ordinary activities)

Class III congestive heart failure (with marked restrictions on ordinary activities)

Class IV congestive heart failure (with severe restrictions on ordinary activities)

clav clavicle

CLB chlorambucil (antineoplastic agent)

CLBBB complete left bundle branch block

CLBP chronic low-back pain

CLC corpus luteum cyst

CL-CP cleft lip, cleft palate

CLD childhood language disorder
chronic liver disease
chronic lung disease
congenital lactase deficiency
Council for Learning Disabilities (913) 492-3840

CLDH choline dehydrogenase

cldy cloudy

CLE centrilobular emphysema (centriacinar emphysema)
congenital lobar emphysema
continuous lumbar epidural

cutaneous lupus
erythematosus

CLF cerebral longitudinal
fissure
Chinese liver fluke
(*Clonorchis sinensis*)
cross-leg flap

CLH cerebral longitudinal
fissure
chronic lobular hepatitis
corpus luteum hormone

CLI corpus luteum
insufficiency

CLIA Clinical Laboratories
Improvement
Amendments (of 1988)

clin clinical (relating to the
bedside observation of
the course and symptoms
of a disease)

CLIP corticotropin-like
intermediate (lobe)
peptide

CLL cholesterol-lowering lipid
chronic lymphatic
leukemia
chronic lymphocytic
leukemia

cl liq clear liquid

CLLs Child Labor Laws

CLM cutaneous larva migrans
(creeping eruption)

CLN caseouslike necrosis
cervical lymph node
Cloquet's lymph node (the
highest of the deep
inguinal lymph nodes)

CLO Caldwell-Luc operation
(surgical opening into
the maxillary sinus from
the mouth)
cod liver oil
congenital lobar
overinflation

ClO$_2$ chlorine dioxide

CL & P cleft lip and palate

CLS capillary-like space
carcinoid-like syndrome

cerebral lateral sulcus

CLS

cerebral
lateral sulcus

CLSH corpus luteum stimulating
hormone

CLT cholesterol-lowering
therapy
chronic lymphocyte
thyroiditis
clotting time

CLV cutaneous leukocytoclastic
vasculitis

CL VOID clean voided specimen

Clysis hypodermoclysis
(replacement fluids into
subcutaneous tissues)

CLZ clozapine (a sedative)

CM cardiac monitor
cardiac muscle
cardiomyopathy
Caucasian male
cell membrane
cervical mucus
chondromalacia
(abnormal softness of
cartilage)
chromosome mapping
chromosome 21
monosomy
chromosome 22
monosomy
chylomicrons
circular muscle
congenital malformation

congestive mastitis
(breast engorgement)
consanguineous marriage
continuous murmur
conus medullaris
(medullary cone; the
tapered end of the
spinal cord)
costal margin
crescendo murmur
Cushieri maneuver

C & M cocaine and morphine

Cm centimeter
curium (a synthetic
radioactive element)

cM centimorgan

cm centimeter

cm² square centimeter

cm³ cubic centimeter

c.m. *causa mortis* [Latin] cause
of death

CMA California Medical
Association
Canadian Medical
Association
carpometacarpal
articulation
certified medical assistant
Chemical Manufacturer's
Association
compound myopic
astigmatism (all
meridians are myopic)
cow's milk allergy

CMADL Controlled Medical
Assistance Drug List

CMAJ *Canadian Medical
Association Journal*

CMAP compound muscle action
potential

C-max maximum concentration
(of agent)

CMB carbolic methylene blue
(Swiss blue)

CMC carpometacarpal (joint)
cell-mediated cytolysis
cell-mediated cytotoxicity
chronic mucocutaneous
candidiasis

chronic myocarditis
congenital megacolon
(Hirschprung's disease)

CMCC chronic mucocutaneous
candidiasis

CMCJ carpometacarpal joint

CMCL carpometacarpal ligament

CMD cerebromacular
degeneration
childhood muscular
dystrophy
congenital muscular
dystrophy
congenital myotonic
dystrophy

CMDRH Center for Medical Devices
and Radiologic Health

CME chloromethyl ether
Code of Medical Ethics
continuing medical
education
crude marijuana extract

CMF chondromyxoid fibroma
(chondromyxoma)
craniomandibulofacial
cyclophosphamide
(Cytoxan) +
methotrexate + 5-
fluorouracil
(combination
chemotherapy)

CMF(P) cyclophosphamide +
methotrexate +
5-fluorouracil +
prednisone (optional)
(combination
chemotherapy)

CMFV cyclophosphamide +
methotrexate +
5-fluorouracil +
vincristine (combination
chemotherapy)

CMFVP cyclophosphamide +
methotrexate +
5-fluorouracil +
vincristine + prednisone
(combination
chemotherapy)

CMG congenital myasthenia

gravis
cystometrography
(recording pressure of
bladder at various
degrees of filling)

CMGN chronic membranous
glomerulonephritis

CMGT chromosome-mediated
gene transfer

CMH congenital malformation
of heart

CMHC community mental
health center

cmH₂O centimeters of water

CMI carbohydrate metabolism
index
carbon monoxide
intoxication
case mix index
cell-mediated immunity
(immune reactions
mediated by cells rather
than by antibodies)
chronically mentally ill
chronic mesenteric
ischemia

CMID cytomegalic inclusion
disease

c/min cycles per minute

CMIR cell-mediated immune
response

CMJ carpometacarpal joint

CMJD carpometacarpal joint
dislocation

CMK congenital multicystic
kidney

CML cell-mediated lympholysis
chronic myelocytic
leukemia
chronic myelogenous
leukemia
chronic myeloid leukemia

CMM cross-modality matching
cutaneous malignant
melanoma

cmm cubic millimeter

CMML chronic myelomonocytic
leukemia

CMN cystic medial necrosis

CMO calculated mean organism
Chief Medical Officer
competitive medical
organization
congenital melanosis oculi

CMOL chronic monocytic
leukemia

C-MOPP cyclophosphamide +
mechlorethamine
(nitrogen mustard) +
vincristine (oncovin) +
prednisone +
procarbazine
(combination
chemotherapy)

CMP carbon monoxide
poisoning
cardiomyopathy
central pontine
myelinolysis
chondromalacia patellae
coal miner's
pneumoconiosis
chondromalacia patellae
comprehensive
medical plan
continue present
management
cow's milk protein
cytidine monophosphate
(cytidylic acid)

CMPB chronic mucopurulent
bronchitis

CMPD chronic myeloproliferative
disorder

CMPF cow's milk, protein-free

CMPGN chronic
membranoproliferative
glomerulonephritis

CMR cerebral metabolic rate
cisplatin + methotrexate
(chemotherapeutic)
regimen

CMRO₂ cerebral metabolic rate of
oxygen (cerebral oxygen
consumption)

CMS chronic maxillary sinusitis
chronic myelodysplastic
syndrome

circulation, muscle
sensation
click murmur syndrome
(left ventricular
abnormality)
custom molded shoe

CMs chylomicrons (minute fat
particles in lymph about
one μ in size)

CMSU clean midstream urine
(specimen)

CMT cancer multistep therapy
cell-mediated toxicity
certified medical
transcriptionist
Charcot-Marie-Tooth
(disease)
Current Medical Terminology

CMTD Charcot-Marie-Tooth
disease (peroneal
muscular atrophy)

CMTF contingency medical
treatment facility

CMTS Charcot-Marie-Tooth
syndrome

CMV cisplatin + methotrexate +
vinblastine (combination
chemotherapy)
continuous mandatory
ventilation
controlled mechanical
ventilation
cytomegalovirus

CMVO continuous mixed venous
oximetry

CN cardiac notch
caudate nucleus
certified nurse
charge nurse
choroidal nevus
Cloquet's node (the
highest of the deep
inguinal lymph nodes)
coagulative necrosis
comparative negligence
compound nevus
compulsive neurosis
concurrent negligence
congenital nephrosis

congenital nystagmus
cortical necrosis
cranial nerve

CN I cranial nerve 1
(olfactory nerve)

CN II cranial nerve II
(optic nerve)

CN III cranial nerve III
(oculomotor nerve)

CN IV cranial nerve IV
(trochlear nerve)

CN V cranial nerve V
(trigeminal nerve)

CN VI cranial nerve VI
(abducent nerve)

CN VII cranial nerve VII
(facial nerve)

CN VIII cranial nerve VIII
(vestibulocochlear nerve)

CN IX cranial nerve IX
(glossopharyngeal nerve)

CN X cranial nerve X
(vagus nerve)

CN XI cranial nerve XI
(accessory nerve)

CN XII cranial nerve XII
(hypoglossal nerve)

Cn complement
component n
cyanide
(extremely toxic)

CNA chart not available
Child Nutrition Act

CNa clearance of sodium

CNAG chronic narrow angle
glaucoma

CNB cutting needle biopsy

CNCbl cyanocobalamin

CNDC chronic nonspecific
diarrhea of childhood

CNE chronic nervous
exhaustion

C3NeF C3 nephritic factor

C. neoformans
Cryptococcus neoformans

CNF chronic nodular fibrosis
cyclophosphamide +
mitoxantrone +
5-fluorouracil

(combination
chemothcrapy)

CNH central neurogenic
hyperpnea

CNHA congenital nonspherocytic
hemolytic anemia

CNI chronic nerve irritation

CNJ cuneonavicular joint

CNK cortical necrosis of kidney

CNL chronic neutrophilic
leukemia

CNM carcinomatous
neuromyopathy
certified nurse-midwife

CNMT certified nuclear medicine
technologist

CNP continuous negative
pressure
cranial nerve palsy
C-type natriuretic peptide

CNPV continuous negative
pressure ventilation

CNS central nervous system
congenital nephrotic
syndrome
cranial nerve syndrome
Crigler-Najjar syndrome

CNSD central nervous system
dysfunction

CNSLD chronic nonspecific
lung disease

CNT connecting tubule
(connects the distal
convoluted tubule of
the kidney to the
collecting duct)
could not test
cyanide-nitroprusside test

CNTF ciliary neurotrophic factor

CNU chloronitrosourea

CNV contingent negative
variation
cutaneous necrotizing
vasculitis

CO calcium oxalate
(insoluble calcium
compound found in acid
urine as crystals and in
urinary stones)

carbon monoxide
cardiac output
caster oil (obtained from
seeds of *Ricinus
communis*)
central obesity
certified orthotist
cervical orthosis
check out
Chiari osteotomy
cochlear occlusion
cochlear ossification
coproporphyrinogen
corneal opacity
corrective osteotomy
court order
cross over
cumulus oophorus
(mass of granulosa cells
surrounding the
developing ovum in the
ovarian follicle)

Co coinsurance

c/o complains of
in care of

CO_2 carbon dioxide

$^{14}CO_2$ radiolabeled carbon
dioxide

Co cobalt (a metallic element;
its ingestion has been
associated with
cardiomyopathy)
coenzyme (a nonprotein
organic compound
which plays an essential
role in the activation
of enzymes)

Co I coenzyme I

Co II coenzyme II

COA coarctation of aorta
condition on admission

CoA children of alcoholics
coarctation of the aorta
(aortic constriction or
narrowing)
coenzyme A

COAD chronic obstructive
airway disease

CoADD Coalition for the

Education and Support of Attention Deficit Disorder

COAG chronic open-angle glaucoma

coag coagulation

COAP cyclophosphamide + Oncovin (vincristine) + ARA-C (cytarabine) + prednisone (combination chemotherapy)

Coarc coarctation

COAS cervico-oculo-acoustic syndrome

CoA-SPC coenzyme A-synthesizing protein complex

COB cisplatin + Oncovin (vincristine) + bleomycin (combination chemotherapy)

chronic obstructive bronchitis

COBT chronic obstruction of biliary tract

COC calcifying odontogenic cyst

cathode opening contraction

combination oral contraceptive

coc coccygeal

COCCID coccidioidomycosis (fungous disease)

coch.amp.

cochleare amplum [Latin] heaping spoonful

coch.mag.

cochleare magnum [Latin] tablespoonful

coch. parv.

cochleare parvum [Latin] teaspoonful

COCM congestive cardiomyopathy

COD cause of death

condition on discharge

Code 99 emergency situation where patient is in respiratory or cardiac arrest

Code blue

cardiac or respiratory

arrest requiring immediate cardiopulmonary resuscitation

CODUC calcium oxalate dihydrate urinary calculi

COE cardiac output estimation

court-ordered examination

coeff coefficient

COFs clubbing of fingers

COFSS cerebro-oculo-facio-skeletal syndrome

COG cognitive (function test)

CoGME Council on Graduate Medical Education

COGTT cortisone oral glucose tolerance test

COH carbohydrate

chronic orthostatic hypotension

CoHb carbonmonoxyhemoglobin

carboxyhemoglobin (test)

COI childhood-onset insomnia

conflict of interest

cutaneous occupational infection

Coke cocaine

COLD chronic obstructive lung disease

coll colloidal

collat collateral

colpo colposcopy (examination of the uterine cervix and vagina by means of a colposcope)

CO₂LT carbon dioxide laser therapy

COM chronic opioid medication

chronic osteomyelitis

chronic otitis media

corpuscle of Meissner

COMC carboxymethylcellulose

commun communicable

COMP cyclophosphamide + Oncovin (vincristine) + methotrexate + prednisone (combination chemotherapy)

Comp complication

	compound
comp	complication
	compound
	compress
comp.	*compositus* [Latin] a compound
Comp A	11-dehydrocorticosterone
Comp B	corticosterone
Comp E	cortisone
Comp F	cortisol
compl	complaint
Comp S	11-deoxycortisol
COMS	cerebro-oculo-muscular syndrome
COMT	catechol-o-methyl transferase (enzyme)
COMUC	calcium oxalate monohydrate urinary calculi
CON	certificate of need
ConA	concanavalin A (hemagglutinating protein)
C-ONC	cellular oncogene
conc	concentration
conf	conference confinement
cong.	*congius* [Latin] a gallon
congen	congenital (present at birth)
conj	conjunctiva
CONQUEST	Computerized Needs-Oriented Quality Measurement Evaluation System
CONPADRI	vincristine + doxorubicin + melphalan (combination chemotherapy)
cons	consultation
cons.	*conserva* [Latin] keep
const	constant
constit	constituent
consult	consultant consultation
cont	containing content continue

	continuous
contag	contagious
contin.	*continuetur* [Latin] let it be continued
contra	contraindicated
cont.rem.	*continuetur remedium* [Latin] continue medication
Contus	contusion (a superficial injury or bruise)
conv	convalescing
COOD	chronic obstruction outflow disease
COP	capillary osmotic pressure colloid osmotic pressure cutoff point (value used to separate positive from negative test results) cyclophosphamide + Oncovin (vincristine) + prednisone (combination chemotherapy)
COPA	cyclophosphamide + Oncovin + prednisone + adriamycin (combination chemotherapy)
COPA CI	cyclophosphamide + Oncovin + prednisone + adriamycin + cytokine interferon (combination chemotherapy)
COPC	community oriented primary care
COPD	chronic obstructive pulmonary disease
COPE	chronic obstructive pulmonary emphysema
COPP	cyclophosphamide + vincristine + procarbazine + prednisone (combination chemotherapy)
COPRO oxidase	coproporphyrinogen oxidase
CoQ	coenzyme Q (ubiquinone)
COR	cardiac output recorder closed observation room

comprehensive outpatient rehabilitation

conditioned orientation reflex

corpuscle of Ruffini

cor	coronary
cor.	*corpus* [Latin] body
CORA	conditioned orientation reflex audiometry
CORD	chronic obstructive respiratory disease
CORF	Comprehensive Outpatient Rehabilitation Facility
corr	corrected
CORT	certified operating room technician
	corticosterone (cortisone)
COS	calcium oxalate stone
	clinically observed seizures
Cosm	osmolal clearance
COSMIS	Computer System for Medical Information Systems
COT	colony overlay test
COTE	complete occupational therapy evaluation
COTH	Council of Teaching Hospitals
COU	chronic obstructive uropathy
coul	coulomb
cov	covariance
COW	circle of Willis (arterial circle of the cerebrum)
COWS	cold opposite, warm same

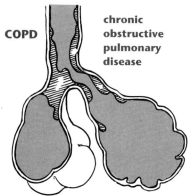

COPD chronic obstructive pulmonary disease

(caloric stimulation response)

COX	Coxsackie virus (name derived from the town of Coxsackie, New York, where it was discovered)
	cyclooxygenase (enzyme that converts arachidonic acid into prostaglandins)
CP	cancer procoagulant
	capillary pressure
	cardiopulmonary
	carotid pulse
	celiac plexus
	cellulitic phlegmasia
	cerebellopontine
	cerebral palsy
	cerebral peduncle
	certified prosthetist
	cervical plexus
	chemically pure
	chemoprophylaxis
	chest pain
	chicken pox

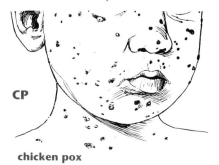

CP

chicken pox

child psychiatry

chondrodysplasia punctata

chronic pain

chronic pharyngitis

chronic pleurisy

chronic polyarthritis

chronic pyelonephritis

cleft palate

colonic polyposis

congenital porphyria

congenital ptosis

cor pulmonale (heart disease caused by

obstruction of pulmonary circulation)

C peptide (the connecting peptide that connects the A chain and B chain of the proinsulin molecule; it splits off as residue during the cleavage of proinsulin to form insulin)

creatine phosphate

creatinine phosphokinase

cryopreservation

cyclophosphamide + Platinol (cisplatin) (combination chemotherapy)

C/P cholesterol-phospholipid (ratio)

C & P chloroquine and primaquine (antimalarial agents)

cystoscopy and pyelography

CP chickenpox

peak concentration

phosphate clearance

cp chemically pure

CPA cardiopulmonary arrest

carotid phonoangiogram

Center for Patient Advocacy

cerebellopontine angle

chlorpropamide

circulating platelet aggregate

costophrenic angle

cyclophosphamide (antineoplastic agent)

CPAH para-aminohippurate clearance (measurement of effective renal plasma flow)

CPAP continuous positive airway pressure

C. parapsilosis

Candida parapsilosis

C. parvum

Corynebacterium parvum

Cryptosporidium parvum

CPAT cerebellopontine angle tumors

CPB cardiopulmonary bypass

CPBA competitive protein-binding assay

CPBP cardiopulmonary bypass

CPBV cardiopulmonary blood volume

CPC chronic pain center

circumferential pneumatic compression

clinicopathologic conference

constrictive pericarditis

CPCL congenital pulmonary cystic lymphangiectasia

CPCR cardiopulmonary cerebral resuscitation

CPD calcium pyrophosphate deposition

cardiopulmonary disease

carnitine palmityltransferase deficiency

cephalopelvic disproportion

childhood polycystic disease

chronic pain disorder

chronic peritoneal dialysis

chronic protein deprivation

chronic psoriasiform dermatitis

citrate-phosphate-dextrose

comparison point decision

compound

congenital polycystic disease

contagious pustular dermatitis

critical-point-drying

cyclopentadiene

Cpd compound

CPDD calcium pyrophosphate desposition disease (pseudogout)

CPE cardiac pulmonary edema

cardiogenic pulmonary edema

centralopathic epilepsy

chronic pulmonary emphysema

cis-platinum diamine-dichloride (antineoplastic agent, cisplatin; Platinol)

corona-penetrating enzyme

CPEO chronic progressive external ophthalmoplegia

CPF cancer-prone family

cardiac pump function

cardiac Purkinje fiber

clot-promoting factor

CPG carotid phonoangiogram

CPGN chronic progressive glomerulonephritis

chronic proliferative glomerulonephritis

CPH Certificate in Public Health

chronic paroxysmal hemicrania

chronic persistent hepatitis

corticotropin-releasing hormone

CPHV Center to Prevent Handgun Violence

CPI congenital palatopharyngeal incompetence

Consumer Price Index

coronary prognosis index

cysteine proteinase inhibitor

CPIB p-chlorophenoxy-isobutyrate

CPID chronic pelvic inflammatory disease

CPIP chronic pulmonary insufficiency of prematurity

CPK creatine phosphokinase (creatine kinase)

CPK-1 creatine phosphokinase MM isoenzyme

CPK-2 creatine phosphokinase MB isoenzyme

CPKD childhood polycystic kidney disease

CPL congenital pulmonary lymphangiectasia

cpl complete

CPM cardiac pacemaker

central pontine myelinolysis

chlorpromazine (Thorazine)

chronic progressive myelopathy

condylar process of mandible

continue present management

coronoid process of mandible

cricopharyngeus muscle

cyclophosphamide

cpm counts per minute

cycles per minute

CPMP Committee on Proprietary Medicinal Products (European Regulatory Committee)

CPMS chronic progressive multiple sclerosis

CPN chronic pyelonephritis

C. pneumoniae

Chlamydia pneumoniae

CPO cellular proto-oncogenes

certified prosthetist and orthotist

C-PORT Cardiovascular Patient Outcomes Research Team (clinical trial directed Johns Hopkins Medical Center)

CPP cancer proneness phenotype

cerebral perfusion pressure

chronic pelvic pain

chronic pigmented purpura

CPPB continuous positive pressure breathing

CPPD calcium pyrophosphate dihydrate

CPPDDD calcium pyrophosphate dihydrate deposition disease

CPPV continuous positive pressure ventilation

CPR cardiac pulmonary reserve
cardiopulmonary resuscitation

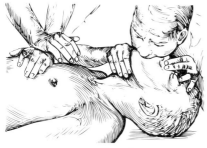

CPR cardiopulmonary resuscitation

cisplatin-paclitaxel (Taxol) regimen (chemotherapy for advanced ovarian cancer)

CPS carbamoyl phosphate synthetase
cardiopulmonary support (system)
cervical pain syndrome
chest pain syndrome
Child Personality Scale
Child Protective Services
chronic prostatitis syndrome
complex partial seizures
Consumer Product Safety Commission
contagious pustular stomatitis
cumulative probability of success

CPs capsular polysaccharides

cps counts per second
cycles per second

CPSA Consumer Product Safety Act

cPSA complexed form of scrum prostate-specific antigen (PSA)

CPSC Consumer Product Safety Commission (800) 638-CPSC

CPSCE ciliated pseudostratified columnar epithelium

CPSP central poststroke pain

CPT cancer pain treatment
carotid pulse tracing
continuous performance test
Current Procedural Terminology

CPT 1 carnitine palmityol transferase (deficiency), type 1

CPTA cerebral percutaneous transluminal angioplasty

CPTH chronic posttraumatic headache

CPU central processing unit (computing part of a computer)

CPUE chest pain of undetermined etiology
chest pain of unknown etiology

CPV chicken pox vaccine

CPW central pocket whorl (fingerprint)

CPX complete physical examination

CPZ chlorpromazine (Thorazine)

CQ chloroquine-quinine

C1Q protein of the complement system

CQA Command Quality Assurance

CQI continuous quality improvement

CR caloric restriction
cardiac resuscitation
cardiac rhythm
cellular receptor
cervical rib (an extra rib similar to, but

independent of, the first rib; usually attached to the seventh cervical vertebra)
chemoreceptor
chest roentgenogram
chief resident
child-resistant (cap on medicine bottle difficult for a child to remove)
chronic rejection
circadian rhythm (biological clock that recurs at about 24-hour intervals)
clinical record
closed reduction (of a fracture)
clot retraction
code red (emergency call designating a fire threat or alarm in an area of the hospital)
complement receptor
complete remission
complete response
conditioned reflex
conditioned response
congenital rubella
Congressional Record (congressional proceedings published each day since 1873)
conjugal rights
controlled release
corona radiata (an investment of granulosa cells remaining attached to the ovum when released by the ovary)
creatinine (a normal metabolic waste widely used as an index of kidney function)
cremaster reflex

CR 1   complement receptor 1
CR 2   complement receptor 2
CR 3   complement receptor 3

C-R   crown–rump (applied to length of fetus)
C/R   closed reduction
C & R   convalescence and rehabilitation
Cr   chromium (a metallic element, considered essential in trace amounts in nutrition)
cranial
creatinine (a normal metabolic waste widely used as an index of kidney function)
cr.   *cras* [Latin] tomorrow
CRA   central retinal artery
chronic respiratory alkalosis
Chinese restaurant asthma
chronic rheumatoid arthritis
colorectal adenoma
CRABP   cellular retinoic acid-binding protein
CRAG   cryptococcus agglutination (test)
cranial I   cranial nerve I (olfactory nerve)
cranial II   cranial nerve II (optic nerve)
cranial III   cranial nerve III (oculomotor nerve)
cranial IV   cranial nerve IV (trochlear nerve)
cranial V   cranial nerve V (trigeminal nerve)
cranial VI   cranial nerve VI (abducent nerve)
cranial VII   cranial nerve VII (facial nerve)
cranial VIII   cranial nerve VIII (vestibulocochlear nerve)
cranial IX   cranial nerve IX (glossopharyngeal nerve)
cranial X   cranial nerve X (vagus nerve)
cranial XI   cranial nerve XI (accessory nerve)
cranial XII cranial nerve XII

(hypoglossal nerve)

CRAO central retinal artery
occlusion

C-RAS-C cortex-reticular activation
system-cortex
activation loop

CRBBB complete right bundle
branch block

CRBSI catheter-related
bloodstream infection

CRC colorectal cancer
colorectal carcinoma
crisis resolution center

CRCA congenital red cell anemia

CrCl creatinine clearance

CR/CO centric relation/centric
occlusion

CRD child-resistant device
(cap on medicine bottle
difficult for a child
to remove)
chronic radiodermatitis
chronic respiratory disease
circadian rhythm disorder
congenital rubella deafness
crown–rump distance
(measurement of fetus)

CRDIP chronic relapsing
demyelinating
inflammatory
polyneuropathy

CRDs Capsaicin-related drugs

CRE cumulative radiation effect

creat creatinine (a normal
metabolic waste widely
used as an index of
kidney function)

Cr-EDTA chromium-labeled
ethylenediaminetetra-
acetate

crep crepitus

CREST calcinosis cutis, Raynaud's
phenomenon,
esophageal dysfunction,
sclerodactyly, and
telangiectasia (syndrome)

CRF cardiorenal failure
cardiorespiratory failure
chronic renal failure
chronic respiratory failure
continuous reinforcement
corticotropin-releasing
factor

CRG chest roentgenogram

CRH corticotropin-releasing
hormone

CRI cardiac risk index
catheter-related infection
chronic respiratory
insufficiency

crie crossed radioimmun-
oelectrophoresis

CRISP Computer Retrieval
of Information on
Scientific Projects

CRL complement receptor
lymphocyte
crown–rump length
(of fetus)

CRLP Center for Reproductive
Law and Policy

CRM chronic rheumatic
myocarditis
crown–rump measurement
(of fetus)

CRMO chronic recurrent
multifocal osteomyelitis

CRN chronic radiation nephritis
colorectal neoplasm

CRNA certified registered
nurse anesthetist

cRNA chromosomal
ribonucleic acid

CRNF chronic rheumatoid
nodular fibrositis

CRNP certified registered nurse
practitioner

CRO cathode ray oscilloscope
centric relation occlusion

CRP cAMP receptor protein
child-resistant packaging
chronic relapsing
pancreatitis
colorectal polyps
C-reactive protein
(abnormal protein found
in the blood serum of
persons in acute stages of

inflammatory diseases such as rheumatic fever)

cyclic AMP receptor protein

CrP creatine phosphate
creatinine phosphate

CRPD chronic restrictive pulmonary disease

CRS catheter-related sepsis
cell recovery system
cervical rib syndrome

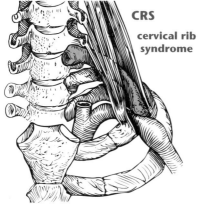

CRS
cervical rib syndrome

cherry-red spot (Tay's sign, a red circular area in the choroid of the eye)

Chinese restaurant syndrome (transient syndrome consisting of chest pains, throbbing of the head, and feelings of tightness of facial muscles after ingesting monosodium glutamate which is used liberally in seasoning Chinese food)

cholinergic receptor site

colorectal surgery

congenital rubella syndrome

CRST calcinosis, Raynaud's phenomenon, sclerosis of fingers, and telangiectasia (syndrome)

CRT capillary refill test
cardiac resuscitation team

cathode-ray tube

collagen replacement therapy

computerized renal tomography

congenital retinal telangiectasia

controlled-release tablet corrected

cranial radiation therapy

CRTT certified respiratory therapy technician

CRV central retinal vein

cr. vesp. *cras vespere* [Latin] tomorrow evening

CRVF congestive right ventricular failure

CRVO central retinal vein occlusion

CRW common ragweed

cryo cryoablation
cryoanalgesia
cryocautery
cryogenic
cryoprecipitate
cryosurgery
cryotherapy

cryoX cryoextraction

Crypto Cryptococcus

crys crystalline

CS calcaneal spur (heel spur)
carcinoid syndrome (argentaffinoma syndrome)
Cardarelli's sign
cardiogenic shock
caries susceptible
carotid sinus
catatonic schizophrenia (catatonia)
cavernous sinus
celiac sprue
celiac syndrome
cerebral seizure (epilepsy)
cerebrospinal
cervical collar
cervical smear
cervical spine
cervical sponge

Cesarean section
Chiari's syndrome
chondroitin sulfate
chondrosarcoma
chronic schizophrenia
Chvostek sign
cigarette smoke
cigarette smoker
climacteric syndrome
clonal selection
coercise sex
conditioned stimulus
congenital syphilis
conscious sedation
conservative surgery
continue same
continuous suture
coronary sclerosis
coronary sinus
corpus spongiosum
cosmetic surgery
Craig splint
craniosynostosis
cross section
Crouzon's syndrome
crush syndrome
cryosurgery
cryptosporidiosis
current smoker
Cushing's syndrome
cystine stone
cytologic smear

C/S   Cesarean section
consult
cycles per second

C & S   calvaria and scalp
culture and sensitvity

CS II   clinical stage two
CS III   clinical stage three
Cs   cesium (a rarc univalent
metallic element)

CSA   cell surface antigen
central sleep apnea
childhood sexual abuse
child sexual abuse
chondroitin sulfate A
colony-stimulating activity
Controlled Substances Act
Council on Scientific

Affairs (of the AMA)
cyclosporine A (used to
prevent rejection of
organ transplant)

CsA   cyclosporine A (used to
prevent rejection of
organ transplant)

CSAA   Child Study Association
of America

CSAB   complete sinoatrial block
CSAP   Center for Substance
Abuse Prevention
chronic stable angina
pectoris

CSAT   Center for Substance
Abuse Treatment

CSAVP   cerebral subarachnoid
venous pressure

CSB   cat-scratch bacillus
Cheyne-Stokes breathing
coil spring brace
contaminated small bowel

CSBF   coronary sinus blood flow
CSBS   contaminated small
bowel syndrome

CSC   chimney-sweeps'
cancer (carcinoma
of the scrotum)
cigarette smoke
condensate
collagen sponge
contraceptive

CSCR   central serous
chorioretinopathy

CSD   calcium store disease
cat-scratch disease
conduction system disease
craniospinal defect
cystine stone disease
cystine storage disease

C S & D   cleaned, sutured,
and dressed

CSDH   chronic
subdural hematoma

CSE   cancer screening
examination
cross-sectional
echocardiography
cytologic smear

examination
C-section Cesarean section
CSEP cortical somatosensory
evoked potential
CSER cortical somatosensory
evoked response
CSF cancer family syndrome
cerebrospinal fluid
clay shoveler's fracture
colony-stimulating factor
CSFE cerebrospinal fluid
examination
CSFP cerebrospinal
fluid pressure
CSFs corticospinal fibers
CSFSs cerebrospinal fluid shunts
CSFV cerebrospinal fluid
voluume
CSH carotid sinus
hypersensitivity
CSHFI cervical spine hyper-
extension-flexion injury
CSI cancer serum index
cavernous sinus infiltration
cervical spine injury
cholesterol saturation
index
chronic smoke inhalation
coital stimulating
instrument
continuous subcutaneous
infusion
cranial spinal irradiation
CSIA confirmatory strip
immunoblot assay
CSII continuous subcutaneous
insulin infusion
CSIIP continuous subcutaneous
insulin infusion pump
CSIN Chemical Substances
Information Network
CSJ costosternal joint
CSK convertible slip knot
CSLU chronic stasis leg ulcer
CSM cerebrospinal meningitis
CSMA chronic spinal muscular
atrophy
CSMB Center for the Study of
Multiple Births

CSME cotton-spot macular edema
CSN congenital sensory
neuropathy
CSNB congenital stationary night
blindness
CSNP corrective septonasoplasty
CSO chronic sclerosing
osteomyelitis
common source outbreak
CSOM chronic serous otitis media
(serous effusion into the
middle ear)
chronic suppurative otitis
media (suppurative
inflammation of the
middle ear)
CSP carotid sinus pressure
carotid sympathetic plexus
cell surface protein
chondroitin sulfate protein
circumsporozoite protein
criminal sexual psychopath
cyclosporin (used to
prevent rejection of
organ transplant)
CSPI Center for Science in the
Public Interest
C-spine cervical spine
CSQ Cognitive Strategies
Questionnaire
CSR central serous retinopathy
Cheyne-Stokes respiration
(breathing characterized
by rhythmic waxing and
waning of respiratory
depth)
continued stay review
corrected
sedimentation rate
cortisol secretion rate
CSS carotid sinus stimulation
carotid sinus syndrome
cavernous sinus syndrome
chronic subclinical scurvy
CSSD closed system sterile
drainage (airtight
drainage)
CST cardiac stress test
cavernous sinus thrombosis

chi-square test
computer scatter
  tomography
contraction stress test
  (exercise test under
  continuous ECG
  monitoring)
convulsive shock therapy
corticoid suppression test

CSTE Council of State and
  Territorial
  Epidemiologists
CSTI Clearinghouse for
  Scientific and Technical
  Information
CSU casualty staging unit
  catheter specimen of
  urinecorpus spongiosum
  urethrae
CSV Coxsackie virus (name
  derived from the town of
  Coxsackie, New York,
  where it was discovered)
CSW current sleep walker
CT calcitonin
  cancer therapy
  cardiac tamponade
  carotid tracing
  carpal tunnel
  cell therapy
  cerebral thrombosis
  cervical traction
  chemotherapy
  cholera toxin
  chordae tendineae
  chorda tympani
  chronic thyroiditis
    (Hashimoto's disease)
  chronotherapeutics
  chymotrypsin
  closed thoracotomy
  clotting time
  collaborative therapy
  collecting tubule
    (in kidney)
  computed tomography
  conjoined twins
  connective tissue
  continue treatment

contraceptive technique
corneal transplant
coronary thrombosis
crista terminalis (tenia
  terminalis)
cryotherapy
C & T color and temperature
ct count
  chest tube
CTA clear to auscultation
  cardiac T assay (to detect
    minor heart damage)
  chemotactic activity
  chemotactic agent
  computed tomographic
    angiography
  cytotoxic assay
CTAC cancer treatment advisory
  committee
c. tant. *cum tanto* [Latin] with the
  same amount
CTAP computed tomography
  angiographic
  portography
  connective tissue
    activating peptide
CTAT computerized transaxial
  tomography
CTB ceased to breathe
CTC circulating tumor cell
  cultured T cells
CTCL convoluted T-cell
  lymphoma
  cutaneous T cell
  lymphomas
CTCP carbon tetrachloride
  poisoning
  clinical toxicology and
  commercial products
CTD central tendon of
  diaphragm
  chest tube drainage
  connective tissue disease
  cumulative trauma
  disorder
C-terminal carboxyl-terminal
C. tetani *Clostridium tetani*
CTF cancer therapy facility
  Colorado tick fever (trans-
    mitted by the wood tick)

cytotoxic factor

CTFS complete testicular feminization syndrome

CT FSH chorionic thyrotropin follicle-stimulating hormone

CTFV Colorado tick fever virus

CTG cervicothoracic ganglion

cidofovir topical gel (used to treat refractory HIV lesions)

cytosine, thymine, and guanine

C/TG ratio cholesterol/triglyceride ratio

CTH chronic tension headache

corticotropic hormone

CTI carbon tetrachloride intoxication

continues to improve

CtI *Chlamydia trachomatis* infection

CTIA cerebral transient ischemic attack

CTICU cardiothoracic intensive care unit

CTJ costotransverse joint

cricothyroid joint

CTL cervico-thoraco-lumbar

chronic tonsillitis

congenital talus luxation (Volkmann's deformity, a congenital tibiotarsal dislocation)

costotransverse ligament

cricothyroid ligament

cytotoxic lymphocyte

cytotoxic T cell

cytotoxic T lymphocyte

CTLC contact transscleral laser cytophotocoagulation (used to treat glaucoma)

CTLM CT laser mammography

CTLN cricothyroid lymph node

CTM cardiotachometer

cricothyroid membrane

cricothyroid muscle

CTMC connective tissue mast cell

CTN calcitonin (thyrocalcitonin)

chorda tympani nerve

CTO cable twister orthosis

carpal-tarsal osteolysis

CTP central tendon of perineum

comprehensive treatment plan

cytidine triphosphate (a nucleotide required for RNA synthesis)

cytosine triphosphate (a component of nucleic acid)

C-TPN cyclic total parenteral nutrition

CTPVO chronic thrombotic pulmonary vascular obstruction

CTR calcaneal tendon reflex

carpal tunnel release

central tumor registry

ctr central

CTRA cardiac T rapid assay

C. trachomatis *Chlamydia trachomatis*

CTS carpal tunnel syndrome (entrapment neuropathy of median nerve at wrist)

Chaddock's toe sign

CTS Chaddock's toe sign

chromosome 21 trisomy syndrome

composite treatment score

computed tomographic scan

corticosteroid
cubital tunnel syndrome
  (entrapment neuropathy
  of ulnar nerve at elbow)
CTs Crutchfield tongs (skull
  tongs; used to exert
  traction on the skull)
CTSH chorionic thyrotropin
CTSO cervical thoracolumbo-
  sacral orthosis
CTT colonic transit time
  critical tracking time
  cytotoxicity test
CT/TT chronic thyroiditis with
  transient thyrotoxicosis
CTU centigrade thermal unit
CTV composite time value
CTW combined testicular weight
CTX chemotaxis
  cyclophosphamide
  (Cytoxan, an antineo-
  plastic agent of the
  nitrogen mustard group)
CTx cardiac transplantation
Ctx contractions
CTXM cerebrotendinous
  xanthomatosis
CTZ chlorothiazide (diuretic)
CU cardiac unit
  cause undetermined
  cause unknown
  cholinergic urticaria
  chyluria (passage of
  chylus into urine)
  cleft uvula
  clinical unit
  cold urticaria (wheal
  formed upon exposure
  to cold)
  contact urticaria (wheal
  formed upon exposure
  to a rapidly absorbable
  urticariogenic agent)
  convalescent unit
Cu copper (cuprum)
cu cubic
CUC chronic ulcerative colitis
  cystourethrocele
cu cm cubic centimeter

CUD cause undetermined
  chancroid ulcer disease
CUDS closed urinary
  drainage system

CUDS
closed urinary drainage system

CUE cumulative urinary
  excretion
  complete upper denture
CUG cystidine, uridine, and
  guanidine
  cystourethrogram
cu in cubic inch
culp culpable
cult culture
cu mm cubic millimeter
CUPN cystoureteropyelonephritis
CUPS cancer of unknown
  primary site
cur cure
curat. *curatio* [Latin] a dressing
CUS carotid ultrasound
  (examination)
  catheterized urine
  specimen
  chronic undifferentiated
  schizophrenia (psychotic
  symptoms that are not
  catatonic, disorganized,
  or paranoid)
CUSA Cavitron ultrasonic
  aspirator

Cavitron ultrasonic
surgical aspiration

CUT carbohydrate
utilization test

CuTS cubital tunnel syndrome

CuWS cockup wrist splint

CV cardiac volume
cardiovascular
carotenoid vesicle
cavernous sinus
cerebrovascular
cervical vertebrae
chorionic villi
closing volume (of lung)
coefficient of variation
contrast ventriculography
coronaviruses
costovertebral (angle)
coxa vera
cubitus valgus (deformity of
the elbow, which deviates
outward, or away from,
the midline of the body
when extended)
cutaneous vasculitis

c.v. *conjugata vera* [Latin]
true conjugate diameter
of pelvic inlet

CVA cardiovascular accident

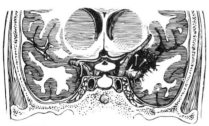

CVA cardiovascular accident

cardiovascular assessment
central visual acuity
cerebrovascular accident
(stroke)
cervicovaginal antibody
costovertebral angle
cyclophosphamide +
vincristine + Adriamycin
(doxorubicin)
(combination

chemotherapy)

CVAE cardiovascular
adverse effects

CVAH congenital virilizing
adrenal hyperplasia

CVAT costovertebral angle
tenderness

CVB chorionic villi biopsy
coxsackievirus group B

CVC cardiovascular
collapse (shock)
central venous catheter
central venous
catheterization
computerized
vectorcardiography

CVCT cardiovascular computed
tomography

CVD cardiovascular disease
cerebrovascular disease
collagen vascular disease
color-vision deviant
compact videodisk

CVF cardiovascular failure
central visual field
cervicovaginal fistula
cervicovaginal fluid
cobra venom factor

CVG contrast ventriculography

CVH central venous hum
cerebroventricular
hemorrhage
cervicovaginal hood
chronic viral hepatitis
combined ventricular
hypertrophy

CVHD chronic valvular heart
disease

CVI cardiovascular insufficiency
central venous infusions
cerebrovascular incident
cerebrovascular
insufficiency
Cervidil vaginal insert
(to soften the cervix prior
to vaginal delivery)
childrens' vaccine initiative
chronic venous
insufficiency

continuous venous infusion

CVID common variable immuno-deficiency

C. virus coxsackievirus (Coxsackie virus)

CVJ costovertebral joint

CVLP coronavirus-like particle

CVM cardiovascular monitor
cyclophosphamide + vincristine + methotrexate (combination chemotherapy)

c.v.o. *conjugata vera obstetrica* [Latin] obstetric conjugate of pelvic inlet

CVOD cerebrovascular obstructive disease
corporal veno-occlusive dysfunction

CVP cell volume profile
central venous pressure
circumvallate papilla (on tongue)
circumvallate placenta
cyclophosphamide + vincristine + prednisone (combination chemotherapy)

cvPO₂ cerebral venous partial pressure of oxygen

CVPP CCNU (lomustine) + vinblastine + procarbazine + prednisone (combination chemotherapy)

CVR cerebral vascular resistance

CVRD cardiovascular-renal disease

CVS cardiovascular surgery
chorionic villi sampling
clean-voided specimen

CVST chorionic villus sampling test

CVT congenital vertical talus

cvu clean voided urine

CVUG cystoscopy with voiding urethrogram

CW cardiac work
case work
cell wall
cerclage wire
chest wall
clockwise
common wart
continuous wave

C/W consistent with

CWA Clean Water Act

CWD cell wall defect
continuous-wave Doppler

CWE cotton-wool exudates (cotton-wool spots, soft-edged opacities in the retina)

CWF cartwheel fracture

CWI cardiac work index

CWL coffee worker's lung
cutaneous water loss

CWOP childbirth without pain

CWP chest wall pain
childbirth without pain
coal worker's pneumoconiosis

CWPEA Childbirth Without Pain Education Association

CWRA Clean Water Restoration Act

CWSs cotton-wool spots (cotton-wool exudates, soft-edged opacities in the retina)

CWT cold water treatment

Cwt hundredweight

CX chest x-ray

Cx cervix
clearance
complaint
convex

CxBx cervical biopsy

CXR chest x-ray

CxTx cervical traction

CY cyclophosphamide (widely used broad-spectrum antitumor agent)
cytochrome (respiratory enzyme capable of undergoing alternate

reduction and oxidation; chemically related to hemoglobin)

CY A   cytochrome A

Cy A   cyclosporine A (helps prevent rejection of organ transplants)

cyath.   *cyathus* [Latin] a glassful

CY B   cytochrome B

CY C   cytochrome C

cyc   cycle

cyclicAMP
cyclic adenosine monophosphate

cyclicGMP cyclic guanosine monophosphate

Cyclo   cyclophosphamide (antineoplastic agent of the nitrogen mustard group)

Cyclo C   cyclocytidine hydrochloride

Cyd   cytidine (a nucleoside consisting of cytosine attached through a ß-glycosidic linkage to ribose)

CYL   casein yeast lactate

cyl   cylinder
cylindrical lens

CYN   cyanide (extremely toxic)

CyP   cyclophilin

CYS   cystoscopy

CyS   half-cystine

Cys   cyclosporine (used to prevent rejection of organ transplants)
cysteine (an amino acid present in most proteins)

CYSTO   cystogram (a roentgenogram of the urinary bladder)

cysto   cystoscope
cystoscopy

Cyt   cytosine (a decomposition product of nucleic acid)

cytol   cytology

CZ   cefazolin (semisynthetic analogue of the antibiotic cephalosporin C)

CZS   cefazolin sodium

CZI   crystalline zinc insulin

CZP   clonazepam (an anticonvulsant agent)

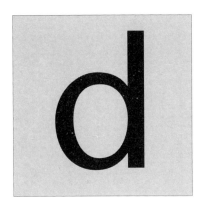

D aspartic acid
dalton
daughter
daunorubicin
day
dead
decamethonium
deceased
deciduous (teeth)
degree
dens
density
dental
depression
dermatology
deuterium
development
deviation
dextrose
diagnosis
diameter
diarrhea
diastolic (the pressure
  when the heart
  muscle relaxes)
died
digit
dilated
dilution
diopter (lens strength)
disease
dispense
displacement
distal

distance
donor
dorsal
dose
douche
drug
duodenum
duration
D1 day one (first day seen
  for treatment)
D3 cholecalciferol (vitamin
  D3)
2-D two-dimensional
3-D three-dimensional
D/3 distal third
D50 50% dextrose injection
d day
deceased
deci (prefix denoting
  decimal factor 10^{-1})
decrease
degree
density
2 'deoxyribo
deuteron (a subatomic
  particle consisting of a
  proton and a neutron)
diameter
died
diopter (lens strength)
diurnal
dorsal
dose
1/d one time a day
2/d two times a day
3/d three times a day
4/d four times a day
d. *dies* [Latin] day
DA dacryoadenitis
  (inflammation of a
  lacrimal gland)
decision analysis
decubitus angina (cardiac
  pain occurring in a
  recumbent position)
degenerative arthritis
delayed action
dental assistant
deoxyadenosine

developmental age

diabetic acidosis

differentiation antigen

direct agglutination

disability assistance

dissecting aneurysm

distended abdomen

dopamine (a compound produced by the decarboxylation of dopa)

dopamine agonist

drug abuse

drug addict

drug addiction

drug allergy

ductus arteriosus (a communicating channel between the pulmonary artery and the aorta in the fetus; it normally obliterates shortly after birth)

duodenal atresia

D/A date of accident

date of admission

D & A dilatation and aspiration

discharge and advise

Da dalton (unit of mass equal to one-twelfth the mass of the carbon-12 atom)

dA deoxyadenosine (nucleoside)

da days

deca (prefix denoting decimal factor x 10)

DAA dementia associated with alcoholism

dream anxiety attack

DAAO diaminoacid oxidase

DAB days after birth

dimethyl-amino-azobenzene (carcinogenic dye)

dysrhythmic aggressive behavior

DABA 2,4-diaminobutyric acid

DAC differentiated adenomatous carcinoma

diffuse alveolar

consolidation

direct-acting carcinogen

DACS data acquisition and control system

DACT dactinomycin (actin omycin D, an anti-neoplastic antibiotic)

DAD delayed after depolarization

depression after delivery

diffuse alveolar damage

dispense as directed

dispensed as directed

DADDS diacetyldiamino diphenyl-sulfone

dADP deoxyadenosine diphosphate

DAF decay accelerating factor

delayed auditory feedback

dag decagram

DAGT direct antiglobulin test

DAH diffuse alveolar hemorrhage

disarticulation of hip

disordered action of heart

DAI diarthrodial joint

diffuse axonal injury

DAK disarticulation of knee

DAL drug analysis laboratory

DALA delta-aminolevulinic acid

DALE Drug Abuse Law Enforcement

DAMA discharged against medical advice

dAMP deoxyadenosine monophosphate

DAO diamine oxidase (copper containing)

DAo descending aorta

DAP delayed-action preparation (time-release preparation)

delayed after depolarization

dextroamphetamine phosphate (abuse may lead to dependence)

diastolic arterial pressure

dihydroxyacetone
 phosphate
direct agglutination
 pregnancy (test)
dorsal artery of penis
draw-a-person
 (psychiatric) test

DAPRE daily adjustable progressive
 resistive exercise

DAPT direct agglutination
 pregnancy test

DAQ diagnostic assessment
 questionnaire

DAR death after resuscitation
 drug-abuse reporting

DARFD Depression Anonymous:
 Recovery from
 Depression

DARP drug abuse rehabilitation
 program

DART Development and
 Reproductive Toxicology
 (bibliographic database)

D/ART depression/awareness,
 recognition and
 treatment

DAS dead-arm syndrome
 delayed anovulatory
 syndrome
 dextroamphetamine
 sulfate (abuse may lead
 to dependence)
 doctor-assisted suicide

DASE dextroamphetamine
 sulfate elixir

DASH distress alarm for the
 severely handicapped

DAST drug abuse screening test

DAT daunorubicin + ARA-C
 (cytarabine) +
 thioguanine
 (combination
 chemotherapy)
 defective anion transport
 (chloridorrhea)
 delayed action tablet
 dementia of the
 Alzheimer type
 diacetylthiamine

diet as tolerated
digital audiotape
diphtheria antitoxin
direct agglutination test
direct antiglobulin test
disaster action team
drop arm test

dATP deoxyadenosine
 triphosphate

DATTA diagnostic and therapeutic
 technology assessment

DAU deazauridine

Dauno daunorubicin (antibiotic
 antineoplastic agent)

DAV Disabled American
 Veterans
 domestic abuse and
 violence

DAVP D-arginine vasopressin
 deamino-arginine
 vasopressin

DAW dispense as written

DAWN Drug Abuse Warning
 Network

DB data base
 date of birth
 deep breath
 diabetes
 diet beverage
 direct bilirubin
 direct bronchoscopy
 disability
 double-blind (study)

Db diabetic

dB decibel (logarithmic
 unit of measure of
 sound pressure)

db date of birth
 decibel (logarithmic
 unit of measure of
 sound pressure)

DBA dibenzanthracene
 (polycyclic hydrocarbon
 capable of producing
 epithelial tumors)

DBC differential blood count
 dye-binding capacity
 double-barrel colostomy

DB & C deep breathing

and coughing

DBCL dilute blood clot lysis

DBCMS *Directory of Board Certified Medical Specialists*

DBCP dibromochloropropane

DBD definite brain damage
diffuse brain damage
disruptive behavior disorder

DBE deep breathing exercise

DBF dashboard fracture

DBH dopamine beta-hydroxylase

DBil direct bilirubin

DBIR *Directory of Biotechnology Information Resources*

dbl double

DBM dibromomannitol

DBMS database management system

DBP diastolic blood pressure
vitamin D-binding protein

DBPT dacarbazine (DTIC) +
BCNU (carmustine) +
Platinol (cisplatin) +
tamoxifen citrate (combi-
nation chemotherapy)
DNA-based predictive test

DBS Denis Browne splint
Diamond-Blackfan syndrome
diminished breath sounds
doctor at bedside
double-blind study
duck-billed speculum

DBT dialectical behavior therapy
double-blind test
double-blind trial
dumbbell tumor

DBV dacarbazine (DTIC) +
BCNU (carmustine) +
vincristine (Oncovin)
(combination chemotherapy)

DBW desirable body weight

DBZ dibenzylchlorethamine
(an alpha-adrenergic blocking agent)

DC death certificate

dendritic cells
dental caries
dermoid cyst

dermoid cyst

diagnostic center
diagnostic code
diagonal conjugate
dietary chaos (bulimia)
differentiated cell
digital clubbing
dilatation catheter
direct Coombs (test)
direct current
discharge
discontinue
Doctor of Chiropractic
dressing change
drug combination
Dupuytren's contracture

D/C discharge
discontinue

D & C dilatation and curettage
dilation and curettage
direct and consensual
drugs and cosmetics

dC deoxycytidine (nucleoside)

dc discharge
discontinue
discontinued

d-c direct current

d/c discontinue

DCA deoxycholic acid (a secondary bile acid)
desoxycorticosterone acetate
dichloroacetate
directional coronary angioplasty
directional coronary atherectomy

DCABG double coronary artery

bypass graft
DCB dichlorobenzidine
DC & B dilatation, curettage, and biopsy
DCBE double-contrast barium enema
DCC day care center
deleted in colon cancer (tumor suppressor gene)
dextran-coated charcoal
disaster control center
dorsal cell column
double-current catheter
dystrophic cardiac calcinosis
DCc double concave
DCCO diffusing capacity of carbon monoxide
DCCT Diabetes Control and Complications Trial
DC'd discontinued
dc'd discontinued
dCDP deoxycytidine diphosphate
DCES direct current electrical stimulation
DCF direct centrifugal flotation (Lane method)
DCG deoxycorticosterone glucoside
dinoprostone cervical gel
DCH day-care home
delayed cutaneous hypersensitivity
DCHN dicyclohexylamine nitrite
DCI dichloroisoproterenol
DCIP 2,6-dichloroindophenol
DCIS ductal carcinoma *in situ*
DCL diffuse cutaneous leishmaniasis
DCLCO diffusing capacity of lung for carbon monoxide
DCLS deoxycholate citrate lactose sucrose
DCM diabetic cardiomyopathy
dichloromethotrexate (antineoplastic agent)
direct cardiac massage
DCML dorsal columnmedial lemniscus

dCMP deoxycytidine monophosphate
DCN depressed, cognitively normal
dorsal cutaneous nerve
D colony dwarf colony
DCP dicalcium phosphate (dibasic calcium phosphate)
disease-causing pathogens
dynamic compression plate
DCP4 deleted in pancreatic cancer (a tumor suppressor gene that causes cancer when it is inactivated or mutated)
DCPN direction changing positional nystagmus
DCR dacryocystorhinostomy
delayed cutaneous reaction
delayed cutaneous reactivity
DCRT Division of Computer Research and Technology (of NIH)
DCS decompression sickness (type 1, bends)
decompression sickness (type 2, chokes)
Del Castillo syndrome
delerium/confusional state
diffuse cortical sclerosis
diffuse cutaneous scleroderma
displaced child syndrome
double-contrast study
dynamic condylar screw
dyskinetic cilia screw
DCSA double-contrast shoulder arthrography
DCT dichloroisoproterenol (beta-adrenergic blocking agent)
direct Coombs' test
distal convoluted tubule (of kidney)
diurnal cortical test
dynamic conformal therapy (irradiation technique)

DCTMA desoxycorticosterone trimethylacetate
dCTP deoxycytidine triphosphate
DCx double convex
DD dandruff
dangerous drug
day of delivery
de Clerambault syndrome
deferent duct

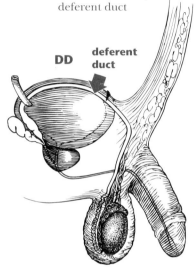

DD   **deferent duct**

degenerated disk
degenerative disease
delivery date
delusional disorder
dental decay
dependent drainage
designer drug
detrusor dyssynergia
developmental disability
developmental dyslexia
developmentally delayed
diaphyseal dysplasia
died of the disease
differential diagnosis
digestive disorder
dignified dying
direct diagnosis
discharged dead
discharge diagnosis
disk diameter
disk drive
distrophic dwarfism

divided dose
drug dependence
dry dressing
dual diagnosis
dual disorder
Duchenne's dystrophy
ductus deferens (vas deferens)
duodenal diverticulum
Dupuytren's disease
dysthymic disorder (dysthymia)
dd dideoxynucleoside
d.d. *detur ad* [Latin] let it be given to
D & D death and dignity
diarrhea and dehydration
dysphagia and dysphonia
dd due date
DDA Dangerous Drugs Act
dementia associated with alcoholism
dideoxyadenosine
ddA dideoxyadenosine
dDAVP desamino D-arginine vasopressin (desmopressin acetate)
DDC dideoxycytidine (zalcitabine)
dicarbethoxydihydro-collidine
diethyldithiocarbamate
distal digital crease
diverticular disease of the colon
ddC dideoxycytidine (zalcitabine)
ddCTP zalcitabine triphosphate
DDD degenerative disk disease
dehydroxydinaphthyl disulfide
dense deposit disease
Denver dialysis disease
derivative of DDT that inhibits adrenocortical function
dihydroxydinaphthyl disulfide
Disability Determination

Division (of Social
Security Administration)
DDE dichlorodiphenylethylene
DDG deoxy-D-glucose
ddG dideoxyguanosine
DDF dideoxy finger-printing
DDH development dysplasia
of hip
DDI dideoxyinosine
(Didanosine)
ddI dideoxyinosine
(Didanosine)
DDIs drug-drug interactions
dDNA denatured DNA
(deoxyribonucleic acid)
DDNTP dideoxynucleoside
triphosphate
DDP diamine-dichloroplatinum
(cisplatin, an
antineoplastic agent)
DDPN deafness, diabetes,
photomyoclonus
and nephropathy
DDRC drug dose-response curve
DDS damaged disk syndrome
Denys-Drash syndrome
depressed DNA synthesis
descriptor differential scale
dialysis disequilibrium
syndrome
diaminodiphenylsulfone
disease-disability scale
Doctor of Dental Surgery
drug delivery system
dystrophy-dystocia
syndrome
DDSI digital damage severity
index
DDSO diaminodiphenylsulfoxide
DDST Denver Development
Screening Test
DDT dichlorodiphenyl-
trichloroethane (toxic
insecticide)
deferent duct tumor
double diffusion test
DDTC diethyldithiocarbamate
Drug Dependence
Treatment Center

DDTP drug dependence
treatment program
ddTTP dideoxythymidine
triphosphate
DDU dermo-distortive urticaria
DDVP dichlorvos (insecticide and
anthelmintic)
D/DW dextrose in distilled water
DDx differential diagnosis
DE dependent edema
dermoepidermal
diagnostic error
digoxin elixir
Doppler effect (the
apparent change in
frequency of sound or
light waves when the
observer and the source
are in relative motion; the
frequency increases when
they approach one
another and decreases
when they move away)
dose equivalent
D & E diet and elimination
dilatation and evacuation
DEA dehydroepiandrosterone
(an androgen)
Drug Enforcement
Administration (Agency)
DEAE diethylaminoethyl
(cellulose)
DEB dystrophic epidermolysis
bullosa
DEBA diethylbarbituric acid
debil debilitation
deb. spis. *debita spissitudine* [Latin] of
the proper consistency
DEC deceased
deoxycholate citrate
diethylcarbamazine
(antifilarial agent)
Doppler echocardiography
dec deceased
deciduous
decreased
DECA nandrolone decanoate (an
anabolic steroid)
DECG Doppler echocardiography

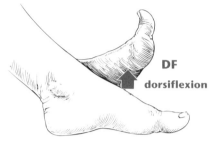

DF dorsiflexion

decomp decompose

decr decreased

decub. *decubitus* [Latin] decubitus position (lying down)

DED date of expected delivery

debrancher enzyme deficiency (type III glycogenosis)

delayed erythema dose

de d.in d. *de die in diem* [Latin] from day to day

DEEG depth electroencephalogram

DEET diethyltoluamide (arthropod repellent)

DEF decayed, extracted, filled (teeth)

def defecation

deficiency

deformity

defib defibrillation

deform deformity

DEG diethylene glycol

Deg degree

deglut. *deglutiatur* [Latin] swallow

dehyd dehydration

DEJ demal-epidermal junction

Del delivery

DEM Demerol (meperidine hydrochloride)

Department of Emergency Medicine

diethylmaleate

dysplasia epiphysalis multiplex

demo demonstration

DEN dermatitis exfoliative neonatorum

device evaluation network

diethylnitrosamine

DEP dependent

diabetic encephalopathy

diesal exhaust particulates

DEPA diethylene phosphoramide

dual energy photon absorptiometry

depr depressed

Dep ST Seg depressed ST segment

DER disulfiram-ethanol (alcohol) reaction (produces an aversion to alcohol in the treatment of chronic alcoholism)

deriv derivative

Derm dermatology

DERV duck embryo rabies vaccine

DES diethylstilbestrol (a synthetic nonsteroidal estrogen; stilbestrol)

diffuse esophageal spasm

disequilibrium syndrome

DES C diethylstilbestrol children

Desc Ao descending aorta

DESI direct egg sperm injection

DET diethyltoluamide (arthropod repellent)

diethyltryptamine (a hallucinogenic substance)

dye excretion test

det. *detur* [Latin] give

detox detoxification

detoxify

d. et s. *detur et signetur* [Latin] let it be given and labeled

DEV duck embryo vaccine (a killed rabies virus vaccine)

dev deviation

DEX dexamethasone (synthetic glucocorticoid)

DEXA dual energy x-ray absorptiometry (predictor of fracture risks)

DF decayed and filled

(permanent teeth)

deferoxamine
(chelating agent)

deficiency factor

dengue fever

Denonvillier's fascia

depressed fracture

dermatofibroma

dietary fiber

dorsiflexion

drug free

duodenal flexure

Dupuytren fracture

Duverney fracture

dysgonic fermenter

dF disseminated foci

df decayed and filled
(deciduous teeth)

dorsiflexion

DFA difficulty falling asleep

direct fluorescent antibody
(test)

DFB dysfunctional bleeding

DFD degenerative facet disease

DFE distal femoral epiphysis

DFF dexfenfluramine (anti-
obesity drug)

distal femoral epiphysis

DFI disease-free interval

DFM dark-field microscopy

decreased fetal movement

DFMC daily fetal movement count

DFMO difluoromethylornithine

DFN disseminated fat necrosis
(metastatic fat necrosis)

DFO deferoxamine (a
chelating agent)

DFP diastoic filling period

diisopropyl
fluorophosphate
(a potent
acetylcholinesterase
inhibitor)

DFPP double filtration
plasmapheresis

DFS dead fetus syndrome

disease-free survival

drop foot splint

DFSP dermatofibrosarcoma

protuberans

DFU dead fetus *in utero*

diabetic foot ulcer

dideoxyfluorouridine

DFW drug-free workplace

DFWP drug-free workplace

DFYR disability-free years
remaining

DFZ drug free zone

DG deoxyglucose (a metabolite
of glucose)

dermographism

diastolic gallop

diglyceride

dominant gene

dry gangrene

D & G deafness and goiter

dG deoxyguanosine (a
nucleoside, guanine beta-
D-deoxyribofuranoside)

dg decigram

DGCM Division of Grants and
Contracts Management

DGCR defective glucose
counterregulation
(failure of the response
mechanism to
hypoglycemia)

dGDP deoxyguanosine
diphosphate

DGE delayed gastric emptying

D gene diversity minigene

DGGE denaturing gradient gel
electrophoresis

DGI dentinogenesis imperfecta

disseminated gonococcal
infection (arthritis-
dermatitis syndrome)

DGLA dihomogamma-
linolenic acid

dgm decigram

dGMP deoxyguanosine
monophosphate

DGN diffuse glomerulonephritis

DGR duodenogastric reflux

DGS diabetic glomerulosclerosis
(intercapillary
glomerulosclerosis)

Di Guglielmo syndrome

(erythroleukemia)

dGTP deoxyguanosine triphosphate

DH definitive host
dehydrogenase
delayed hypersensitivity
dental hygienist
dermatitis herpetiformis
dermatoheliosis
diaphragmatic hernia
disseminated histoplasmosis
dissociative hysteria
dowager's hump (a protuberance on the upper back, seen in the elderly, especially among women, usually due to osteoporosis)
drug hypersensitivity
dry heaves (respiratory disturbance resulting from reduced elasticity of the bronchioles and alveoli)

DHA dehydroepiandrosterone (dehydroisoandrosterone)

DHA-P dihydroxyacetone phosphate

DHAS dehydroepiandrosterone sulfate

DHBV duck hepatitis B virus

DHC dehydrocholesterol

DHCA deep hypothermic cardiac arrest

DHCC dihydroxycholecalciferol (group of active metabolites of vitamin D_3)

DHCS dehydrocorticosterone

DHD doghouse disease

DHE 45 dihydroergotamine mesylate (an antiadrenergic)

DHEA dehydroepiandrostenedione (an androgen)
dehydroepiandrosterone (dehydroisoandrosterone, an androgen)

DHEAS dehydroepiandrosterone sulfate (important prehormone for DHEA and ovarian testosterone)

DHEASO₄
dehydroepiandrosterone sulfate (important prehormone for DHEA and ovarian testosterone)

DHEC dihydroergocryptine

DHF dengue hemorrhagic fever
diastolic heart failure

DHF/DSS
dengue hemorrhagic fever/dengue shock syndrome

DHFR dihydrofolate reductase (oxidoreductase enzyme)

DHFRD dihydrofolate reductase deficiency (genetic disorder of folate metabolism)

DHg Doctor of Hygiene

DHGG deaggregated human gammaglobulin

DHHS Department of Health and Human Services

DHI deafness, hyperprolinuria and ichthyosis

DHIA dehydroisoandrosterone

DHIC dihydroisocodeine

DHL diffuse histiocytic lymphoma

DHM dihydromorphine
doll-head maneuver

DHMA dihydroxymandelic acid

DHP dehydropeptidase (aminoacylase)
dihydroprogesterone

DHPA dihydroxypropyl adenine

DHPG dihydroxy-propoxymethyl guanine (Gancyclovir)

DHPR dihydropteridine reductase

DHR delayed hypersensitivity reaction

DHS delayed hypersensitivity
diabetic hyperosmolar state
duration of hospital stay
dynamic hip screw

DHSM dihydrostreptomycin
DHT dihydrotachysterol (AT-10)
dihydrotestosterone (a
  powerful androgenic
  hormone)
DHTP dihydrotestosterone
  propionate
DI date of injury
dentinogenesis imperfecta
dento-infuser
diabetes insipidus
diagnostic imaging
digitalis intoxication
drug-induced
drug intoxication
dry ice (solid CO_2)
dyskaryosis index
DIA diabetes
diazepam (tranquilizer)
Drug Information
  Association
DIAA drug-induced aplastic
  anemia
diag diagnosis
diam diameter
diaph diaphragm
DIAPPERS
delirium, infection,
  atrophic urethritis,
  pharmaceuticals,
  psychologic depression,
  excessive urination,
  restricted mobility, and
  stool impaction (causes
  of transient urinary
  incontinence)
DIAS diastolic
dias diastolic
DIAS BP diastolic blood pressure
DIAZ diazepam
  (a benzodiazepine
  tranquilizer)
DIB diagnostic interview for
  borderlines (of
  personalities)
disability insurance
  benefits
duodenoileal bypass
DIC differential interference

contrast (microscopy)
diffuse intravascular
  coagulation
direct illumination
  component
disseminated intravascular
  coagulation
  (consumption
  coagulation)
drip infusion
  cholangiography
drug-induced constipation
dict dictionary
DIDA diisopropyl iminodiacetic
  acid
DIDD dense intramembranous
  deposit disease
DIDL diffuse intermediately
  differentiated lymphatic
  lymphoma
DIDMOAD
diabetes insipidus +
  diabetes mellitus + optic
  atrophy + deafness
  (Wolfram syndrome)
DIDs drug-induced disorders
DIE died in emergency (room)
dieb. alt. *diebus alternis* [Latin] every
  other day
DIED died in emergency
  department
DIER died in emergency room
DIF diffuse interstitial fibrosis
direct immuno-
  fluorescence
DIFF differential (blood count)
diff difference
differential
differential count
diffusate
diff diag differential diagnosis
DIFP diffuse interstitial fibrosing
  pneumonitis
DIG digitalis (purple foxglove)
digoxin (a cardiotonic
  glycoside)
drug-induced glaucoma
digit I big toe
first digit
thumb

digit II   index finger
second digit
second toe

digit III   long finger
middle finger
third digit
third toe

digit IV   fourth digit
fourth toe
ring finger

digit V   fifth digit
little finger
little toe

DIH   died in hospital
drug-induced headache

DIHE   drug-induced hepatic
encephalopathy

DIHPPA   diidohydroxyphenylpyruvic
acid

DIL   Dilantin (phenytoin)

dil   dilute

dilat   dilatation
dilated

DILD   diffuse infiltrative lung
disease
diffuse interstitial lung
disease

DILE   drug-induced lupus
erythematosus

dim   diminish

dim.   *dimidus* [Latin] one-half

DIMD   drug-induced movement
disorder

DIMS   disorders of initiating and
maintaining sleep

d. in p. aeq.
divide in partes aequales
[Latin] divide into
equal parts

DIP   desquamative interstitial
pneumonia (marked by
thickening of the walls of
distal air passages and
desquamation of large
alveolar cells)
distal interphalangeal
(joint)
drip-infusion pyelography

dip   diploid

DIPB   deep infrapatellar bursa

DIPD   diagnostic interview for
personality disorders

DIPF   diffuse interstitial
pulmonary fibrosis
diisopropylphospho-
fluoridate

diph   diphtheria (an acute contagious disease caused
by a bacillus, *Coryne-
bacterium diphtheriae*)

DIPJ   distal interphalangeal joint

DIR   deep inguinal ring
diurnal insulin resistance

Dir   director

dir.   *directione* [Latin] directions

DIRD   drug-induced renal disease

DIRLINE   Directory of Information
Resources OnLine

DIS   digital imaging
spectrophotometer

dis   disability
disease
dislocation

DISA   digital intravenous
subtraction angiography

disc   discontinue

disch   discharge

dischg   discharge

DISH   diffuse idiopathic skeletal
hyperostosis (ankylosing
vertebral hyperostosis)

DISI   dorsiflexed intercalated
segment instability

disl   dislocation

disp   dispensary
dispense

dist   distal

distal/3   distal third

distal RTA
distal renal tubular acidosis

DIT   deferoxamine infusion test
diet-induced
thermogenesis (thermic
effect of food)
diiodotyrosine (a precursor
of the thyroid hormone
thyroxine)
drug-induced
thrombocytopenia

dITP   deoxyinosine triphosphate

DIVA	digital intravenous angiography
DJD	degenerative joint disease (osteoarthritis)

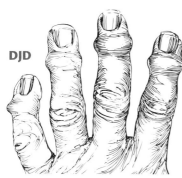

DJD

degenerative joint disease

DJJ	duodenojejunal junction
DJOA	dominant juvenile optic atrophy
DJS	Dubin-Johnson syndrome (a familial chronic form of nonhemolytic jaundice)
DK	diabetic ketoacidosis
	diseased kidney
	don't know
DKA	diabetic ketoacidosis
DKB	deep knee bends
DL	danger list
	diagnostic laparotomy
	diffuse lymphoma (lymphosarcoma)
	direct laryngoscopy
	disabled list
	doxorubicin and lomustine (combination chemotherapy)
dL	deciliter (1/10 liter)
dl	deciliter (1/10 liter)
DL&B	direct larygoscopy and bronchoscopy
DLC	differential leukocyte count
	double-lumen catheter
DLD	date of last (alcoholic) drink
DLE	dialyzable leukocyte extract

	discoid lupus erythematosus
	disseminated lupus erythematosus
DLF	digitalislike factor
	dorsolateral funiculus
DLIS	digoxin-like immunoreactive substance
DLMP	date of last menstrual period
DLNMP	date of last normal menstrual period
DLP	dislocation of patella (kneecap)
	dorsal lithotomy position
DLPT	dorsolateral pontomesencephalic tegmentum
D5LR	5% dextrose in lactated Ringer's (solution)
DLS	digitalis-like substance
DLT	double lumen tube
	double-lung transplantation
DLTS	digoxin-like immunoreactive substance
DLVD	diastolic left ventricular dysfunction
DLW	double loop whorl (fingerprint)
DM	defensive medicine
	dermatomyositis
	Descemet's membrane (one of the five layers of the cornea)
	diabetes mellitus
	diabetic mother
	diastolic murmur
	diffuse myalgia
	distal metastases
	distolic murmur

DM

diastolic murmur

	dopamine
	dura mater
dM	decimorgan
dm	decimeter
DMA	denervated muscle atrophy
	dimethylamine
	dimethoxyamphetamine
	direct memory access
DMAB	dimethylaminobenz-aldehyde
DMAE	dimethylaminoethanol
DMAPN	dimethylamino propionitrile
DMARDs	disease-modifying antirheumatic drugs
DMAT	disaster medical assistance team
DMBA	dimethylbenz anthracene (highly carcinogenic hydrocarbon)
DMC	dactinomycin + methotrexate + cyclophosphamide (combination chemotherapy)
	diffuse myocarditis
	diphtheritic myocarditis
DMCD	Dyggve-Melchior-Clausen dysplasia
DMCT	demethylchlortetracycline
DMD	distal muscular dystrophy
	Doppler method of diagnosis
	Duchenne's muscular dystrophy
DMDZ	desmethyldiazepam
DME	degenerative myoclonus epilepsy
	dexamethasone elixir
	durable medical equipment
DMF	decayed, missing, filled (permanent teeth)
	diphasic milk fever
dmf	decayed, missing, filled (deciduous teeth)
DMFO	eflornithine
DMG	dimethylglycine
DMI	diaphragmatic myocardial

	infarction
D/min	disintegrations per minute
DMKA	diabetes mellitus ketoacidosis
DMN	dimethylnitrosamine
	dorsal motor nucleus
	dysplastic melanocytic nevus
DMNA	dimethylnitrosamine
DMNVN	dorsal motor nucleus of vagus nerve
DMO	dimethadone
DMOOC	diabetes mellitus out-of-control
DMP	dimercaprol (antidote to poisoning by arsenic and mercury)
	dimethyl phthalate (insect repellent)
DMPA	depo-medroxy-progesterone acetate
DMPE	3,4-dimethoxyphenyl-ethylamine
DMPP	dimethylphenyl-piperazinium
DMPS	dysmyelopoietic syndrome
DMS	dermatomyositis
	dexamethasone suppression
	dimethylsulfoxide
	Directory of Medical Specialists
	dysmyelopoietic syndrome
DMSA	dimercaptosuccinic acid
DMSO	dimethyl sulfoxide (powerful solvent)
DMT	dimethyltryptamine (hallucinogenic substance)
	disseminated *Mycobacterium tuberculosis*
DMVA	direct mechanical ventricular actuator
DN	delphian node (a midline node encased in fascia and lying on the isthmus of the thyroid gland)
	diabetic nephropathy
	diabetic neuropathy

dicrotic notch

dinitrocresol

double-negative

DNA deoxyribonucleic acid (the genetic material of all cellular organisms)

DNA **deoxyribonucleic acid**

diabetes nutritional assessment

did not answer

does not apply

DNA PA deoxyribonucleic acid ploidy analysis

DNA PP DNA probe patterns

DNAR do not attempt resuscitation

DNA SA DNA sequence analysis

DNase deoxyribonuclease

DNA-TV deoxyribonucleic acid tumor virus

DNB destructive nerve block (injection of alcohol to deaden nerve)

dinitrobenzene (poisonous substance)

DNC did not come

DNCB dinitrochlorobenzene (sensitizing agent)

DND died a natural death

DNFB dinitrofluorobenzene (sensitizing agent)

DNG diffuse nontoxic goiter

DNH *Directory of Nursing Homes*

DNHL diffuse non-Hodgkin's lymphoma

DNI do not intubate

DNIG *de novo* inflammatory growth

DNK did not keep (appointment)

DNKA did not keep appointment

DNLL dorsal nucleus of lateral lemniscus

DNM dilator naris muscle

DNOC dinitro-*o*-cresol (insecticide)

dinitro-orthocresol

DNP did not pay

dinitrophenyl

do not publish

DNPM dinitrophenylmorphine

DNR daunorubicin (daunomycin, an antineoplastic antibiotic)

did not respond

do not resuscitate (order)

dorsal nerve root

D/N ratio dextrose (glucose)-nitrogen ratio (in urine)

DNS deviated nasal septum

dextrose in normal solution

did not show (for appointment)

dysplastic nevus syndrome

D5NS 5% dextrose in normalsaline (solution)

DNSc Doctor of Nursing Science

DNT did not test

DNT cells double-negative T cells

DNTM disseminated nontuberculous mycobacterial (infection)

dorsal nucleus of vagus nerve

DO diamine oxidase

dissolved oxygen

Doctor of Optometry

Doctor of Osteopathy

doctor's orders

drug overdose

drug oxidation

D$_2$O deuterium oxide (heavy water)

DO$_2$ oxygen delivery

d/o day old

DOA date of admission

dead on arrival

detrusor overactivity

duration of action

DOA-DRA
dead on arrival despite
resuscitation attempt

DOB date of birth
dobutamine (a synthetic
catecholamine)

DOC date of conception
deoxycholate
deoxycorticosterone
(a mineralocorticoid
produced by the
adrenal cortex)
diabetes out of control
died of other causes
drug of choice

DOCA deoxycorticosterone
acetate

DOCG deoxycorticosterone
glucoside

DOCLINE
Documents OnLine

DOCS deoxycorticoids

DOCSO₄ deoxycorticosterone
sulfate

DOD date of death
date of discharge
dentino-osseous dysplasia
Directory of Online Databases
drug overdose

DOE date of examination
dyspnea on exertion

DOES disorders of excessive
somnolence (sleepiness)

DOFOS disturbance of function
occlusion syndrome

DOH Department of Health

DOI date of illness
date of implant
date of injury
date of investigation

DO₂I oxygen delivery index

dol. *dolor* [Latin] pain

DOM Department of Medicine
dimethoxy-
methylamphetamine
(hallucinogenic
compound, popularly
called STP)

dominance

DOMA dihydroxymandelic acid

DOMS delayed-onset
muscular soreness

DON determination of need
diazo-oxo-norleucine
director of nursing

don. *donec* [Latin] until

DOOR deafness, onycho-
osteodystrophy, (mental)
retardation

DOP dopamine

DOPA dihydroxyphenylalanine
dopamine

dopa dihydroxyphenylalanine
dopamine

DOPAC 3,4-dihydroxyphenyl-
acetic acid

DOPC determined osteogenic
precursor cell

DOPEG 3,4-dihydroxyphenyl-
ethyleneglycol

DOPET 3,4-dihydroxyphenyl-
ethanol

DOPS diffuse obstructive
pulmonary syndrome

DORA *Directory of Rare Analyses*
(lists clinical tests that are
not commonly ordered
and the laboratories
performing them)

DORV double outlet right
ventricle

DORx date of treatment

DOS date of surgery
deoxystreptamine
dialysis osteomalacia
syndrome
disk operating system
dysosteosclerosis

dos dosage

DOSS dioctyl sodium
sulfosuccinate (docusate
sodium, used as a fecal
softener)

DOT died on (operating room)
table

DOW died of wounds

DOX doxorubicin (broadly

active antitumor
antibiotic)

DOXO doxorubicin (broadly
active antitumor
antibiotic)

DP data processing
demand pacemaker
dementia paralytica
dementia praecox
dental plaque
diastolic pressure
diazepam (Valium)
displaced person
distal pancreatectomy
distal phalanx
Doctor of Pharmacy
donor's plasma
dorsalis pedis (pulse
taking site)
double pneumonia
dying pateint

Dp dyspnea

DPA dual-photon
absorptiometry
durable power of attorney

DPAC ductal pancreatic
adenocarcinoma

DP & AD depressive personality and
allied disorders

DPB days postburn

DPBP diphenylbutylpiperidine
(antipsychotic agents)

DPC days post coitum
direct platelet count
distal palmar crease

DPCRT double-blind placebo-
controlled randomized
clinical trial

DPD delayed pigment
darkening
dependent personality
disorder
diffuse pulmonary disease
dual photon densitometry

DPDL diffuse poorly
differentiated
lymphocytic lymphoma

DPG 2,3-diphosphoglycerate
diphosphoglyceric acid

displacement
placentogram

DPGN diffuse proliferative
glomerulonephritis

DPH diphenhydramine
(antihistaminic)
diphenylhydantoin
(Dilantin, an
anticonvulsant and
cardiac depressant)
Doctor of Public Health

DPI daily permisssible intake
Doppler perfusion index
(ratio of total liver blood
flow to hepatic arterial
blood flow)

DPIF *Drug Products*
Information File

DPL diagnostic peritoneal
lavage
dipalmitoyl lecithin

DPLN diffuse proliferative
lupus nephritis

DPM discontinue previous
medication
Doctor of Podiatric
Medicine
dopamine

DPMD Duchenne's progressive
muscular dystrophy

DPN diabetic polyneuropathy
diabetic proximal
neuropathy
diphosphopyridine
nucleotide
(now called NAD)

DPNase NAD nucleosidase

DPNH reduced diphos-
phopyridine nucleotide
(now called NADH)

DPP dimethoxyphenyl
penicillin
Directory of Published
Proceedings
doctor-patient privilege
dorsalis pedis pulse (dorsal
artery of foot)
dysrhythmia
pneumophrasia (in

speech, defective breath grouping)

DPPC dipalmitoyl phosphatidylcholine (test to evaluate fetal lung maturity and predictor of respiratory distress syndrome)

double-blind placebo-controlled (trial)

DPS descending perineum syndrome

dysesthetic pain syndrome

DPT Demerol (meperidine hydrochloride), Phenergan (promethazine hydrochloride), Thorazine (chlorpromazine hydrochloride)

diphosphothiamine (thiamine diphosphate)

diphtheria-pertussis-tetanus (vaccine)

dumping provocation test

DPTA diethylenetriamine penta-acetic acid

DPTPM diphtheria, pertussis, tetanus, poliomyelitis and measles (vaccine)

DPU delayed pressure urticaria

DPUD duodenal peptic ulcer disease

DPUS *Directory of Physicians in the United States*

DPV disabling positional vertigo

dorsal penis vein

DQ developmental quotient

DQS de Quervain syndrome

DR date rape

delivery room

deoxyribose

detached retina

diabetic retinopathy

diagnostic radiology

diaper rash

dorsal root

drug receptor

drug residue

drug resistance

ductus reuniens

D & R desquamation and regeneration

Dr doctor

dr dram (4 ml)

DRA drug-related admission

DRADA Depression and Related Affective Disorders Association

DRAM de-epithelialized rectus abdominis muscle

dynamic random access memory

DRAT differential rheumatoid agglutination test

DRB daunorubicin (antibiotic used as an antineoplastic agent)

DRD dorsal root damage

drug-related dementia

DRD2 D2 dopamine receptor

DRE digital rectal examination

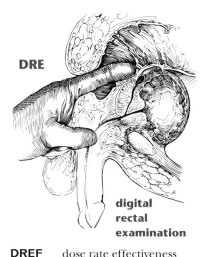

DRE

digital rectal examination

DREF dose rate effectiveness factor

DREZ dorsal root entry zone

DRF Deafness Research Foundation

dose-reduction factor

DRG diagnosis-related group

diagnostic-related group

dihydrofoliate
reductase gene

Division of Research
Grants (of NIH)

dorsal respiratory group

dorsal root ganglion

duodenal-gastric reflux
gastropathy

drg   drainage

DRGE   drainage

DRGs   diagnosis-related groups

dRib   deoxyribose

D5RL   dextrose 5% with
Ringer's lactate

DRM   donor-recipient matching

DRME   Division of Research in
Medical Education

DRMS   drug reaction
monitoring system

3-D RODEO MRI

3-dimensional rotating
delivery excitation off-
resonance magnetic
resonance imaging
(provides higher
resolution than
conventional MRI)

DRP   drug-related problem

dystrophin-related protein

DRQ   diagnostic radiographic
quality

discomfort relief quotient

DRR   Division of Research
Resources (of NIH)

dorsal root reflex

DRS   disability rating scale

Division of Research
Services (of NIH)

Duane's retraction
syndrome (Stilling-Turk-
Duane syndrome)

drsg   dressing

DRT   dermal regeneration
template

distal renal tubular acidosis

DRUJ   distal radioulnar joint

dRVVT   dilute Russel viper
venom time

DS   decompression

sickness (bends)

deep sedative

deep sleep
(slow-wave sleep)

delayed sensitivity

dendritic spines
(gemmules)

depolarizing shift

depressive stupor

desynchronized sleep

deviated septum

diastolic murmur

diffuse scleroderma

digital signal

dilute strength

discharge summary

disequilibrium syndrome

disorganized schizophrenia
(hebephrenia)

disseminated sclerosis

donor's serum

Doppler sonography

double strength

Down's syndrome

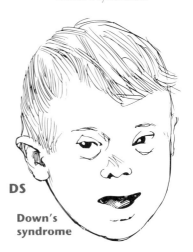

DS

**Down's
syndrome**

Dressler's syndrome
(postmyocardial
infarction syndrome)

drug screening

dry socket

dumping syndrome
(postgastrectomy
syndrome; jejunal

syndrome)
Duncan's syndrome
duration of systole

D5S 5% dextrose in
saline solution

D15S 15% dextrose in
saline solution

DSA digital subtraction
angiography (technique
that subtracts the
background of bones and
soft tissues to better
visualize blood vessels
after injection of
contrast medium)

D-SACT direct sinoatrial
conduction time

DSAP disseminated superficial
actinic porokeratosis

Dsbl disabled

DSBT donor-specific blood
transfusion

DSc Doctor of Science

DSCT dorsal spinocerebellar tract

DSD discharge summary
dictated
dry sterile dressing

dsDNA double-stranded DNA
(deoxyribonucleic acid)

DSE diffuse spasm of esophagus
dry skin eczema

DSF diffuse sound field

DSG dry sterile gauze

dsg dressing

DSH deliberate self-harm

DSHR delayed skin
hypersensitivity reaction

DSHS deliberate self-harm
syndrome

DSI Depression Status
Inventory
digital subtraction imaging

DS-IgA-ELISA
double sandwich IgA
enzyme-linked
immunosorbent assay

DS-IgM-ELISA
double sandwich IgM
enzyme-linked/

immunosorbent assay

DSIP delta sleep-inducing
peptide

dslv dissolve

DSM diamond-shaped murmur

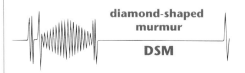

diamond-shaped
murmur
DSM

disk sensitizing method

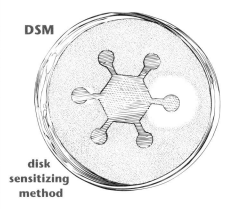

DSM

disk
sensitizing
method

disposable surgical mask
drink skim milk

DSM-IV *Diagnostic and Statistical
Manual of Mental Disorders*
(fourth edition)
(American Psychiatric
Association)

DSMD dilated submandibular
duct

DSMMD *Diagnostic and Statistical
Manual of Mental Disorders*

DSO distal subungual
onchomycosis

DSP decreased sensory
perception
delayed sleep phase
digital subtraction
phlebography

DSPD delayed sleep phase
disorder

D-spine dorsal (thoracic) spine

DSR	dry sterile dressing
DSRCT	desmoplastic small round-cell tumor
DS-REO	deafness-sensorineural, recessive early-onset
dsRNA	double-stranded RNA (ribonucleic acid)
DS-RP	deafness sensorineural, recessive profound
DSS	dengue shock syndrome
	dioctyl sodium sulfosuccinate (stool softener)
	disability status scale
	discharge summary sheet
DST	desensitization test
	dexamethasone suppression test (to diagnose Cushing's syndrome and useful for the diagnosis of melancholic depression)
	distal straight tubule (kidney)
	donor-specific (blood) transfusion
DSTs	drug susceptibility tests
DSU	day surgery unit
DSUH	direct suggestion under hypnosis
DSWI	deep surgical wound infection
DSWS	disorders of sleep-wake schedule
DT	Darwin tubercle (marker)
	delirium tremens
	desmoid tumor
	detoxification
	diet therapy
	digitoxin
	diphtheria and tetanus (vaccine)
	diphtheria toxoid
	discharge tomorrow
	diuretic therapy
	dog tick
	dominant trait
	drawer test
	drug therapy
	drug toxicity

	duration of tetany
D/T	date of treatment
	due to
D & T	dependence and tolerance
dT	deoxythymidine (thymidine)
DTA	differential thermal analysis
DTaP	diphtheria and tetanus toxoids combined with acellular pertussis vaccine
DTC	distal transverse crease (hand crease)

DTC

distal transverse crease

dTc	d-tubocurarine
DT CFP	*Drug Therapeutics: Concepts for Physicians*
dTDP	deoxythymidine diphosphate
DTE	desiccated thyroid extract
DTG	diffuse toxic goiter
DTH	delayed-type-hypersensitivity
dThd	thymidine
DTIC	dacarbazine (dimethyl triazene imidazole carboxamide, a cytotoxic alkylating agent)
DTICH	delayed traumatic intracerebral hematoma
	delayed traumatic intra-cerebral hemorrhage
DTIP	detoxification inpatient
DTL	dynamic tetracycline

labeling

DTM dermatophyte test medium

dTMP deoxythymidine
monophosphate

DTNB dithionitrobenzoic acid

DTOP detoxification outpatient

d. tox. *dosis toxica* [Latin]
toxic dose

DTP diphtheria, tetanus,
pertussis (triple vaccine)

distal tingling
on percussion

distal tingling on pressure

DTPA diethylenetriamine
pentacetic acid
(pentetic acid)

dTPM deoxythymidine
monophosphate

DTR deep tendon reflex

DTS donor specific transfusion

DTs delirium tremens

DTT diphtheria-tetanus toxoid

dTTP deoxythymidine
triphosphate

DTUS diathermy, traction,
and ultrasound

DTV due to void

DTW duty to warn

DTX detoxification (treatment
to free an addict from
his drug habit)

DTZ diatrizoate (x-ray contrast
medium)

DU decubitus ulcer
(pressure sore)

deoxyuridine

diabetic ulcer

diagnosis undetermined

duodenal ulcer

dU deoxyuridine

DUA dorsal uterine artery

DUB dysfunctional uterine
bleeding

DUCT differential ureteral
catherization test

DUD duodenal ulcer diet

dUDP deoxyuridine dephosphate

DUDS duplex ultrasound
Doppler study

DUET drug use education tips

DUF drug use forecast

DUI driving under the
influence

DUID driving under the
influence of drugs

DUL diffuse undifferentiated
lymphoma

dUMP deoxyuridine
monophosphate

DUN dialysate urea nitrogen

duod duodenum

DuPr due process

DUR drug use review

dur. dolor.

durante dolore [Latin] while
the pain lasts

DUS distal urethral stenosis

DUST Doppler ultrasound
technique

DUT defective urate transport
(hypouricemia)

dUTP deoxyuridine triphosphate

DV defective virus

detached vitreous
(vitreous body of eye)

dilated veins

dilute volume

diploic vein

distemper virus

domestic violence

double vision

ductus venosus (the major
blood vessel through the
embryonic liver
transmitting venous
blood from the umbilical
vein to the inferior
vena cava)

D & V diarrhea and vomiting

DV2 DynaVox 2 (nonverbal
communication aid)

DVA developmental venous
anomaly

distance visual acuity

US Department of
Veterans Affairs

DVB divinylbenzene

DVC direct visualization of vocal
cords

dVDAVP diamino-valine-D-arginine

vasopressin

DVH Domestic Violence Hotline
(800) 799-SAFE

DVIS digital vascular imaging
system

DVIU direct visualization internal
urethrotomy

DVM Doctor of Veterinary
Medicine

DVN dorsal vagal nucleus

DVPA doxorubicin + vincristine +
prednisone +
asparaginase
(combination
chemotherapy)

DVR Doctor of Veterinary
Radiology
double valve replacement

DVS Division of Vital Statistics
(US government)
Doctor of Veterinary
Surgery

DVSA digital venous subtraction
angiography

DVT deep vein thrombosis
deep venous thrombosis

DW deworming
distilled water
doing well
dry weight

D/W dextrose in water

DV

ductus
venosus

D5W 5% dextrose in water

D10W 10% dextrose in water

D50W 50% dextrose in water

DWC distal wrist crease

DWCC differential white
cell count

DWD died with disease

DWDL diffuse well-differentiated
lymphocytic lymphoma

DWI driving while impaired
driving while intoxicated

DWL detergent worker's lung

DWS Dandy-Walker syndrome
double whammy syndrome

DWT duck waddle test

Dx diagnosis
diagnostic
disease

DXA dual-energy x-ray
absorptiometry

Dxd discontinue
discontinued

DXM dexamethasone (synthetic
glucocorticoid)

DXRT deep x-ray therapy

DXT dextrose (glucose; blood
sugar)

dXTP deoxyxanthine
triphosphate

Dy dysprosium (rare
earth element)

dysp dyspnea (difficult
breathing usually
associated with serious
disease of the heart
or lungs)

DZ diazepam
disease
dizygotic (twins)
dizziness
dozen

DZP diazepam (Valium; an
antianxiety agent; also a
useful adjunct in the
treatment of muscular
spasms)

DZT dizygotic (fraternal) twins
(twins derived from two
separate zygotes)

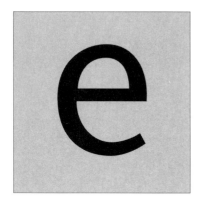

E edema
electric charge
electrode potential
electron
embryo
emmetropia
endogenous
endoplasm
enema
energy
enzyme
eosinophil
ephelis (freckle)
epinephrine
error
erythrocyte
esophagus
esophoria
ester
estradiol
ethanol
ethyl
etiology
evaluation
examination
expired
extract
eye
glutamic acid
kinetic energy
redox potential
E1 estrone
E2 estradiol
E3 estriol

E4 estetrol
e electric charge
electron
erythrocyte
base of natural logarithms,
with a numerical value
of 2.7
e– electron
e+ positron
EA early amniocentesis
early antigen
Eaton agent
economic analysis
edetic acid
educational age
egg albumin
elder abuse
electro-acupuncture
electro-anesthesia
embryonic antibody
endometrial ablation
Endometriosis
Association
enteral alimentation
epidural abscess
epithelioid angiomatosis
erythrocyte amboceptor
erythrocyte antibody
erythrocyte antiserum
esophageal achalasia
esophageal atresia
ethacrynic acid
etiologic agent
E & A evaluate and advise
ea each
EAA electro-acupuncture
analgesia
essential amino acid
extraarticular ankylosis
extrinsic allergic alveolitis
EAB Ethics Advisory Board
EAC energy absorption capacity
epithelioma adenoides
cysticum
erythrocyte amboceptor
complement
eythrocyte, antibody, and
complement
external auditory canal

EACA epsilon-aminocaproic acid (potent anti-fibrin-olytic agent)

EACD eczematous allergic contact dermatitis

EACOA endometrioid endocarcinoma of ovary

EAD early after-depolarization
exogenous antigen disease

EA-D early antigen – diffuse

ead. *eadem* [Latin] the same

EAE edetic acid eugenics
experimental allergic encephalitis
experimental allergic encephalomyelitis

EAEC enteroadherent *Escherichia coli*

EAF extra-articular fracture

EAG electroarteriography

EAHF eczema-asthma-hay fever

EAI Emphysema Anonymous, Inc.

EAM external auditory meatus

EAP ectopic abdominal pregnancy
employee assistance program
epiallopregnanolone (corticoid hormone present in pregnancy urine)
etoposide + Adriamycin (doxorubicin) + Platinol (cisplatin) (combination chemotherapy)
evoked action potential

EA-R early antigen – restricted

EAS external anal sphincter

EAST external rotation, abduction, stress test

EAT ectopic atrial tachycardia
epidermolysis acuta toxica
exercise-associated tinnitus

EB elementary body
endometrial biopsy
epidermolysis bullosa
Epstein-Barr (virus)
escape beat (an automatic heart beat following an interval longer than the dominant cycle, i.e. after the normal beat has defaulted)
esophageal balloon
estradiol benzoate
excisional biopsy

EBA epidermolysis bullosa acquisita (seen in adults with evidence of genetic transmission)

EBBA Eye Bank Association of America

EBC esophageal balloon catheter
extension body cast

EBD epibulbar dermoid
epidermolysis bullosa dystrophica (dermatolytic bullous dermatosis)
exploration of bile duct

EBDCs ethylene bis dithiocarbamates

EBDP endoscopic balloon dilation prostate

EBF epidural bladder function
erythroblastosis fetalis (hemolytic disease of newborn)

EBI

erythroblastic island

EBG	electroblepharogram		ejection click
EBI	electron beam		electrocautery
	instrumentation		electrode catheter
	erythroblastic island		embolectomy catheter
	(reticulum cells of the		endemic cretinism
	bone marrow surrounded		endocervical
	by red blood cell		endothelial cell
	precursors at various		endotracheal catheter
	stages of development)		enteric coated
EBL	endoscopic band ligation		entering complaint
	estimated blood loss		epithelial cancer
eBL	endemic Burkitt's		epithelial cell
	lymphoma (African		*Escherichia coli*
	lymphoma)		esophageal chalasia
EBL/S	estimated blood loss		excitation-contraction
	during surgery		exfoliative cytology
EBM	expressed breast milk		expiratory center
EBN	erythroblastosis		external conjugate
	neonatorum		extracellular
	(hemolytic disease		eyes closed
	of newborn)	**EC0157**	*Escherichia coli* 0157
EBNA	Epstein-Barr (virus)		(virulent strain of the
	nuclear antigen (test)		usual harmless bacterium
EBP	estradiol-binding protein		*E. coli*, responsible for
EbR	erythroblast receptor		thousands of cases of
EBRT	electron beam		severe food-borne illness)
	radiotherapy	**ECA**	echinococcus antibody
EBS	elastic back strap		electrocardioanalyzer
	emergency bypass surgery		electrode catheter ablation
	epidermolysis bullosa		endocervical aspiration
	simplex		endocervical aspirator
	equal breath sounds		endometrial-conceptus
EBT	early bedtime		asynchrony
EBV	Epstein-Barr virus (herpes		enteric coated aspirin
	virus 4; a virus that has		enterobacterial
	specificity for B		common antigen
	lymphocytes and causes		epicranial aponeurosis
	infectious		external carotid artery
	mononucleosis)	**E-CABG**	endarterectomy and
	estimated blood volume		coronary artery
EBv	Epstein-Barr virus (herpes		bypass graft
	virus 4)	**ECAVS**	extracorporeal
EBV-1	Epstein-Barr virus type 1		arteriovenous shunt
EBV-2	Epstein-Barr virus type 2	**ECBF**	extracorporeal blood flow
EB virus	Epstein-Barr virus (herpes	**ECBV**	effective circulating
	virus 4)		blood volume
EC	ectopia cordis (congenital	**ECC**	echinococcus cyst
	displacement of		ectopic calcification
	the heart)		conjunctiva

electrocorticogram
embryonal cell carcinoma
emegency cardiac care
endocervical canal
endocervical conization
endocervical curettage
estimated creatinine
　clearance
external cardiac
　compression
extracorporeal circulation

ECCE extracapsular cataract
　extraction

ECCE c IOL
　extracapsular cataract
　extraction with
　intraocular lens
　implantation

ECD epithelial corneal
　dystrophy

ECDO virus
　enteric cytopathogenic dog
　orphan virus

E cells expiratory neurons

ECF effective capillary flow
　eosinophilic chemotactic
　factor
　epicondyle fracture
　extended care facility
　extracapsular fracture
　extracellular fluid

ECF-A eosinophilic chemotactic
　factor of anaphylaxis

ECFC eosinophilic chemotactic
　factor complement

ECFS extracellulr fluid spaces

ECFV extracellulr fluid volume

ECG echocardiogram
　echocardiography

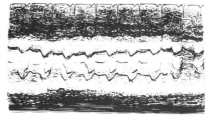

ECG echocardiogram

electrocardiogram
electrocardiograph
electrocardiography
endocrine gland

eCG equine chorionic
　gonadotropin

ECGA electrocochleographic
　audiometry

ECGF endothelial cell
　growth factor

ECGM electrocardiagraphic
　monitoring

ECH endocardial hemorrhage
　epicardial hemorrhage
　episodic cluster headache
　extended care hospital

ECHO echocardiogram

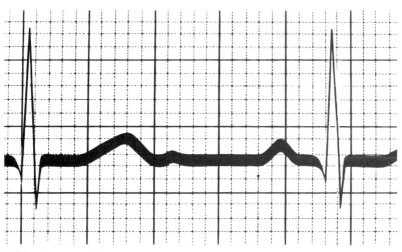

ECG electrocardiogram

echocardiography
echoencephalogram
enteric cytopathogenic
human orphan (virus)
etoposide +
cyclophosphamide +
Adriamycin
(doxorubicin) + Oncovin
(vincristine)
(combination
chemotherapy)

EchoCG echocardiography
EchoEG echoencephalography
ECI extracorporeal irradiation
ECIB extracorporeal irradiation
of blood
EC-IC extracranial to intracranial
(arterial bypass)
ECIL extracorporeal irradiation
of lymph
ECL extent of cerebral lesion
ECM enchondromatosis
erythema chronicum
migrans (deep form of
gyrate erythema at the
site of a bite by an
ixodid tick)
esophagocardiomyotomy
external cardiac massage
extracellular mass
extracellular matrix
ECMO extracorporeal
membrane oxidation
extracorporeal
membrane oxygenator
ECN extended care nursery
ECO endochondral ossification
ECochG electrocochleography
ECoG electrocorticography
E. coli *Escherichia coli*

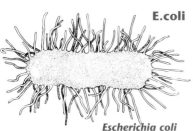

E.coli

Escherichia coli

ECOS extracardiac obstructive
shock
ECP emitter current
programmer
eosinophil cationic protein
erythrocyte
coproporphyrin
estradiol cyclopentane
propionate
external cardiac pressure
ECPD external counterpressure
device
ECPO enteric cytopathic porcine
orphan (virus)
ECPR external cardiopulmonary
resuscitation
ECRB extensor carpi radialis
brevis (muscle)
ECRL extensor carpi radialis
longus (muscle)
ECRN enzyme catalogue
reference number
ECS elective cosmetic surgery
electrocerebral silence
electroconvulsive shock
ECSWL extracorporeal shock-wave
lithotripsy

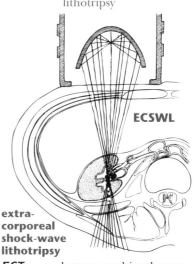

ECSWL

extra-
corporeal
shock-wave
lithotripsy

ECT electroconvulsive therapy
electroconvulsive
treatment
emssion computed
tomography

enhanced-computed tomography
enteric-coated tablet
euglobulin clot test (euglobulin lysis test)

ECTR endoscopic carpal tunnel release

ECU electrocautery unit
environmental control unit
extended care unit
extensor carpi ulnaris (muscle)

ECV epithelial cell vacuolization
extracellular volume

ECW extracellular water

ED eardrum
eating disorder
ectodermal dysplasia
ectopic depolarization
education
effective dose
Ehlers-Danlos (syndrome)
elbow disarticulation
elbow dislocation
electrodialysis
ejaculatory dysfunction
elbow disarticulation
emergency department
emotionally disturbed
entering diagnosis
enzyme deficiency
epidural
Erb disease
erectile dysfunction
erythema dose
esophageal diverticulum
estrogen deficiency
evidence of disease
exertional dyspnea
exfoliative dermatitis

ED50 median effective dose

ed edema

EDA electrodermal audiometry
electronic dental anesthesia
epidermal abscess
epidural anesthesia

EDAC early defibrillation/ advanced care

EDAS encephalo-duro-arteriosynangiosis

EDB ethylene dibromide (pesticide)
extensor digitorum brevis (muscle)

EDC ectodermal cell
end-diastolic counts
epidermal cancer (malignant epithelioma of the skin)
epidural catheter
estimated date of conception
estimated date of confinement
ethylene dichloride (solvent; 1,2, dichloroethane ethidine chloride)
expected date of confinement
extensor digitorum communis (muscle)

ED & C electrodessication and currettage

EDD effective drug duration
end diastolic dimension
estimated due date
expected date of delivery

edent edentulous (toothless)

EDF eosinophil differentiation factor
electrodermography

EDH epidural hematoma

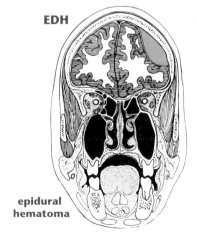

EDH

epidural hematoma

EDI endosseous dental implant
E-diol estradiol
EDL end-diastolic load
extensor digitorum longus (muscle)
ED-LD emotionally disturbed and learning disabled
EDM early diastolic murmur
EDMA ethylene glycol dimethacrylate
EDN eosinophil-derived neurotoxin
EDNA Emergency Department Nurses Association
EDO epididymoorchitis
EDP electronic data processing
emergency department physician
end-diastolic pressure
EDPVCs end-diastolic premature ventricular contractions
EDQ extensor digiti quinti (extensor digiti minimi) (muscle)
EDR early diastolic relaxation
edrophonium (anticholinesterase agent)
effective direct radiation
electrodermal response
enzyme-dependent reaction
EDRF endothelium-derived relaxing factor
EDS Ehlers-Danlos syndrome (hyperelastic skin and

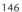

EDS

Ehlers-Danlos syndrome

hypermobile joints)
energy-dispersive spectrometry
epidural space
epigastric distress syndrome
excessive daytime sleepiness
EDSS expanded disability status scale
EDT end-diastolic thickness
EDTA ethylenediaminetetra-acetic acid (edetic acid)
EDU eating disorder unit
EDV end diastolic volume
epidermodysplasia verruciformis
EDVI end-diastolic volume index
EDW estimated dry weight
EDXA energy-dispersive x-ray analysis
EE energy expenditure
equine encephalitis
esterified estrogen
ethinyl estradiol (potent semisynthetic derivative of estradiol)
external ear
E & E eye and ear
EEA electroencephalic audiometry
end-to-end anastomosis
EEAS end-to-end anastomosis stapler
EEC enteropathogenic *Escherichia coli*
EECG electroencephalography
EECO endometroid endocarcinoma of ovary
EED eosinophilic endomyocardial disease (Loeffler's endocarditis)
erythema elevatum diutinum
EEE eastern equine encephalitis
eastern equine encephalomyelitis
edema, erythema, and exudate

EEEP   end-expiratory esophageal pressure

EEE virus
     eastern equine encephalomyelitis virus

EEG   echo-encephalography
     electroencephalogram

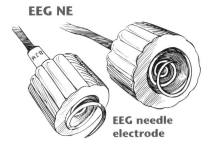

EEG electroencephalogram

     electroencephalograph
     electroencephalography

EEGA   electroencephalographic audiometry

EEG NE   EEG needle electrode

EEG NE

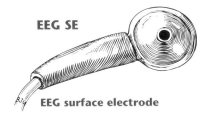

EEG needle electrode

EEG SE   EEG surface electrode

EEG SE

EEG surface electrode

EELS   electron energy loss spectrometry

EELV   end-expiratory lung volume

EEM   erythema exudativum multiforme

EEME   ethinylestradiol methyl ether

EEMG   evoked electromyogram

EENT   eyes, ears, nose and throat

EEP   end-expiratory pause
     end-expiratory pressure

EERP   extended endocardial resection procedure

EES   erythromycin ethylsuccinate (salt of erythromycin)

EEUA   end-to-end ureteral anastomosis

EEV   Eastern equine virus

EF   edema factor
     ejection fraction
     electric field
     embryo fibroblasts
     emergency facilities
     emotional factor
     endurance factor
     enteric fistula
     eosinophilic fasciitis
     epicondylar fracture
     erythroblastosis fetalis
     extended field (irradiation)
     extrinsic factor

EFA   efferent glomerular arteriole
     enhancing factor of allergy
     Epilepsy Foundation of America
     essential fatty acids

EFAD   essential fatty acid deficiency

EFAS   embryo-fetal alcohol syndrome

EFD   episode free day
     Erlenmeyer flask deformity

EFE   endocardial fibroelastosis

EFF   effacement (the temporary obliteration of the cervix

just prior to giving birth)
efficiency
electromagnetic
field focusing
EFM elderly fibromyalgia
electronic fetal monitoring
external fetal monitoring
EFMM external fetal maternal
monitoring
EFP early follicular phase
EFR effective filtration rate
EFT erythrocyte fragility test
essential-familial tremor
EFU evaluation and follow-up
EFV extracellular fluid volume
EFVC expiratory flow-
volume curve
EFW estimated fetal weight
EG endometrial carcinoma
eosinophilic granuloma
estrogen gel
exfoliation glaucoma
external genitalia
e.g. *exempli gratia* [Latin] for
example
EGA estimated gestational age
EGB eosinophilic granuloma
of bone
EGC early gastric carcinoma
early glottic carcinoma
epiglottic cartilage
EGCS extragonadal germinal cell
syndrome
EGD Erb-Goldflam disease
esophagogastroduodeno-
scopy
EGDF embryonic growth and
development factor
EGE eosinophilic gastroenteritis
EGF epidermal growth factor
EGFR epidermal growth factor
receptor
EGG electrogastrography
EGJ esophagogastric junction
EGL eosinophilic granuloma of
the lung
EGLT euglobin lysis time
EGME ethylene glycol monoethyl
ether

EGNB enteric gram negative
bacteria
EGOT erythrocyte glutamic
oxaloacetic transaminase
EGP endoluminal graft
procedure
epiphyseal growth plate
EGRA equilibrium-gated
radionuclide angiography
E. granulosus *Echinococcus granulosus*
(causative agent of
echinococcosis)
EGS electrogalvanic stimulation
empty glenoid sign
EGT experimental gene therapy
EGTA egtazic acid
esophageal gastric
tube airway
EGVs esophagogastric varices
EH endometrial hyperplasia
enlarged heart
epidermolytic
hyperkeratosis
epidural hematoma
essential hypertension
external hemorrhoids
E & H environment and heredity
euchromatin and
heterochromatin
EHAA epidemic hepatitis
associated antigen
EHB elevate head of bed
EHBA extrahepatic biliary atresia
EHBD extrahepatic bile duct
EHBF estimated hepatic blood
flow
EHBO extrahepatic biliary
obstruction
EHBP essential high blood
pressure
EHC enterohepatic circulation
enterohepatic clearance
essential
hypercholesterolemia
extended health care
EHD environmental
hypersensitivity disease
epizootic hemorrhagic
disease

EHDP	ethane-hydroxy-diphosphonate (etidronate)
EHDV	epizootic hemorrhagic disease virus
EHEC	enterohemorrhagic *E. coli*
EHF	epidemic hemorrhagic fever (acute, febrile viral disease)
	exophthalmos-hyperthyroid-factor
EHH	esophageal hiatal hernia
EHIP	Employee Health Insurance Plan
E. histolytica	
	Entamoeba histolytica
EHL	electrohydraulic lithotripsy
	endogenous hyperlipidemia
	essential hyperlipemia
	extensor hallucis longus (muscle)
EHNA	erythrohydroxynonyl-adenine
EHO	extrahepatic obstruction
EHP	extrahigh potency
EHPH	extrahepatic portal hypertension
EHS	ectopic-hypercalcemia syndrome
	employee health service
EHT	essential hypertension
EHV	equine herpes virus
EI	ectopic implantation
	electrolyte imbalance
	emotional intelligence
	emotionally impaired
	environmental illness
	enzyme inhibitor
	eosinophilic index
	erythema infectiosum
E/I	expiration-inspiration ratio
EIA	early infantile autism
	electroimmunoassay
	enzyme immunoassay
	enzyme-linked immunosorbent assay
	exercise-induced asthma
EIB	electrophoretic immunoblotting

	exercise-induced bronchospasm
EIC	epidermal inclusion cyst
	epidermoid inclusion cyst
	extensive intraductal carcinoma
	extensive intraductal component
EID	electroimmunodiffusion
	electronic infusion device
	emergency infusion device
EIDC	extreme intervertebral disk collapse
EIDD	epileptic intentional deficit disorder
EIEC	enteroinvasive *E. coli*
EIEE	early infantile epileptic encephalopathy
EIEN	endometrial intraepithelial neoplasia
EIF	early infantile autism
	erythrocyte initiation factor
EIMI	exercise-induced myocardial ischemia
EIN	endometrial intraepithelial neoplasia
	excitatory interneuron
EIP	end-inspiratory pressure
	extensor indicis proprius (muscle)
EIPS	endogenous inhibitor of prostaglandin synthase
eIPV	enhanced potency inactivated poliovirus (vaccine)
EIQ	emotional IQ (emotional social skills)
EIT	erythrocyte iron turnover
EITB	enzyme-linked immunoelectrotransfer blot
EIV	external iliac vein
EJ	elbow jerk (elbow reflex test)
	external jugular (vein)
ejec	ejection
EJN	external jugular vein
EJP	excitatory junction potential

ejusd.	*ejusdem* [Latin] of the same
EJV	external jugular vein
EK	erythrokinase
EKC	epidemic keratoconjunctivitis (shipyard keratoconjunctivitis)
EKG	electrocardiogram (ECG) electrocardiograph electrocardiography
EKO	echoencephalogram
EKS	epidemic Kaposi's sarcoma
EKY	electrokymogram
EL	ectopia lentis emergency laparotomy epidemic listeriosis excimer laser exercise limit exploratory laparotomy
el	elixir (a clear, sweetened solution of alcohol and water, used as a vehicle for medicine taken orally)
ELAD	extracorporeal (situated outside the body) liver-assist device
ELAM-1	endothelial-leukocyte adhesion molecule 1
ELAS	extended lymphadenopathy syndrome
ELB	early-labeled bilirubin early light breakfast
ELBW	extremely low birth weight
ELC	expression-linked copy
ELD	emergency laparotomy drain endolymphatic duct
elec	elective electric
elecs	electrolytes
elev	elevated
ELF	etoposide + leucovorin + 5-fluorouracil (combination chemotherapy) elective low forceps Essex-Lopresti fracture
ELH	endolymphatic hydrops

	(accumulation of endolymph in the inner ear)
ELIA	enzyme-linked immunoassay
ELIEDA	enzyme-linked immunoelectron diffusion assay
ELIFA	enzyme-linked immunofiltration assay
ELISA	enzyme-linked immunosorbent assay
elix	elixir (a clear, sweetened solution of alcohol and water, used as a vehicle for medicine taken orally)
ELM	external limiting membrane (the third of ten layers of the retina)
ELN	encapsulated lymph node
ELND	elective lymph node dissection (excision)
ELO	enteroviral leukemic oncogene
ELOS	estimated length of stay
ELOSA	enzyme-linked oligonucleotide sorbent assay
ELP	electrophoresis
ELPS	excessive lateral pressure syndrome
ELS	Eaton-Lambert syndrome (a myasthenia-like syndrome) endolymphatic sac (of inner ear)

ELS

endo-lymphatic sac

extracorporeal life support

ELSI ethical, legal and social
implications

ELSS Emergency Life
Support System

ELT endoscopic laser therapy
euglobulin lysis test
(euglobulin clot test)
euglobulin lysis time

ELV efferent lymphatic vessel

EM early melanoma
ejection murmur
electromagnetic
electron micrograph
electron microscope

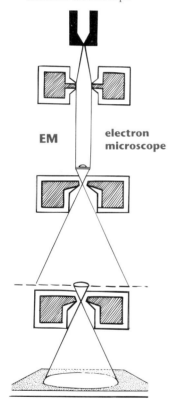

EM **electron
microscope**

electron microscopy
electrophoretic mobility
emergency medicine
emmetropia (the normal
condition of the
refractive system of the

eye in which light rays
entering the eyeball focus
exactly on the retina)
erythema migrans (benign
migratory glossitis)
erythema multiforme
erythrocyte mass
external monitor
extracellular matrix

Em emmetropia (the normal
condition of the
refractive system of the
eye in which light rays
entering the eyeball focus
exactly on the retina)

EMA electronic microanalyzer
epithelial membrane
antigen

EMA-CO etoposide + methotrexate +
Actinomysin D
(dactinomycin) +
cyclophosphamide +
Oncovin (vincristine)
(combination
chemotherapy)

EMAP evoked muscle action
potential

EMB embryology
endometrial biopsy

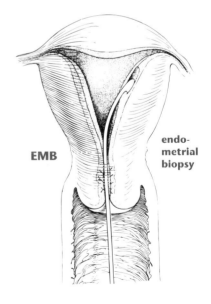

EMB **endo-
metrial
biopsy**

endomyocardial biopsy
eosin-methylene blue

emb embryo (life from the time
of conception to the end
of the second month in
the uterus)

EMC emergency medical care
encephalomyocarditis
endometrial cancer
endometrial carcinoma
endometrial curettage
essential mixed
cryoglobulinemia

EMCB endomyocardial biopsy

EMCV encephalomyocarditis virus

EMD electromyocardial
dissociation
esophageal myotonia
dystrophica

EMF elastomyofibrosis
electromagnetic field
(electric and
magnetic field)
electromagnetic force
electromotive force
electronic fetal monitoring
endomyocardial fibrosis
erythema multiforme
(Stevens-Johnson
syndrome)
erythrocyte maturation
factor

emf electromotive force

EMG electromyelogram
electromyelography
electromyogram

electromyogram (of muscle cramp)

electromyography
essential monoclonal
gammopathy
exophthalmos,
macroglossia, gigantism

EMG BF electromyography
biofeedback

EMGdi diaphragmatic
electromyography

EMGn extramembranous
glomerulonephritis

EMH endometrial hyperplasia

E-3M2H E-3-methyl-2-hexenoic acid
(human odor component
secreted by apocrine
glands under the arms)

EMI elderly and mentally
infirmed
electromagnetic
interference
emergency medical
identification
Emergency Medical
Information
endometriosis interna

EMIC emergency maternity and
infant care
Environmental Mutagen
Information Center
(bibliographic database)

EMICBACK
Environmental Mutagen
Information Center
Backfile

EMIS emergency medical
identification symbol

EMI scan Electric and Musical
Industries scan (first
computerized
tomographic
device developed
in England)

EMIT enzyme-multiplication
immunoassay technique
enzyme-multiplied
immunoassay technique

EML erythema nodosum
leprosum

EMLA eutectic (easily dissolved)

mixture of local
anesthetics

EMLNG external mammary lymph
node group

EMP electromagnetic pulse
extraocular muscle palsy

emp. *emplastrum* [Latin] plaster

e.m.p. *ex modo prescripto* [Latin]
in the manner prescribed

EMPS exertional muscle
pain syndrome

EMR educable mentally retarded
electromagnetic radiation
endoscopic mucosal
resection

EMS early morning specimen
early morning stiffness
electromagnetic spectrum
emergency medical
services
endoscopic mucosectomy
eosinophilia myalagia
syndrome

EMSS emergency medical
services system

EMSU early morning specimen
of urine

EMT emergency medical team
emergency medical
technician
ergonovine maleate test
(for detection of
coronary artery disease)

EMTA endomethylene
tetrahydrophthalic acid

EMT-A emergency medical
technician-ambulance

EMU early morning urine
electromagnetic unit
epilepsy monitoring unit

EMUS early morning urine
specimen

EMV eyes, motor, verbal
(Glasgow coma scale
grading score)

EMW electromagnetic waves

EN efferent nerve
endoscopy
enteral nutrition

enteritis necroticans
entrapment neuropathy
erythema nodosum
essentially negative

En enema

ENA Emergency Nurses
Assciation
extractable nuclear
antigen/antibody

ENB esthesioneuroblastoma
(radiosensitive glioma
seen in the nasal cavity)

ENBS early neurobehavioral
score

END early neonatal death

ENDO endocrinology
endodontics
endoscope
endoscopy
endotracheal

Endocrin endocrinology

ENDOR electron-nuclear double
resonance (spectroscopy)

ENE ethylnorepinephrine
(synthetic adrenergic)

ENF epineural fibrosis

ENG electroneurography
electronystagmogram
electronystagmography

ENK enkephalin
(neurotransmitter or
neuromodulator)

ENL erythema nodosum
leprosum

Eno enolase (an enzyme)

ENOG electroneurography

ENSC emergency nonoperative
surgical care

ENT ears, nose and throat

ENU enuresis (involuntary
discharge of urine)

enz enzyme

EO elbow orthosis
eosinophil
ethylene oxide
(bactericidal agent)
expected outcome
external otitis
eyes open

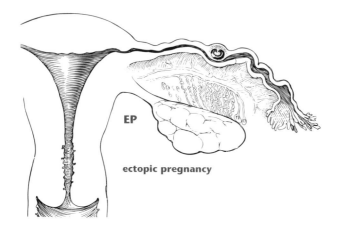

EP

ectopic pregnancy

Eo	eosinophil
EOA	erosive osteoarthritis
	esophageal obturator airway
	examination, opinion and advice
	external oblique aponeurosis
	external ostomy appliance
EOB	exstrophy of bladder
EOBC	early-onset breast cancer
EOC	early ovarian cancer
	enema of choice
	epiphyseal ossification center
	epithelial ovarian cancer
EOCA	early onset cerebellar ataxia
EOD	end-organ dysfunction
	extent of disease
eod	every other day
EOEC	early-onset endocarditis
EOG	electro-oculogram
EOJ	extrahepatic obstructive jaundice
EOLC	end-of-life care
EOM	extraocular movement
EOMs	extraocular muscles
EOOC	early-onset ovarian cancer
EOP	endogenous opioid peptide
	external occipital protuberance

EORA	elderly onset rheumatoid arthritis
Eos	eosinophils
eosin	eosinophils
EOT	effective oxygen transport
EP	ectopic pacemaker
	ectopic pregnancy
	edematous pancreatitis
	electrophoresis
	emergency physician
	emergency procedure
	endogenous pyrogen (induces fever by acting on the hypothalamus)
	endoperoxide
	endorphin (capable of producing effects similar to those of opiates)
	cntcropcptidasc (enterokinase)
	eosinophilic pneumonia
	epithelium
	Erb paralysis
	ergot poisoning
	erythrocyte protoporphyrin
	erythroid proliferation
	erythropoietic porphyria
	erythropoietin
	escape pacemaker
	estrogen patch
	evoked potential
E & P	estrogen and progesterone

Ep	epilepsy
EPA	extrinsic plasminogen activator
	U. S. Environmental Protection Agency
EPAP	expiratory positive airway pressure
EPB	extensor pollicis brevis (muscle)
EPC	elevated plasma cholesterol
	epilepsia partialis continua
	external pneumatic (calf) compression
	endoscopic pancreatocholangiography
EPDP	extrapulmonary disseminated pneumocystosis
EPE	erythropoietin-producing enzyme
EPEC	enteropathogenic *E. coli*
EPF	early pregnancy factor
	endothelial proliferating factor
	external pin fixation
EPG	electropneumogram
EPH	edema, proteinuria, and hypertension
	episodic paroxysmal hemicrania
	extensor proprius hallucis (muscle)
	extrapyramidal hypertonia
EPI	ectoparasite infestation (mites, ticks, lice, fleas, flies, tongue worms and leeches)
	epinephrine
	epithelium
	evoked potential index
	exocrine pancreatic insufficiency
EPIC	etoposide + ifosfamide + cisplatin (combination chemotherapy)
Epid	epidural
Epig	epigastric
epil	epilepsy
epis	episiotomy

epith	epithelium
EPL	extensor pollicis longus (muscle)
	extracorporeal piezoelectric lithotriptor
EPLp(a)	elevated plasma lipoprotein (a)
EPM	electronic pacemaker
	epipapillary membrane
EPO	eosinophil peroxidase
	epoetin alpha (recombinant human erythropoietin)
	erythropoiesis
	erythropoietin
	exclusive provider organization
Epo	epoetin alpha (recombinant human erythropoietin)
EPP	end-plate potential
	epiphyseal plate (growth plate)
	equal pressure point
	erythropoietic protoporphyria
EPPB	end positive-pressure breathing
EPR	electron paramagnetic resonance
	electrophrenic respiration
	endoplasmic reticulum
	estradiol production rate
EPRS	electron pulse radiolysis system
EPRs	estrogen-progesterone receptors
EPS	elastosis perforans serpiginosa
	electrophysiologic study
	enzyme pancreatic secretion
	exophthalmos-producing substance
	expressed prostatic secretions
	extracellular polysaccharide
	extrapyramidal syndrome

extrapyramidal system

EPs ectopic pregnancies

EPSA elevated prostate-specific antigen

EPSAL elevated prostate-specific antigen level

EPSP excitatory postsynaptic potential

EPSPC extraovarian peritoneal serous papillary carcinoma

EPSS E point to septal separation

EPT early pregnancy test

electric pulp test

estrogen-progesterone therapy

estrogen-progestin therapy

extrapulmonary tuberculosis

EPt elderly patient

EPTE existed prior to entry

EPV external pudendal vein

EQ encephalization quotient

educational quotient

Eq equivalent

Eqn equation

equil equilibrium

equiv equivalent

ER electroresection

emergency room

endoplasmic reticulum (an extensive network of fine parallel membranes interspersed throughout the cytoplasm of the cell)

equivalent roentgen

erythrocyte receptor

escape rhythm (a completely blocked or depressed rhythm of the heart occurring when the sinoatrial node fails to initiate impulses)

esophageal reflux

estradiol receptor

estrogen receptor

evoked response

external rotation

Er erbium (a rare metallic element)

ERA estradiol receptor assay

estrogen receptor assay

evoked response audiometry

exercise-related anaphylaxis

ERA/PRA estrogen receptor assay/ progesterone receptor assay

ERA/PRA/DNA estrogen receptor assay/ progesterone receptor assay/DNA methodology

ERAS endogenous renin-angiotensin system

ERBF effective renal blood flow

ERC endoscopic retrograge cholangiography

erythropoietin-responsive cell

ERCP endoscopic retrograde cholangiopancreatography

ERD early retirement for disability

ERE external rotation in extension

ERF external rotation in flexion

ERG electroretinogram

ERG

electro-retino-gram

ERHD	exposure-related hypothermic death
ERIA	electroradioimmunoassay
ERIC	Educational Resources Information Center
ERICA	estrogen receptor-immunocytochemical assay
ERM	epiretinal membrane
	extended radical mastectomy
ERMS	exacerbating-remitting multiple sclerosis
ERP	early receptor potential
	effective refractory period
	emergency room physician
	endoscopic retrograde pancreatography
	enzyme-releasing peptide
ERPF	effective renal plasma flow
	estimated renal plasma flow
ERS	emergency response system
	endoscopic retrograde sphincterotomy
ERs	estrogen receptors
ERT	emergency room triage (sorting out to determine priority of need)
	enzyme replacement therapy
	estrogen replacement therapy
	extended-release tablets
	external radiation therapy
ERU	endorectal ultrasound
ERV	expiratory reserve volume
ERY	erysipelas (acute superficial cellulitis)
Er:YAG	erbium: yttrium-aluminum-garnet (laser)
erythro	erythrocyte (red blood cell)
ES	Eisenmenger syndrome
	ejection sound (early systole following first heart sound)
	elastic stockings
	electrical stimulation

	electroshock
	embryonic stem (cell)
	emission spectroscopy
	emotional stress
	endometritis-salpingitis
	enterospasm (intestinal spasm or colic)
	entotic sound (sound that originates within the ear)
	epileptic syndrome
	epiphyseal stapling
	Epsom salt (magnesium sulfate)
	esophageal spasm
	esophageal stenosis
	esophageal stricture
	esophoria (condition in which the eyes have a tendency to turn inward)
	esterase (any enzyme that promotes the hydrolysis of an ester)
	Ewing's sarcoma
	extrasystole (interpolated premature contraction of the heart)
Es	einsteinium (a synthetic radioactive element)
e.s.	*enema saponis* [Latin] soapy enema
ESA-IRS	European Space Agency, Information Retrieval Service
esap	evoked sensory (neurons) action potential
ESAT	extrasystolic atrial tachycardia
ESB	electrical stimulation to brain
ESC	end systolic counts
	erythropoietin-sensitive stem cell
ESCC	epidural spinal cord compression
ESD	emission spectrometric device
	extrinsic sleep disorder
ESE	electron spin echo
ESEOC	early-stage epithelial

ovarian cancer

ESEP extreme somatosensory evoked potential

ESES electrical status epilepticus during sleep

ESF erythropoiesis-stimulating factor (erythropoietin)

ESG estrogen

ESI epidural steroid injection

ESIMV expiratory synchronized intermittent mandatory ventilation

ESIN elastic stable intramedullary nailing

ESKD end-stage kidney disease

ESL extracorporeal shockwave lithotripsy

ESLD end-stage liver disease

ESLF end-stage liver failure

ESLP electric shocklike pain

ESM ejection systolic murmur
endometrial stromal meiosis
erector spinae muscle(s)

ESN estrogen-stimulated neurophysin

ESO electrospinal orthosis
esophagus
esophoria

eso esophagus

ESP effective systolic pressure
electric shock protector
endometritis, salpingitis, and peritonitis
end-systolic pressure
especially
evoked synaptic potential
extrasensory perception

esp especially

ESPA electrical stimulation–produced analgesia

ESR electron spin resonance
erythrocyte sedimentation rate

ESRD end stage renal disease (late stages of chronic renal failure)

ESRD-DM
end stage renal disease –

attributable to diabetes mellitus

ESRF end stage renal failure

ESRT erythrocyte sedimentation rate test

ESS empty sella syndrome
endometrial stromal sarcoma
endoscopic sinus surgery
erythrocyte-sensitizing substance
euthyroid sick syndrome

ess essential

EST endodermal sinus tumor
electroshock therapy
electrostimulation treatment
endoscopic sphincterectomy
Entri Star tube
esterase (any enzyme that promotes the hydrolysis of an ester)
eversion stress test
exercise stress test

Est estradiol
estrogen

est estimation

Est-ring estradiol (vaginal) ring

ESU electrosurgical unit

ESV end-systolic volume

ESVI end-systolic volume index

ESVS epiurethral suprapubic vaginal suspension

ESWL extracorporeal shock wave lithotripsy
electroshock wave lithotripsy

ET educational therapy
Einthoven's triangle
ejection time
electrophoretic type
embryo transfer
endocrine therapy
endothelins
endothelium
endotoxin
endotracheal
endotracheal tube

end-tidal
enterotoxin
epidemic threshold
epithelial tumor
ergotamine therapy
essential thrombocythemia
essential thrombocytosis
essential tremor
ethanol
etiology
eustachian tube
  (auditory tube)
Ewing's tumor
exchange transfusion
exercise test
exercise treadmill
expiratory time

ET3 erythrocyte
  triiodothyronine

E(T) intermittent esotropia at
  infinity

E(T') intermittent esotropia at
  near

E & T excitability and threshold

Et etiology

ETA endotracheal airway
endotracheal anesthesia
estimated time of arrival
ethionamide
  (antibacterial agent)

ET-A enterotoxin A

ETAB extrathoracic assisted
  breathing

et al. *et alii* [Latin] and others

ETB exudative tuberculosis

ET-B enterotoxin B

ETC electron transport chain
essential
  thrombocytopenia
  (idiopathic
  thrombocytopenic
  purpura)
estimated time of
  conception

ET-C1 enterotoxin C1

ET-C2 enterotoxin C2

ET-C3 enterotoxin C3

etc. *et cetera* [Latin] and
  so forth

ETCO₂ end tidal carbon dioxide

ETD eustachian tube
  dysfunction

ET-D enterotoxin D

ET-E enterotoxin E

ETEC enterotoxigenic
  Escherichia coli

ETF electron tranfer
  flavoprotein
epidemic typhus fever
exchange transfusion

ETH elixir terpin hydrate
ethanol (ethyl alcohol)

eth ether

ETH/C elixir terpin hydrate
  with codeine

ETI endotracheal intubation

ETI
endotracheal intubation

ejection time index

ETIC Environmental Teratology
  Information Center

ETICBACK
  Environmental Teratology
  Information Center
  Backfile (bibliographic
  database)

ETIG equine tetanus immune
  globulin

ETIO etiocholanolone (reduced
  form of testosterone

excreted in the urine)

etiol	etiology
ETKM	every test known to man
ETM	erythromycin (intermediate spectrum antibiotic)
ETN	erythrityl tetranitrate
ETO	eustachian (auditory) tube obstruction
EtO	estimated time of ovulation ethylene oxide
ETOA	estimated time of arrival
EtOH	ethyl alcohol (ethanol) electron transport particle
ETOP	etoposide (antineoplastic agent)
ETOX	ethylene oxide
ETP	entire treatment period ephedrine, theophylline and phenobarbital
ETR	emergency treatment record
ETS	encephalotrigeminal syndrome (Sturge-Weber disease) endotracheal suction environmental tobacco smoke (second hand smoke)
ETSPSA	elevated total serum prostate-specific antigen (PSA)
ETT	endotracheal tube epinephrine tolerance test exercise tolerance test exercise treadmill test
ETU	emergency trauma/ treatment unit
EU	Ehrlich unit emergency unit emotionally unstable endotoxin unit enzyme unit esterase unit etiology unknown excretory urogram
Eu	europium (a rare element, used as a laser dopant and to absorb neutrons

in research)

E & U	erosion and ulcer
EUA	examination under anesthesia
EUG	excretory urography
EUM	external urethral meatus
EUP	extrauterine pregnancy
EUROTOX	European Committee on Chronic Toxicity Hazards
EUS	endoscopic ultrasound (evaluation) external urethral sphincter
EV	Ebola virus echovirus emissary vein enteroviruses esophageal varices estradiol valerate extravascular
eV	electron-volt (energy acquired by an electron moving through a potential difference of 1 volt)
EVA	echo virus antibody etoposide +vinblastine + Adriamycin (doxorubicin) (combination chemotherapy)
Evac	evacuation
eval	evaluate
EVAP	etoposide + vinblastine + ARA-C (cytarabine) + Platinol (cisplatin)

E. vermicularis

Enterobius vermicularis

(combination
chemotherapy)

EVB esophageal variceal
bleeding

EVCS Ellis-van Creveld syndrome

EVD Ebola virus disease

E. vermicularis
Enterobius vermicularis
(pinworm)

EVF enterovaginal fistula

EVG electroventriculography

EVL endoscopic variceal
ligation

EVMC enteroviral meningitis in
childhood

EVP enteric viral pathogens
episcleral venous pressure
evoked visual response
extroverted personality

EVRS early ventricular
repolarization syndrome

EVT external vacuum therapy
(nonsurgical way to
produce an erection
among impotent men)

EW earwax
emergency ward

ew elsewhere

EWB estrogen withdrawal
bleeding

EWHO elbow-wrist-hand orthosis

EWL estimated weight loss

EWT erupted wisdom teeth
(3rd molars)

Ex excision

ex examination
examined
example
except
exchange
excision
exemplary
exercise
exposure
express
extra
extraction

EXAFS extended x-ray absorption
fine structure

exam examination

exc excision

exer exercise

exhib. *exhibeatur* [Latin] let
it be given

EXL elixir (a sweetened
solution of alcohol and
water that is used as a
vehicle for medicine
taken orally)

exp lap exploratory laparotomy

EXO exophoria

exog exogenous

exoph exophthalmos

exos exostosis

EXP exploratory

exp expectorant
experienced
experiment
expired
exploratory
exposed

expect expectorant

ExPGN extracapillary proliferative
glomerulonephritis

expir expiration
expiratory

exp lap exploratory laparotomy

expt experiment

ExS ex-smoker
extra strength

ext extensive
external
extract
extraction
extremity

ext. *extende* [Latin] spread

extens extension
extensor

ext mon external monitor

extr extremity

extrav extravasation

ext rot external rotation

EXTUB extubation

EXU excretory urogram

exud exudate

exx examples

EZ erogenous zone

Ez eczema

EZD Ellison-Zollinger disease

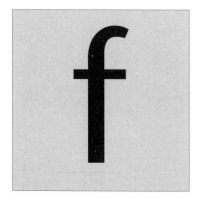

F
factor
Fahrenheit
failure
false
family
farad
fascia
fasting
fat
fecalith
feces
felon (whitlow)
female
femur
fertility
fertilization

fetal
fever
fibroblast
fibula
filament
finger
flexion
floaters
flow
fluorine
focus
folacin
fontanel
foramen
force
formula
fossa
fracture
fragment
French (name of catheter)
7 French (size and name of catheter)
frequency
fundus
phenylalanine
visual field

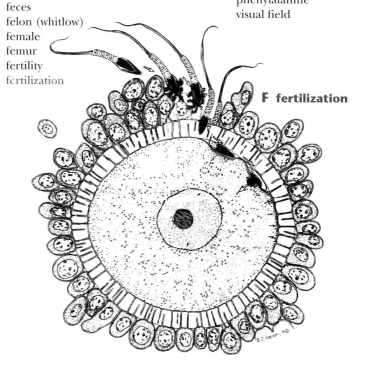

F fertilization

F1 first filial generation
F I factor I (fibrinogen)
F2 second filial generation
F II factor II (prothrombin)
F V factor V (proaccelerin)
F IX factor IX (Christmas factor)
F X factor X (Stuart-Prower factor)
F XI factor XI (plasma thromboplasma antecedent)
F XII factor XII (Hageman factor)
LF XIII factor XIII (fibrinase)
f fasting
    femto (prefix denoting decimal factor 10^{-15})
    fluid
    focal length
    frequency
FA false aneurysm
    Families Anonymous
    Fanconi anemia
    far advanced
    fatty acid
    febrile antigens
    femoral artery
    fetal age
    fibrinolytic activity
    fibroadenoma
    filtered air
    first aid
    fludarabine (antiviral agent)
    fluorescein angiography
    fluorescent antibody
    folic acid (folacin)
    food additive
    food allergy
    forearm
    Friedreich ataxia
FAA febrile antigen agglutination
    formaldehyde, acetic acid, and alcohol
FAAT fluorescent antinuclear antibody test
FAB antigen binding fragments

fast-atom spectrometer
fibroadenoma of breast (most common benign tumor of the female breast)
formalin ammonium bromide
functional arm brace
Fab antigen-binding fragment (monovalent)
    fragment, antigen-binding (monovalent)
FABER flexion in abduction and external rotation
FABP fatty acid-binding protein
FAC fatty acid cyclooxygenase
    5-fluorouracil + Adriamycin (doxorubicin) + Cytoxan (cyclophosphamide) (combination chemotherapy)
    foamy alveolar cast
Fac factor
fac. *facere* [Latin] to make
Facb fragment, antigen, and complement binding
FACC Fellow of the American College of Cardiologists
FACO Fellow of the American College of Otolaryngology
FACOG Fellow of the American College of Obstetricians and Gynecologists
FACOSH Federal Advisory Committee on Occupational Safety and Health
FACP 5-fluorouracil + Adriamycin (doxorubicin) + cyclophosphamide + Platinol (cisplatin) (combination chemotherapy)
FACS fluorescence-activated cell sorter (flow cytometer)
FACSM Fellow of the American

College of Sports
Medicine

FACT functional assessment of
cancer therapy

F-actin fibrous actin

FAD familial Alzheimer's
dementia
familial Alzheimer's
disease
familial autonomic
dysfunction
flavin adenine dinucleotide
(oxidized form of
the coenzyme)
Frohlich adiposogenital
dystrophy

FADH2 flavin adenine dinucleotide
(reduced form of the
coenzyme)

FADIR flexion in adduction and
internal rotation

FADN flavin adenine dinucleotide

FAE fetal alcohol effects

FAEEs fatty acid ethyl esters
(esters of fatty acids and
ethanol)

FAF fibroblast-activating factor

Fahr Fahrenheit (scale/
thermometer)

FAI folic acid injection
food allergy insomnia
functional aerobic
impairment
functional assessment
inventory

FAIDS fear of AIDS

FAJ fused apophyseal joint

FAK floating arm keyboard

FALP fluoro-assisted lumbar
puncture

FAM fibroangiomyxoma
5-flpuorouracil +
Adriamycin
(doxorubicin) +
mitomycin C
(combination
chemotherapy)

FAMA fluorescent antibody to
membrane antigen

FAMe 5-fluorouracil +
Adriamycin
(doxorubicin) + methyl
CCNU (semustine)
(combination
chemotherapy)

FAM-M familial atypical mole and
melanoma (syndrome)

FAMS 5-fluorouracil +
Adriamycin
(doxorubicin) +
mitomycin C +
streptozotocin
(combination
chemotherapy)

FANA fluorescent antinuclear
antibody

FAP familial adenomatous
polyposis
familial amyloid
polyneuropathy
fixed action potential

FAR Federal Acquisition
Regulations

FARE Federation of Alcoholic
Rehabilitation
Establishments

FARS fatal accident
reporting system

FAS fatty acid synthetase
fetal alcohol syndrome
(prevalent cause of
defective cerebral
development)
fetal aminopterin
syndrome

FASC fasciculation (small local
contraction of muscles)

fasc. *fasciculus* [Latin] bundle

FASEB Federation of American
Societies for
Experimental Biology

FAS/FAE fetal alcohol syndrome/
fetal alcohol effects

FasL Fas ligand (protein that
causes apoptosis in
targeted T cells)

FAST fluorescent
allergo-sorbent test

fluorescent antibody
  staining technique
FAT 5-fluorouracil +
  Adriamycin
  (doxorubicin) + trazinate
  (combination
  chemotherapy)
fluorescent-antibody test
FATF fatty-acid transfer factor
fax facsimile
FB feedback
fever blister (herpes
  febrilis)
fiberoptic bronchoscopy
film badge
fingerbreadth (measured
  distance)
followed by
footling breech
foreign body
frostbite
fb fingerbreadth
FBA fecal bile acid
FBC flexion body cast
FBCP familial benign chronic
  pemphigus
FBD foreign born doctor
functional bowel disorder
FBE full blood examination
FBF football finger
FBG fasting blood glucose
fibrinogen
FBHH familial benign
  hypocalciuric
  hpercalcemia
FBI foodborne illness
FBN Federal Bureau of
  Narcotics
FBP femoral blood pressure
footling breech
  presentation
frank breech presentation
FBR foreign body reaction
FBS failed back syndrome
fasting blood sugar
feedback system
fetal blood sample
fetal blood sampling
fetal bovine serum

fibrocystic breast syndrome
flabby back syndrome
  (disuse hypoplasia)
foreign-body sarcoma
functional bladder
  syndrome
FBSS failed back surgery
  syndrome
F. buski *Fasciolopsis buski*
  (an intestinal fluke that
  generally causes nausea
  and diarrhea)
FBW fasting blood work
FC facial canal
fasciculus cuneatus
fat cell
febrile convulsion
fibrocyte
finger clubbing
finger counting
flail chest
flow cytometry
fluorocarbon
Fogarty catheter
Foley catheter
follicular cyst

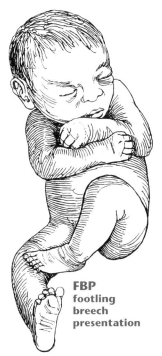

**FBP
footling
breech
presentation**

foramen cecum
foster care
fovea centralis
free cholesterol
French catheter
functional constipation
funnel chest (pectus
    excavatum)

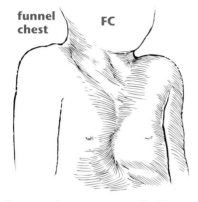

funnel chest   **FC**

Fc   fragment, crystallizable
F & C   fever and chills
      foam and condom
5-FC   flucytosine
      (antifungal agent)
Fc   crystallizable fragment
      (non-Fab part of
      immunoglobulin)
      footcandle
FCA   fluorescent cytoprint assay
      Freund's complete
      adjuvant
Fcath   Foley catheter
FCBD   fibrocystic breast disease
FCC   follicular center cell
      fracture, compound
      (opened) and
      comminuted (crushed)
FCCL   follicular center cell
      lymphoma (B-cell
      lymphoma)
FCD   fatal childhood diarrhea
      fibrocystic disease
      fibrocystic dysplasia
FCDB   fibrocystic disease of breast
      fibrocystic disorder of
      breast

FCE   5-fluorouracil + cisplatin
      (Platinol) + etoposide
      (derivative of
      podophyllotoxin)
      (combination
      chemotherapy)
FCF   fasciocutaneous flap
FCH   FDA Consumer Hotline,
      (800) FDA-4010
FCHL   familial combined
      hyperlipidemia
FCI   flow cytometric
      immunophenotyping
      food chemical intolerance
fCi   femtocurie
FCIS   Flint Colon Injury Scale
FCL   fibular (lateral) collateral
      ligament (of knee)
FCM   flow cytometry
FCMC   family centered maternity
      care
FCMVS   fetal cytomegalovirus
      syndrome
FCO   fibrocytoma of ovary
FCR   flexor carpi radialis
      (muscle)
      fractional catabolic rate
FCS   fecal containment system
      fetal cocaine syndrome
      fever, chills, and sweating
      foot compartment
      syndrome
FCSNVD   fever, chills, sweating,
      nausea, vomiting and
      diarrhea
FCST   Fellow of the College of
      Speech Therapists
FCT   ferric chloride test
      foramen cecum of tongue
FCU   flexor carpi ulnaris
      (muscle)
FCx   frontal cortex
FD   Fabry's disease
      (X-linked disorder)
      facial dyskinesias
      Fairbanks dysostosis
      familial dysautonomia
      (Riley-Day syndrome)
      fatal dose

Felix's disease
fetal death (stillbirth)
fetal distress
fibrous dysplasia
floppy disk
focal distance
folate deficiency
footdrop
forceps delivery
Fothergill's disease
freeze drying

FD50 median fatal dose

Fd ferredoxin (nonheme iron-containing protein)

FDA Food and Drug Administration
frontodextra anterior (right frontoanterior fetal position)

FDB first-degree burn

FDBLP familial dysbetalipoproteinemia

FDC first-dollar coverage (no deductible)
follicular dendritic cell

FD&C Food, Drug, and Cosmetic (Act)

FDE final drug evaluation

FD/EI field desorption/electron impact

FDF fast death factor

FDG fluorodeoxyglucose

Fdg feeding
fibroblast-derived growth factor

FDGPET fluorodeoxyglucose positron-emission tomography

FDH familial dysalbuminemic hyperthyroxinemia
focal dermal hypoplasia (Glotz syndrome)

FDIU fetal death *in utero*

FDL flexor digitorum longus (muscle)

FDLMP first day of last menstrual period

FDM fetus of diabetic mother

FDNB fluorodinitrobenzene

FDOP fibrodysplasia ossificans progressiva

FDP fibrin degradation product
fibrinogen degradation product
flexor digitorum profundus (muscle)
fronto-dextra posterior (right frontoposterior fetal position)
fructose-1,6-diphosphate

FDPase fructose-1,6-diphosphatase

FDQB flexor digiti quinti brevis (muscle)

FDR first dose reaction (initial dose reaction)

FDS flexor digitorum superficialis (flexor digitorum sublimis) (muscle)
for duration of stay
forced duction test

FDT foot-dorsiflexion test
Friend disease virus
fronto-dextra transversa (right frontotransverse fetal position)

FdUMP fluorodeoxyuridine monophosphate (inhibitor of thymidylate synthase)

FdUTP fluorodeoxyuridine triphosphate (breaks DNA strands)

FDZ fetal danger zone

FE fat embolism
fertilized egg
forced expiration

Fe iron (*ferrum*)

FEAU fluoroethylarabinosyl uracil (potent selective inhibitor of herpes viruses)

FEB free erythrocyte protoporphyrin

feb. dur. *febre durante* [Latin] while the fever lasts

FEBP fetal estrogen-binding protein

FÉC	forced expiratory capacity
	free erythrocyte coproporphyrin
FECG	fetal electrocardiogram
FECP	free erythrocyte coproporphyrin
FECT	fibroelastic connective tissue
FeD	iron deficiency
FEDRIP	Federal Research in Progress (OnLine)
FEED	fiberoptic endoscopic evaluation of deglutition (swallowing)
FEF	forced expiratory flow
FEFmax	maximal forced expiratory flow
FEG	female external genitalia
FEGN	focal embolic glomerulonephritis
FEGO	International Federation of Gynecology and Obstetrics
FEHBP	Federal Employees Health Benefit Program
FEI	fluid-electrolyte imbalance
FEL	familial erythrophagocytic lymphohistiocytosis
	free-electron laser
FeLV	feline leukemia virus
fem	femoral
	femur
FEMA	Federal Emergency Management Agency
FENa	fractional excretion of sodium
fen-phen	fenfluramine-phentermine
FEP	fibroepithelial polyp
	free erythrocyte protoporphyrin
FEPB	functional electronic peroneal brace
FEPCA	Federal Environmental Pesticide Control Act
FER	flexion, extension, and rotation
ferv.	*fervens* [Latin] hot; boiling
FES	fat embolism syndrome
	forced expiratory

	spirogram
	functional electrical stimulation
FeSO$_4$	iron sulfate
FESS	functional endoscopic sinus surgery
FET	forced expiratory time
FETS	forced expiratory time in seconds
FEUO	for external use only
FEV	forced expiratory volume
FEV1	forced expiratory volume in one second (of expiration)
FEV1"	forced expiratory volume in one second (of expiration)
FEV3"	forced expiratory volume in three seconds (of expiration)
fev	fever
FEV1/FVC%	
	forced expiratory volume timed to forced vital capacity ratio
FEVR	familial exudative vitreoretinopathy
FF	fat free
	fatigue factor
	fatigue fracture
	fecal frequency
	fertility factor
	fibula fracture
	filtration fraction
	finger-to-finger (test)
	flat feet (pes planus)
	fog fever
	follicular fluid
	force fluids
	fortified food
	freeze-fracturing
ff	following
FFA	free fatty acids
FFA-AC	free fatty aicds-albumin complex
FFaU	fundus (of pregnant uterus) firm at umbilicus
FFB	flexible fiberoptic bronchoscopy

FFC	fixed flexion contracture
	free from chlorine
FFCP	forme fruste of chickenpox
FFD	fat-free diet
FFG	free fat graft
FFI	fatal familial insomnia
	free from infection
FFIH	familial fat-induced hyperlipemia (familial hyperlipoproteinemia, type I)
FFL	floral variant of follicular lymphoma
FFN	fetal fibronectin
FFP	filiform papilla (on tongue)
	fresh frozen plasma
	fungiform papilla (on tongue)
FFR	freedom from relapse
FFROM	free and full range of motion
FFS	fee-for-service
	flexible fiberoptic sigmoidoscopy
FFT	finger-to-finger test (for coordinated movements of the arms)
	flicker fusion threshold
FG	fasciculus gracilis
	fibrinogen
	free gingiva
FGAH	first-generation antihistamine
FGAR	formylglycinamide ribonucleotide
FGC	fiberglass cast (light cast)
	fibrinogen gel chromatography
FGF	fibroblast derived growth factor
	fibroblast growth factor
FGG	focal global glomerulosclerosis
FGL	fasting gastrin level
FGLU	fasting glucose
FGM	female genital mutilation
	focal glomerulonephriis
FGS	focal glomerulosclerosis

FGT female genital tract

FGT

female genital tract

	fluorescent gonorrhea test
FGV	fasting glucose value
FH	familial hypercholesterolemia
	family history
	fasting hemoglobin
	femoral hernia
	fetal heart
	fetal hemoglobin
	follicular hyperplasia
FH+	positive family history
FH–	negative family history
FH2	dihydrofolate
FH4	tetrahydrofolate
	tetrahydrofolic acid
FHA	familial hypoplastic anemia
FHC	familial hypercholesterolemia
	familial hypertrophic cardiomyopathy
	family health center
FHCM	familial hypertrophic cardiomyopathy
FHCS	Fitz-Hugh Curtis syndrome (perihepatitis)
FHD	familial histiocytic dermatoarthritis
FHDLD	familial high-density lipoprotein deficiency
FHE	fatal hyponatremic encephalopathy
FHF	fulminant hepatic failure
	forward heart failure

FHG	fibrous hyperplasia of gingiva		fibula
fHG	free hemoglobin	**FIC**	Federal Information Center (800) 347-1997 (assistance in locating the appropriate U. S. government agency for queries)
FHH	familial hypocalciuric hypercalcemia (benign disorder)		
	fetal heart heard (and recorded)		Fogarty International Center (of NIH)
FHHBP	Federal Employees' Health Benefits Program	**FICO$_2$**	fraction of inspired carbon dioxide
FHL	flexor hallucis longus (long flexor muscle of big toe)	**FICU**	fetal intensive care unit
		FID	fungal immunodiffusion
		FIF	fibroblast interferon
	functional hearing loss		forced inspiratory flow
FHNH	fetal heart not heard	**FIFO**	first in, first out
FHR	fetal heart rate	**Fig**	diagram
FHRA	fetal heart rate acceleration		figure (with identifying number)
FHRV	fetal heart rate variability	**FIGD**	familial idiopathic gonadotropin deficiency
FHS	fetal heart sounds		
	fetal hydantoin syndrome	**FIGlu**	formiminoglutamic acid
FHSLA	Federal Hazardous Substances Labeling Act	**FIGO**	International Federation of Gynecology and Obstetrics
FHT	fetal heart		
FHTG	familial hypertriglyceridemia	**FIH**	fat-induced hyperglycemia
		fil	filial (of or relating to a daughter or son)
FHX	familial hypercholesterolemic xanthomatosis		
		FIM	functional independence measure
FHx	family history		
FHx+	positive family history	**FIN**	fine intestinal needle
FHx–	negative family history	**FINCC**	familial idiopathic nonarteriosclerotic cerebral calcification
FI	fecal impaction		
	fecal incontinence		
	fever caused by infection	**FiO$_2$**	forced inspiratory oxygen
	fibula		fraction of inspired oxygen (inspired oxygen concentration)
	firearm injury		
	food intolerance		
	forced inspiration	**FIP**	familial intestinal polyposis
	Frieberg infarction	**FIPV**	infectious peritonitis virus
	fructose intolerance	**FIQ**	full scale IQ
	fulminating infection	**FIS**	floppy infant syndrome
	fungal infection		forced inspiratory spirogram
FIA	fluoroimmunoassay		
	focal immunoassay	**FISH**	fluorescence *in situ* hydridization
FIAC	fluoroiodoarabinosyl cytosine	**fist**	fistula
fib	fibrillation	**FITC**	fluorescein isothiocyanate
	fibrinogen	**FIUO**	for internal use only

FIV	forced inspiratory volume
FIV1	forced inspiratory volume in one second
FIVC	forced inspiratory vital capacity
FJ	finger joint
FJN	familial juvenile nephrophthisis
FJP	familial juvenile polyposis
FJRM	full joint range of motion
FJS	facet joint syndrome
	finger joint size
FK	ferrokinetics
	floating kidney (hypermobile kidney)
	fused kidney
FKBP	FK binding proteins
FKE	full knee extension
FKPS	Foster-Kelly-Patterson syndrome
FL	face lift
	false labor
	farmer's lung
	fascia lata (deep fascia)
	fatty liver
	fetal length
	fluid
	follicular lymphoma (nodular lymphoma)
	foodborne listeriosis
	foramen lacerum
	frontal lobe
fL	femtoliter
fl	fluid
FLA	fluorescent-labeled antibody
	fronto-laeva anterior (left frontoanterior fetal position)
flac	flaccid
flav.	*flavus* [Latin] yellow
FLC	fatty liver cell
	frontal lobe of cerebrum
FLD	fibrotic lung disease
	full lower denture
fld	field
	fluid
fld rest	fluid restriction
FLEX	Federal Licensing

	Examination
flex	flexion
flex sig	flexible sigmoidoscopy
FLK	funny looking kid (derogatory; should not be used)
FLKS	fatty liver and kidney syndrome
FLLD	familial lipoprotein lipase deficiency
floc	flocculation
fl oz	fluid ounce
FLP	frog-leg position
	fronto-laeva posterior (left frontoposterior fetal position)
FLS	Fanconi-Lignac syndrome
	fatty liver syndrome
FLSA	follicular lymphosarcoma
FLT	first-line therapy
	fronto-laeva transversa [Latin] left frontotransverse (fetal position)

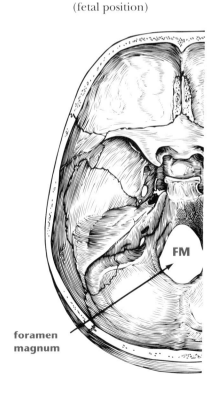

foramen magnum

FM

Flt	floating
flu	influenza
flu A	influenza A virus
fluoro	fluorometry
	fluoroscopy
FLV	Friend leukemia virus (causes malignant reticulopathy in mice)
FLZ	flurazepam hydrochloride (a hypnotic)
FM	face mask
	familial melanoma
	feedback mechanism
	fetal medicine
	fetal membranes
	fetal monitor
	fetal monitoring
	fetal movements
	fibromuscular
	fibromyalgia
	Flint's murmur
	fluorescent microscopy
	foramen magnum
	forensic medicine
	furuncular myiasis
F & M	firm and midline (pregnant uterus)
Fm	fermium (radioactive element)
fm	femtometer
FMAU	fluoromethylarabinosyl uracil (potent selective inhibitor of herpes viruses)
FMC	fetal movement count
	focal macular choroidopathy
	fulminating meningococcemia
FMD	familial metaphyseal dysplasia (Pyle disease)
	family medical doctor
	foot-and-mouth disease (viral disease of domestic and wild animals)
FMDV	foot and mouth disease virus
FME	fetal-maternal exchange
	full-mouth extraction

fMet	formylmethione
FMF	familial Mediterranean fever (familial paroxysmal polyserositis)
	fetal movement felt
	forced midexpiratory flow
FMG	foreign medical graduate
FMH	family medical history
	fetomaternal hemorrhage
	fibromuscular hyperplasia
FmHx	family history
FML	flail mitral (left atrioventricular) leaflet
	Fluorometholone (trade name for a synthetic glucocorticoid)
FMLP	formyl-methionyl-leucyl-phenylalanine
FMM	familial malignant melanoma
FMN	first malignant neoplasm
	flavin mononucleotide (acts as a coenzyme for a number of oxidative enzymes)
fmol	femtomole
FMP	first menstrual period
	fructose monophosphate
FMR	fetal movement record
FMS	fibromyalgia syndrome
	5-fluorouracil + mitomycin + streptozocin (combination chemotherapy)
	full mouth series (x-rays)
FMTC	familial medullary thyroid carcinoma
FMU	first morning urine
FMV	5-fluorouracil + MeCCNU (semustine) + vincristine (combination chemotherapy)
FMX	full mouth x-ray
FN	facial nerve (7th cranial nerve)
	false-negative
	familial nephrosis
	febrile neutropenia
	finger-to-nose (test)

F-N	finger-to-nose (test)
F & N	fetus and neonate
FNA	fine-needle aspiration (cytologic or biopsy)
FNAB	fine-needle aspiration biopsy
FNAC	fine-needle aspiration cytology
FNC	fatty nutritional cirrhosis
FNCJ	fine needle catheter jejunostomy
FND	febrile neutrophilic dermatosis
	fungal nail disease
FNE	false-negative error (type II error)
	free nerve ending
Fneg	false negative (denoting a test result that wrongly indicates that a person does not have the attribute or disease for which the test is conducted)
FNEs	free nerve endings
FNF	finger-to-nose-to-finger test (for coordinated movements of the arms)
FNH	familial neonatal hypoglycemia
	focal nodular hyperplasia
FNHR	febrile nonhemolytic reaction
FNM	focal nodular myositis (syndrome)
fNE	free normetanephrine
FNP	family nurse practitioner
	frontonasal process
FNS	functional neuromuscular stimulation
FNT	finger-to-nose test (for coordinated movements of the arms)
FNTC	fine needle transhepatic cholangiography
FNTT	femoral nerve traction test
FNZ	flunitrazepam (a hypnoic and induction agent in anesthesia)

FO	fiberoptic
	foramen ovale
F/O	fiberoptic
fo	forearm
FOB	father of baby
	fecal occult blood (might indicate colorectal cancer)
	feet out of bed
	fiberoptic bronchoscopy
FO8B	figure-of-8 bandage
FOBS	fiberoptic bronchoscope
FOBT	fecal occult blood test (Hemoccult)
FOC	father of child
	fronto-occipital circumference
FOCMA	feline oncornavirus cell membrane antigen
FOD	familial osseous dystrophy (Morquio's syndrome)
	free of disease
FOG	Fluothane (halothane)+ oxygen + gas (nitrous oxide)
FOH	familial orthostatic hypotension
FOHx	family ocular history
FOIA	Freedom of Information Act
FOL	fiberoptic laryngoscopy
FOM	floor of mouth
	5-fluorouracil + Oncovin (vincristine) + mitomycin (combination chemotherapy)
Font	fontanel
FOOB	fell out of bed
FOP	fibrodysplasia ossificans progressiva
	forensic pathology
FOPS	fiberoptic proctosigmoidoscopy
For	forensic
form	formula
FOS	fiberoptic sigmoidoscopy
	Frank orthogonal system
	fiber optic sigmoidoscope
	fiber optic sigmoidoscopy

FOV	field of view
FP	facial pain
	false-positive
	familial polyposis (familial intestinal polyposis)
	family physician
	family planning
	family practice
	fat pad
	feeding pump
	fetal presentation
	fibrinopeptide
	filiform papilla
	filter paper
	fixation protein
	flavin phosphate
	flavoprotein
	foliate papilla (on tongue)
	food poisoning
	foot pad
	Frejka pillow (abduction pillow splint)
	frozen plasma
	fungiform papilla
F-6-P	fructose-6-phosphate
fp	freezing point
FPA	fibrinopeptide A
	fluorophenylalanine
FPB	femoropopliteal bypass (treatment for inguinal occlusive disease)
	flexor pollicis brevis (muscle)
FPBG	fingerprick blood glucose
FPC	familial polyposis coli
	fish protein concentrate
FPD	feto-pelvic disproportion
	fixed partial denture
FPE	false-positive error (type I error)
	fatal pulmonary embolism
FPFDA	Federal Pure Food and Drug Act
FPG	fasting plasma glucose
FPGN	focal proliferative glomerulonephritis
FPH	flat-plate hemodialyzer
FPIA	fluorescence-polarization immunoassay

FPK	fructose phosphokinase
FPL	fasting plasma lipids
	flexor pollicis longus (muscle)
FPNA	first pass nuclear angiocardiography
FPOR	follicular puncture for oocyte retrieval
FPPH	familial primary pulmonary hypertension
FPR	false positive rate
	Familial Polyposis Registry
FPRA	first pass radionuclide angiogram
fps	foot-pound-second (system of units)
fPSA	free form of serum prostate-specific antigen (PSA)
fPt	fasting patient
FPVB	femoral popliteal vein bypass
FPZ	fluphenazine
FPZ-E	fluphenazine enanthate
FR	failure rate
	father
	flocculation reaction (Sachs-Georgi test)
	flow rate
	fluid restriction
	fluid retention
	foramen rotundum
	fractional reabsorption
	free radical
	frequency of respiration
F & R	force and rhythm (of pulse)
Fr	fracture
	francium (a radioactive element)
	French (size of catheter or tube)
FRA	fibrinogen-related antigen
	fluorescent rabies antibody
Frac	fracture
frac	fracture
fract dos.	*fracta dosi* [Latin] in divided doses
frag	fragility

FRAP	fluoride-resistant acid phosphatase
FRAT	free radical assay technique
FRAX	fragile X (chromosome)
	fragile X (syndrome)
FRC	Federal Radiation Council
	frozen red (blood) cells
	functional residual capacity
FRCS	Fellow of the Royal College of Surgeons
FRD	fat-restricted diet
	fiber-rich diet
FRDC	fixed-ratio drug combination
FRDT	flexion-rotation drawer test
free PSA	free prostate-specific antigen
FREIR	Federal Research on Biologic and Health Effects of Ionizing Radiation
freq	frequency
FRF	Fertility Research Foundation
	follicle-stimulating hormone releasing factor
FRG	filtration-resistant glaucoma
FRH	follicle regulatory hormone
	FSH-releasing hormone
FRI	firearm-related injury
FRJM	full range of joint movement
FROM	full range of motion
	full range of movements
FRP	follicle regulatory protein
	functional refractory period
FRS	fecal reducing substance
	female reproductive system
	fetal radiation syndrome
	fetal rubella syndrome
FRT	full recovery time
Fru	fructose (fruit sugar; the sweetest of the simple sugars)
Frx	fracture
FS	Fanconi syndrome

	(a functional disturbance of the proximal kidney tubules)
	Felty syndrome (rheumatoid arthritis + leukopenia + enlargement of the spleen)
	fetoscope (special stethoscope for listening to the fetal heart beat)
	fibromyalgia syndrome
	flexible sigmoidoscopy
	fluorescence spectroscopy
	foramen spinosum
	foreskin
	fracture site
	Frolich's syndome (adiposogenital dystrophy)
	frozen section
	frozen shoulder
F & S	fatigue and sleep
FSB	fetal scalp blood
FSBG	fingerstick (fingerprick) blood glucose
FSC	facet synovial cyst
	flexible sigmoidoscopy
FSD	fish-slime disease
	focal-skin distance
FSE	fetal scalp electrode
FSF	fibrin-stabilizing factor
FSG	family support group
	fasting serum glucose
	focal segmental sclerosis
FSGN	focal sclerosing glomerulonephritis
	focal segmental glomerulonephritis
FSGS	focal segmental glomerulosclerosis (focal glomerular sclerosis)
FSH	focal and segmental hyalinosis
	follicle-stimulating hormone
FSH-LH	follicle-stimulating hormone-luteinizing hormone

FSH/LRRH
follicle-stimulating hormone and luteinizing hormone releasing hormone

FSH MD facioscapulohumeral muscular dystrophy (Landouzy-Dejerine dystrophy)

FSH-RF follicle-stimulating hormone-releasing factor

FSH-RH follicle-stimulating hormone-releasing hormone

FSI foam stability index
Food Sanitation Institute
foreign substance inhalation

FSNE flower-spray nerve ending

FSP familial spastic paraplegia
fibrin-split products

FSS fetal scalp sampling
fetal solvent syndrome
fetal syphilis syndrome
focal segmental sclerosis
frequency-selective saturation

FST foam stability test

FSV fat-soluble vitamins

FT Fallot's tetralogy (pulmonary stenosis + interventricular septal defect + aortic dextroposition + right ventricular hypertrophy)
family therapy

FTG

full-thickness graft

fast twitch
fecal trypsin
fibrous tissue
filum terminale
finger tip
fissured tongue
fluoride treatment
follow through
free testosterone
free thyroxine
full term
functional test

FT$_3$ free triiodothyronine

FT$_4$ free thyroxine

Ft ferritin (a protein rich in iron found mainly in the liver, spleen and intestinal mucosa)

ft foot
feet

ft. *fiat* [Latin] make

FTA fluorescent titer antibody
fluorescent treponemal antigen (test)

FTA-ABS fluorescent treponemal antibody-absorption (test)

FTAAT fluorescent treponemal antibody absorption test

FTB full-thickness burn

FTBD full term born dead

FTBE focal tick-borne encephalitis

FTC fallopian (uterine) tube carcinoma
Federal Trade Commission

FTD failure (of fetus) to descend

FTE full-time equivalent

FTF finger-to-finger (test for coordinated movements of the arms)

FT$_4$F free thyroxine fraction (test)

FTG free tendon graft
full-thickness graft

FTI free thyroxine index

FT$_3$I free triiodothyronine index

FT$_4$I free thyroxine index

F TIP	finger tip
FTKA	failed to keep appointment
FTLB	full term living birth
FTLR	fallopian tube ligation ring
FTM	fractional test meal
ft. mist.	*fiat mistura* [Latin] make a mixture
FTN	finger to nose (test for coordinated movements of the arms)
FTNB	full-term newborn
FTND	full term normal delivery
FTO	fructose-terminated oligosaccharide
FTOP	first trimester of pregnancy
FTOS	full-time outservice
FTP	failure to progress (labor)
	fallopian tube papilloma
	finger-trap phenomenon
	full-term pregnancy
FTR	for the record
	fractional tubular reabsorption
FTRS	full-text retrieval system
FTS	fallopian tube sarcoma
	feminizing testis syndrome
	fetal tobacco syndrome
	fissured tongue syndrome
FTS-ABS	fluorescent treponema antibody-absorption (test)
FTSD	full-term spontaneous delivery
FTSG	full-thickness skin graft
FTT	failure to thrive
	fat tolerance test
	free tissue transfer
FTTD	full-time training duty
FTTS	failure to thrive syndrome
FTU	fluorescence thiourca
FTUPLD	full-term uncomplicated pregnancy, labor, and delivery
FTW	fish tapeworm (*Diphyllobothrium latum*)
FU	fecal urobilinogen
	fetal urobilinogen
	fluorouracil (an antineoplastic agent)
	follow up
	fractional urinalysis
	fundus (of uterus) at umbilicus
5-FU	5-fluorouracil (an antineoplastic agent)
FUB	functional uterine bleeding
FUD	full upper denture
FUDR	floxuridine (inhibitor of thymidylate synthase)
FudR	floxuridine (inhibitor of thymidylate synthase) fluorodeoxyuridine
FUE	fever of undetermined etiology
5FU/FA	5-fluorouracil + folinic acid (leucovorin) (combination chemotherapy)
Fulg	fulguration (destruction of living tissue by electric sparks)
5FU/LV	5-fluorouracil and leucovorin (antineoplastic agents)
FUMP	fluorouridine monophosphate
FUN	follow-up note
FUO	fever of undetermined origin
	fever of unknown origin
FUOV	follow-up office visit
FUR	fluorouracil riboside
	fluorouridine
FUT	fibrinogen uptake test
	fimbriae of uterine tube
FUTP	fluorouridine triphosphate (interferes with function of RNA)
FV	facial vein
	femoral vein
	fluid volume
FVBG	free vascularized bone graft
FVC	false vocal cord
	forced vital capacity
FVE	forced volume expiration
FVH	focal vascular headache

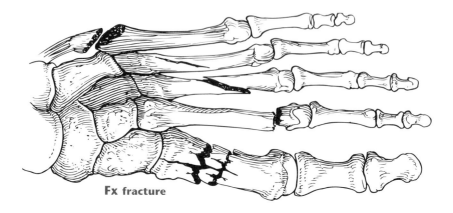

Fx fracture

FVL	femoral vein ligation
	flexible video laparoscope
FVN	familial visceral neuropathy
FVO	femoral valgus osteotomy
FVS	floppy valve syndrome
FVV	fossa of vestibule of vagina
FW	fragment wound
fw	fresh water
FWB	full weight-bearing
FWLS	fever without localizing signs
FWR	Felix-Weil reaction (Weil-Felix test for diagnosis of typhus and other rickettsial diseases)
FX	fluoroscopy
Fx	fracture
Fx-dis	fracture-dislocation
FXF	Fragile X Foundation
FXR	fracture
FXS	fragile X syndrome (defect in the X chromosome)
FY	fiscal year
FYI	for your information
FYS	five-year survival
FZ	focal zone
FZRC	frozen red cells (blood cells)
FZS	frontozygomatic suture

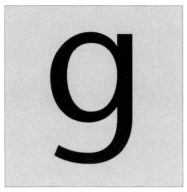

G	force of gravity
	gallop
	gap
	gas
	gastrulation
	gauge
	gauss
	gender
	gingiva
	gland
	glucose (Glc is preferred)
	glycine (Gly is preferred)
	glycogen
	gram (15 grains)
	granulocyte
	gravida
	guanine
	guanosine
G	Gibbs energy
G–	gram negative
G+	gram positive
G$_1$	gap-1 in cell cycle (long active segment of cell cycle from the end of mitosis to the next round of DNA synthesis)
G2	gap-2 in cell cycle (short relatively inactive segment of cell cycle between the end of DNA synthesis and mitosis)
g	gauge
	gender
	gram

	gravitational constant
	gravity
	group
GA	galea aponeurotica
	Gamblers Anonymous
	gastric acid
	gastric analysis
	general anesthesia
	general appearance
	genome analysis
	geriatric assessment
	gestational age
	global aphasia
	glucuronic acid
	glutaric aciduria
	gouty arthritis
Ga	gallium (a rare metallic element)
ga	gauge
GAAT	glacial acetic acid test
GABA	gamma-aminobutyric acid
GABHS	group A beta-hemolytic streptococci
GAC	gastric adenocarcinoma
	glucose-alanine cycle
G-actin	globular actin
GAD	general adaptation syndrome
	general anxiety disorder
	glutamate decarboxylase
	glutamic acid decarboxylase
GAE	granulomatous amebic encephalitis
GAG	glycosaminoglycan (class of compounds of high molecular weight linear heteropolysaccharides)
Gal	galactose
gal	gallon
Gald-P	glyceraldehyde phosphate
GAL-1-PUT	
	galactose-1-phosphate uridyl transferase
GALT	galactose-1-phosphate uridyl transferase
	gut-associated lymphoid tissue

GAM	great adductor muscle
gang	ganglion
GAP	glycolic acid peel
	GTPase-activating protein
GAPD	glyceraldehyde-3-phosphate dehydrogenase
GAR	gonococcal antibody reaction
garg	gargle
garg.	*gargarisma* [Latin] gargle
GAS	Gainesville anesthesia stimulator
	general adaptation syndrome
	Global Assessment Scale
GASA	growth-adjusted sonographic age
gast fl	gastric fluid
Gastro	gastroenterology
gastroc	gastrocnemius (muscle)
GAU	geriatric assessment unit
GB	gallbladder
Gb	gallbladder
GBA	ganglionic blocking agent
GBBHS	group B beta-hemolytic streptococcus
GBC	glassblower's cataract
GBG	glycine-rich beta-glycoprotein
	gonadal steroid-binding globulin
GBH	gamma benzene hexachloride (the insecticide Lindane)
	graphite-benzalkonium-heparin
GBL	glucose-blood level
GBM	glioblastoma multiforme (anaplastic astrocytoma)
	glomerular basement membrane
GBMI	guilty but mentally ill
GBP	gastric bypass
GBS	gallbladder series
	gallbladder stones
	gas-bloat syndrome
	gastric bypass surgery
	group B streptococci

	Guillain-Barré syndrome (acute inflammatory disease of the peripheral nervous system)
GB series	gallbladder series
GBT	Gordon's biological test (test for Hodgkin's disease)
GBW	general body weakness
GC	ganglion cells
	gas chromatography
	genetic code (pattern of three adjacent nucleotides in a DNA molecule that controls protein synthesis)
	genetic counseling
	geriatric care
	Ghon complex
	glandular cancer (adenocarcinoma)
	glucocorticoid
	glycocalyx
	goblet cells
	Golgi complex (Golgi apparatus)
	gonococci
	gonorrheal cervicitis
	good condition
	guanine cytosine
	guanylate cyclase
	guanylyl cyclase
	guide catheter
G–C	gram-negative cocci
G+C	gram-positive cocci
GCA	germinal cell aplasia
	giant-cell arteritis
g-cal	gram calorie
GCC	germ cell cancer
	glassy cell carcinoma
GCCC	glassy cell carcinoma of cervix
G cells	gastrin cells
GCFs	geniculocortical fibers
GCGA	gamma carboxyl glutamic acid
GCHB	greater cornu of hyoid bone
GCI	gestational carbohydrate intolerance

GCIIS	glucose control insulin infusion system
GCL	gastrocolic ligament
GCLO-2	gastric campylobacter-like organism, type 2
GC/MS	gas chromatography/mass spectroscopy
GCP	giant cell pneumonia (Hecht's pneumonia) granulocytopenia (deficiency of granulocytes in the blood)
GCPs	Good Clinical Practices (regulations to protect humans who are volunteers in clinical research)
GCRCs	general clinical research centers
GCRG	giant cell reparative granuloma
GCS	gas chemical sterilization giant-cell sarcoma Glasgow Coma Scale glossitis + cheilosis + stomatitis gluteus compartment syndrome
G-CSF	granulocyte colony-stimulating factor
GCT	giant cell tumor
GCU	gonococcal urethritis
GCV	great cephalic vein granulosa cell tumor
GD	Gaucher's disease (glucosylceramide lipidosis; a rare enzyme deficiency disorder) gauze dressing genetic disorder gestational diabetes Gierke's disease Gilbert's disease gonadal dysgenesis (Turner's syndrome) Goodpasture's disease (anti-basement membrane antibody-mediated nephritis) Gorham disease (osteolysis) granular dystrophy Graves' disease (hyperthyroidism) growth deformity
G & D	growth and development
Gd	gadolinium (a rare element)
GDA	gastroduodenal artery germine diacetate
GDB	Genome Database guide dog for the blind
GDC	Guglielmi detachable coil (to treat inoperable intracranial aneurysms)
GDD	glucosephosphate dehydrogenase deficiency guide dog for the deaf
GdDTPA	gadolinium-diethylene-triamine-pentaacetic acid
GDF	gel diffusion precipitin Guidaut defibrillator (sends pacing signals to restore normal rhythm when heart beat is irregular)
GDH	glutamate dehydrogenase (enzyme)
GDID	genetically determined immunodeficiency disease
GDM	gestational diabetes mellitus
Gdn	guanidine (poisonous base)
GDO	gastroduodenostomy (surgical anastomosis between stomach and duodenum)
GDP	gel diffusion precipitin guanosine diphosphate
GDR	Gaucher Disease Registry
GDS	geriatric depression scale gradual dosage schedule
GE	gainfully employed gas embolism gastric emptying

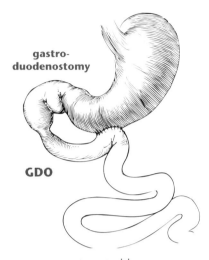

gastro-duodenostomy

GDO

	gastroenteritis
	gastroenterology
	gastrointestinal endoscopy
	gel electrophoresis
	gene expression
	genetic expression
	glycolytic enzyme
	golfer's elbow
G/E	granulocyte-erythroid ratio
Ge	germanium
GEAG	gastroepiploic artery graft
GEC	glomerular epithelial cell
GED	genetically engineered drug
GEF	gastroesophageal fundoplication
	glycosylation-enhancing factor
GEFs	glossoepiglottic folds
GEJ	gastro-esophageal junction
GELN	gastro-epiploic lymph node
GEN	gender
	general (anesthesia)
	generic
	genetics
	genital
gen	genus
genet	genetics
GENETOX	
	Genetic Toxicology (data bank)
genit	genitalia

gen'l	general
GENPS	genital neoplasm-papilloma syndrome
GENT	gentamicin (antibiotic)
GENTA/P	gentamicin-peak
GEP	gastroenteropancreatic
GEPH	gestational edema with proteinuria and hypertension
GEQ	generic equivalent
GER	gastroesophageal reflux (heartburn)
	gene expression regulation
	geriatrics
	granular endoplasmic reticulum (rough endoplasmic reticulum)
GERD	gastroesophageal reflux disorder
GEreflux	gastroesophageal reflux (scan)
Geront	gerontology
GES	glucose-electrolyte solution
GEST	gestation
GET	gastric emptying time
GETA	general endotracheal anesthesia
GeV	giga electron volt
GEX	gas exchange
GF	Galeazzi fracture
	gastric fistula
	gastric fluid
	germ free
	gingival fibromatosis
	glandular fever (mononucleosis)
	glenoid fossa (glenoid cavity)
	glomerular filtration
	gluten free
	Graafian follicle (ovarian follicle)
	greenstick fracture
	growth factor
	growth failure
GFAC	glucose-fatty acid cycle
GFAP	glial fibrillary acidic protein
GFB	gas-forming bacteria

GFCL giant follicular cell lymphoma

GFD Galeazzi fracture-dislocation

gluten-free diet

GFL germ-free life

giant follicular lymphoma

GFN ganglion of facial nerve

genitofemoral nerve

GFP gamma-fetoprotein

GFR glomerular filtration rate

growth factor receptors

GFS glaucoma filtering surgery

GG gamma globulin

gamma globulinemia

gas gangrene (often accompanies lacerated wounds and due to Clostridium bacteria)

gestational glaucoma

glycogenosis

GG-I glycogenosis, type I

GG-III glycogenosis, type III

GG-VIII glycogenosis, type VIII

GGA general gonadotropic activity

GGC glutamate-glutamine cycle

GGCS gamma-glutamyl cysteine synthetase

GGE general glandular enlargement

gradient gel electrophoresis

GGG glycine-rich gammaglycoprotein

GGM genioglossus muscle

glucose-galactose malabsorption

GGT gamma-glutamyl transferase

gestational glucose tolerance

GGTP gamma-glutamyl transpeptidase

GGU glucoglycinuria

GH general health

general hospital

genetic hypertension

genital herpes

gestational hypotension

gingival hyperplasia

globus hystericus (subjective sensation of a lump in the throat)

growth hormone

GHB gamma hydroxybutyrate

glycosylated hemoglobin

GHb glycosylated hemoglobin

GHBA gamma-hydroxybutyric acid

GHC Group Health Cooperative

GHD growth hormone deficiency

GHDs good health days

growth hormone deficiencies

GHHV gray heron hepatitis virus

GHIH growth hormone inhibiting hormone

GHJ glenohumeral joint

GHL glenohumeral ligament

GHM geniohyoid muscle

GHP gingival hyperplasia

GHQ general health questionnaire

GHR granulomatous hypersensitivity reaction

GH-RF growth hormone releasing factor

GH-RH growth hormone-releasing hormone (somatocrinin)

GH-RIF growth hormone-release-inhibiting factor

GH-RIH growth hormone-release-inhibiting hormone (somatostatin)

GHT geniculohypothalamic test

glycosylated hemoglobin test

GHz gigahertz

GI gas insufflation

gastrointestinal

gelatin infusion

genomic imprinting

gingival index

globulin insulin

glucose intolerance

gold inlay

granuloma inguinale
gym itch
GIA gastrointestinal
anastomosis
gastrointestinal anthrax
GIB gastrointestinal bleeding
GIBA gastrointestinal bleeding
from aspirin
GIBF gastrointestinal bacterial
flora
GIC gastrointestinal cancer
general
immunocompetence
GICA gastrointestinal cancer
GID gastrointestinal disease
gastrointestinal disorder
gender-identity disorder
GIE glomerular infective
endocarditis
gluten-induced
enteropathy
GIF gastrointestinal fistula
giant intestinal fluke
(*Fasciolopsis buski*)
glycosylation inhibition
factor
growth hormone-inhibiting
factor
GIFT gamete intrafallopian
(uterine tube) transfer
GIGO garbage in, garbage out
(computer science)
GIH gastrointestinal
hemorrhage
growth hormone release-
inhibiting hormone
(somatostatin)
growth inhibiting
hormone
GIK glucose, insulin, potassium
GIM gastrointestinal myiasis
GIN Golgi type I neuron
GIIN Golgi type II neuron
ging gingiva
GIO gastrointestinal obstruction
GIP gastric inhibitory peptide
gastric inhibitory
polypeptide

giant cell interstitial
pneumonia
GIR gastroileal reflux
gastrointestinal reflux
GIRI gastrointestinal reflux
infant
GIS gas in stomach
GI series gastrointestinal series
GIT gastrointestinal tract
gastrointestinal
tuberculosis
gonorrheal invasive
peritonitis
GITT glucose-insulin
tolerance test
GJ gastric juice
GJO gastrojejunostomy
(surgical anastomosis
between stomach and
jejunum)
GK galactokinase
glycerol kinase
GKD glycerol kinase deficiency
GKT gamekeeper's thumb
(skier's thumb)
GL gastric lavage
genomic library
germ line
gland
glycolipid
granulomatous lymphoma
(Hodgkin's disease)
Gl glucinium
gl. *glandula* [Latin] gland
g/l grams per liter
GLA galactosidase A
(lysosomal enzyme)
Giardia lamblia antigen
Gla carboxyglutamic acid
G.lamblia *Giardia lamblia*
(common parasite)
GLC gas-liquid chromatography
granulosa lutein cell
Glc glucose
glc glaucoma
GLC-MS gas-liquid chromatography
– mass spectrometry
Glc-1-P glucose-1-phosphate

Glc-6-P	glucose-6-phosphate		grand mal (major epilepsy)
GLD	granulomatous lung disease	**GM–**	gram-negative
		GM+	gram-positive
GLDH	glutamate dehydrogenase	**gm**	gram(s) (15 grains)
GLH	generalized lymphoid hyperplasia	**g-m**	gram-meter
		GMA	gas metal arc
	giant lymph node hyperplasia		glyceryl methacrylate
		GMC	granulomatous myocarditis
GLI	glucagon-like immunoreactivity	**GMCD**	grand mal convulsive disorder
GLIO	glioma	**GM-CFU**	granulocyte-macrophage colony forming unit
GLL	Gay-Lussac's law		
GLM	genetic linkage map	**GM-CSF**	granulocyte-macrophage colony-stimulating factor
Glm	glutamine		
GLN	gastric lymph node	**GMD**	glutamate dehydrogenase
Gln	glucagon		Gowers' muscular dystrophy
	glutamine		
GLNH	giant lymph node hyperplasia	**GME**	graduate medical education
glob	globulin	**GML**	gut mucosa lymphocyte
GLP	glycolipoprotein	**gm/l**	grams per liter
GLP-1	glucagon-like peptide-1 (regulates appetite)	**g/ml**	grams per milliliter
		GMM	gluteus maximus muscle
GLS	generalized lymphadenopathy syndrome	**g-mol**	gram-molecule
		GMP	glucose monophosphate
			guanosine monophosphate (guanylic acid)
	granulosa layer of skin		
GLTT	glucose-lactase tolerance test	**GMP140**	granule membrane protein -140
Glu	glucose (Glc is preferred)	**GMS**	Gomori methenamine silver (stain)
	glutamate (chief substance used by the brain to excite actvity between nerve cells)		grand mal seizure
		GMTC	geometric mean titer of controls
		GMW	gram-molecular weight
	glutamic acid	**GN**	gaze nystagmus
	glutamine		glomerulonephritis (inflammation of the renal glomeruli)
glu	glucose		
GluA	glucuronic acid		
glud	glutamate dehydrogenase		gouty nephropathy
Gly	glycine (principal amino acid present in sugar cane; the simplest of the amino acids)		gouty node (a concretion of sodium biurate generally occurring in the vicinity of joints in individuals with gout)
GLYC Hb	glycosylated hemoglobin		
GM	gastric mucosa		graduate nurse
	Geiger-Muller (counter)		gram-negative
	geriatric medicine	**G/N**	glucose-nitrogen ratio
	German measles (rubella)	**G1N**	Golgi type 1 neuron
	giant myxoma		

G2N	Golgi type 2 neuron
Gn	gonadotropin
GNB	ganglioneuroblastoma
	gram-negative bacilli
	gram-negative bacteria
GNBM	gram-negative bacillary
	meningitis
GNC	gram-negative cocci
	general nursing care
GNDC	gram-negative diplococci
GNI	gram-negative infection
GN & PH	
	glomerulonephritis and
	pulmonary hypertension
GNR	gram-negative rods
GNS	gram-negative sepsis
GnRF	gonadotropin-releasing
	factor
GnRH	gonadotropin-releasing
	hormone (luteinizing
	hormone-releasing
	hormone; LHRH)
Gn-RHa	gonadotropin-releasing
	hormone analog
GnSAF	gonadotropin surge
	attenuating factor
GO	glucose oxidase
Go	gonion
GOAT	Galveston orientation and
	amnesia test
GOD	glucose oxidase
GOG	Gynecologic Oncology
	Group
GOH	geroderma
	osteodysplastica
	hereditaria (Walt Disney
	dwarfism)
GOK	God only knows
GOM	gelatinous otolithic
	membrane
GON	gonococcal ophthalmia
	neonatorum (hyperacute
	purulent conjunctivitis
	occurring during the first
	ten days of life)
GOO	gastric outlet obstruction
	giant osteoid osteoma
	(osteoblastoma)
GOR	general operating room

GORD	gastroesophageal
	reflux disease
GOS	Glasgow Outcome Scale
GOT	glucose oxidase test
	glutamic-oxaloacetic
	transaminase (the
	enzyme aspartate
	aminotransferase)
	goal of treatment
GOTM	glutamic-oxaloacetic
	transaminase,
	mitochondrial
gov't	government
GP	gangliocytic paraganglioma
	gastric polyp
	general paralysis
	general paresis
	general physician
	general practitioner
	globus pallidus
	glucose phosphorylation
	glutathione peroxidase
	glycophorins
	glycopeptide
	glycoprotein
	gonorrheal prostatitis
	Goodpasture syndrome
	gram-positive
	growth plate
	gutta percha
G6P	glucose-6-phosphatase
gp	glycoprotein
GPA	gravida, para and abortus
	(each followed by a
	numeral indicating the
	number of pregnancies,
	deliveries and abortions)
G6Pase	glucose-6-phosphatase
GPB	gram-positive bacilli
	gram-positive bacteria
GPC	gastric parietal cell
	giant papillary
	conjunctivitis
	giant pyramidal cell
	(Betz cell)
	gram-positive cocci
G6PD	glucose-6-phosphate
	deficiencies
	glucose-6-phosphate

G6PDD dehydrogenase (common X-linked disorder)

G6PDD glucose-6-phosphate dehydrogenase deficiency (common X-linked disorder)

G6PDH glucose-6-phosphate dehydrogenase (reduced)

GPe external globus pallidus

GPF glomerular plasma flow
greater palatine foramen

GPG Gould polygraph (to measure gastric motility)

GPI gingival-periodontal index
glucose phosphate isomerase
growth plate injury

GPID glucose phosphate isomerase deficiency

GPIMH guinea pig intestinal mucosal homogenate

GPL gastrophrenic ligament

GPM giant pigmented melanosome
greater pectoral muscle

GPN glossopharyngeal nerve (9th cranial nerve)
glossopharyngeal neuralgia
graduate practical nurse

GPRVS giant prosthetic reinforcement of visceral sac

GPS Goodpasture's syndrome
gray platelet syndrome

GPSD glycoprotein storage disorder

GPT glutamic pyruvic transaminase (alanine aminotransferase)

GpTh group therapy

GPU glomerular proteinuria

GPUT galactose phosphate uridyl transferase

GPx glutathione peroxidase

GR gastric resection
genetic recombination
genu recurvatum
glucocorticoid receptor
glutathione reductase

grand rounds

gr grain (60 milligrams)

gr. *granum* [Latin] grain

GRA gonadotropin-releasing agent

grad gradient

grad. *gradatim* [Latin] gradually (by degrees)

GRAE generally regarded as effective

gram-neg
gram-negative

gram-pos
gram-positive

GRAS generally regarded as safe (food additive substances)

grav gravid

grav I gravid one (primigravida)

GRC Gerontology Research Center (of the National Institute on Aging)

GRD gastroesophageal reflux disorder

GRE gradient-recalled echo
Graduate Record Examination

GRF gastrin-releasing factor
gonadotropin releasing factor
growth hormone-releasing factor

GRFG gelatin-resorcin-formalin glue (tissue glue)

GRG glycine-rich glycoprotein

GRH growth hormone releasing hormone

GRIF growth hormone-inhibiting factor

GrN gram-negative

Grn glycerone (a ketone derived from glycerol)

GRP gastrin-releasing peptide

GrP gram-positive

Grp group

Grp Rx group therapy

GRT graduate respiratory therapist

GS gallstone

Gardner's syndrome
genetic screening
ghost surgery
Gilbert syndrome
glomerular sclerosis
glucagonoma syndrome
glutamine synthetase
glycogen synthesis
Goodpasture's syndrome
(combination of alveolar
hemorrhage and
glomerular hemorrhage)
gram stain
granulocytic sarcoma
Grebe syndrome
ground substance

Gs gauss
GSA Genetics Society
of America
Gerontological Society of
America
group-specific antigen
GSBG gonadal steroid-binding
globulin
GSC gas-solid chromatography
gamma scintillation
camera
GSD genetically significant dose
glycogen storage disease
(glycogenosis)
glycogen synthetase
deficiency
gunstock deformity
(cubitus varus)
GSD-I glycogen storage disease,
type I (von Gierke's
disease; most common
form of glycogenosis)
GSD-IV glycogen storage disease,
type IV (amylopectinosis)
GSD-VI glycogen storage disease,
type VI (Hers' disease)
GSE genital self-examination
Gianturco spring embolus
(placed within damaged
blood vessel to arrest
bleeding)
gluten-sensitive
enteropathy

GSF galactosemic fibroblast
greater sciatic foramen
greenstick fracture
gunshot fracture
GSH glutathione (a tripeptide
composed of glutamate,
cysteine and glycine)
growth-stimulating
hormone
GSH-Px glutathione peroxidase
GSHV ground squirrel
hepatitis virus
GSI gestational stress
incontinence
GSL gastrosplenic ligament
glycosphingo lipids
GSN greater sciatic notch

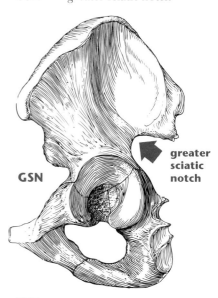

GSN

greater
sciatic
notch

GSR galvanic-skin response
glutathione reductase
GSS Gerstmann-Straussler-
Scheinker syndrome
(rare hereditary
spinocerebellar
degeneration)
GSSG-R glutathione reductase
GST genetic screening test
glucosesuppression test
gold sodium thiomalate
gravity stress test

G-suit	antigravity suit
GSW	gunshot wound
GSW-A	gunshot wound – abdominal
GT	gait training
	gamekeeper thumb
	gastric tonometry
	gastrostomy tube
	gene therapy
	genetic transduction
	gene transcription
	geographic tongue (erythema migraine)
	glucose tolerance
	glucose transport
	glutamyl transpeptidase
	glyceryl trinitrate (nitroglycerin)
	granulation tissue
	greater trochanter
	group therapy
	guaiac test
gt	great
gt.	*gutta* [Latin] a drop (0.05 ml)
GTA	gene transfer agent
GTB	gastrointestinal tract bleeding
GTC	gestational trophoblastic carcinoma
GTCS	generalized tonic-clonic seizure
GTD	gestational trophoblastic disease
GTF	glucose tolerance factor
GTG	glycerol tolerant gel
GTH	gonadotropic hormone
GTHR	generalized thyroid hormone resistance
GTI	Genetic Therapy, Inc.
	great toe implant (replacement of 1st metatarsophalangeal joint)
GTM	generalized tendomyopathy
GTN	gestational trophoblastic neoplasm
	glomerulotubulonephritis

GTO	Golgi tendon organ
GTP	glutamyl transpeptidase
	guanosine triphosphate (nucleotide)
GTP-CH	guanosine triphosphate cyclohydrolase
GTR	granulocyte turnover rate
GTS	Gilles de la Tourette syndrome
GTT	gestational trophoblastic tumor
	glucose tolerance test
gtt.	*guttae* [Latin] drops
GU	gastric ulcer
	giant urticaria (angioedema)
	genitourinary
	glucose uptake
	gonococcal urethritis (clap)
	gravitational ulcer
Gua	guanine (a fundamental constituent of DNA and RNA)
GUI	genitourinary infection
GUL	genital ulcer-lymphadenopathy
GUS	genitourinary system

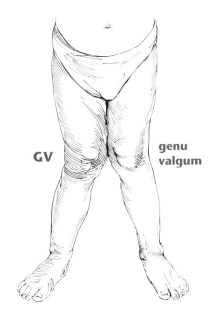

GV   **genu valgum**

GUT genitourinary tract
GV gentian violet
genu valgum (knock knee)
genu varum (bowleg)
germinal vesicle
gingivectomy
gonorrheal vaginitis
G. vaginalis
Gardnerella vaginalis
GVC gold-veneer crown
GVF good visual fields
GVG greater vestibular gland
(Bartholin's gland)
GVH graft-versus-host (disease or
reaction)
GVHD graft-versus-host disease
GVHR graft-versus-host reaction
GVS gastric vertical stapling
GVTY gingivectomy

GW genital warts
gradual withdrawal
gymnast's wrist
GWDS generalized work distress
scale
GWE glycerol and water enema
GWS Gigli wire saw
Gram-Weigert stain
Gulf war syndrome
GWT Gardner-Wells tongs (skull
tongs; used to exert
traction on the skull)
GXD graded
GXT graded exercise test
Gy gray (unit in radiation
therapy)
GYN gynecology
GZTS Guilford-Zimmerman
temperament survey

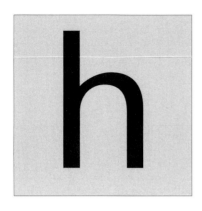

H hair
hallucis (big toe)
handage (bandage glove)
H-band
H-disk
head
heart
heavy
height
hemisphere
hemolysis
hemorrhoids
henry
heparin
hernia
heroin
high
histidine
histoplasmosis
hives (urticaria)
horizontal
hormone
hospice
hospital
hot
hour
Humalog
human
humerus
Humulin
hydrogen
hydrolysis
hygiene
hyperopia

hyperphoria
hypertension
hypodermic
H-zone

H+ hydrogen-ion
concentration

¹H protium (hydrogen-1)

²H deuterium (heavy
hydrogen; hydrogen-2)

H2 histamine

³H tritium (hydrogen-3)

h heat transfer coefficient
hecto- (prefix denoting
decimal factor 10^2)
height
horizontal
hour
hundred
secondary constriction

h Planck constant

HA halothane anesthesia
(potent inhalational
anesthetic)
headache
hearing aid
hemadsorbent
hemagglutinating antibody
hemolytic anemia
hepatic agenesis
hepatic cyst
hepatitis A
hepatitis-associated
high anxiety
hippuric acid
histamine
histocompatibility antigen
hospital admission
human albumin
hyaluronic acid
hydroxyapatite
hyperactivity
hypersensitivity alveolitis
hypothalmic amenorrhea

H/A headache

Ha hahnium (a transuranic
element)

HAA hearing aid amplifier
hemolytic anemia antigen
hepatitis-associated antigen

	hepatitis-associated aplasia
HAAb	hepatitia A antibody
HAAg	hepatitis A antigen
HABA	hydroxybenzeneazo-benzoic acid
HABF	hepatic artery blood flow
HAC	hanging arm cast
	hyperactive child
	hyperadrenocorticism
HACE	high-altitude cerebral edema
HACEK group	
	Haemophilus influenzae, H. aphrophilis, H. paraphrophilis, H. influenzae, Actinobacillus actinomycetemcomitans, Cardiobacterium hominis and Kingella group (fastidious organisms)
HACS	hyperactive child syndrome
HAD	hemadsorption
	heterologous antibody disease
hADA	human adenosine deaminase
HADD	hydroxyapatite deposition disease
HAE	hearing aid evaluation
	hepatic artery embolism
	hereditary angioedema
	hereditary angioneurotic edema
HaF	Hageman factor
HAFOE	high air flow oxygen enrichment
hAFP	human alpha-fetoprotein
HAG	heat-aggregated globulin
HAGG	hyperimmune antivariola gamma globulin
HAGH	hydroxyacyl-glutathione hydrolase
HAI	hemagglutination inhibition
	hospital-acquired infection
HAL	hyperalimentation
	hypoplastic acute leukemia
HALO	halothane
	halogen(nonmetallic

	elements of group 7, i.e. bromine, chlorine, fluorine, iodine and the radioactive element astatine)
halluc	hallucinations
HALP	hyperalphalipo-proteinemia
HAM	home apnea monitoring
	hospital-acquired meningitis
	HTLV-1-associated myelopathy
	HTLV-1-associated myopathy
	hypoparathyroidism, Addison's disease, and mucocutaneous candidiasis (syndrome)
hAM	human alveolar macrophage
HAM-A	Hamilton Anxiety (scale)
hAMA	human anti-murine antibodies
HAM-D	Hamilton Depression (scale)
HAN	heroin-associated nephropathy
	hyperplastic alveolar nodule
HANE	hereditary angioneurotic edema
HAO	hip osteoarthritis
HAP	heredopathia atactica polyneuritiformis
	histamine phosphate acid
	hospital-acquired pneumonia
	hydroxyapatite (a mineral compound found in the matrix of bones and teeth)
HAPC	hospital-acquired penetration contact
HAPD	home-automated peritoneal dialysis
HAPE	high-altitude pulmonary edema
HAPS	hepatic arterial perfusion

scintigraphy
HAQ Headache Assessment
Questionnaire
Health Assessment
Questionnaire
HAR high-altitude retinopathy
HARH high-altitude retinal
hemorrhage
HARI hospital-acquired
respiratory infection
HARM heparin assay rapid
method
hypertension, anemia,
renal, malabsorption
HAS hepatic angiosarcoma
high altitude syncope
high Apgar score
highest asymptomatic
(dosage)
Holmes–Adie syndrome
hyperalimentation solution
hypertensive
arteriosclerosis
HASCVD hypertensive
arteriosclerotic
cardiovascular disease
HASHD hypertensive
arteriosclerotic
heart disease
HAT heparin-associated
thrombocytopenia
hospital arrival time
hypoxanthine,
aminopterin
and thymidine
HATT heparin-associated
thrombocytopenia and
thrombosis
HATTS hemagglutination
treponemal test for
syphilis
haust. *haustus* [Latin] a drink
HAV hemi-azygos vein
hepatitis A virus
HB bundle of His
heart block
heartburn
(gastroesophageal reflux)
hemoglobin

hepatitis B
His bundle
hold breakfast
hospital bed
housebound
hunchback (kyphosis)
hyoid bone

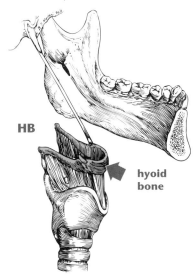

HB

hyoid
bone

1° HB first-degree heart block
2° HB second-degree heart block
3° HB third-degree heart block
Hb deoxygenated hemoglobin
hemoglobin
HbA adult hemoglobin
hemoglobin A
Hb A$_{1c}$ glycosylated hemoglobin
(an integrated measure
of fasting and postmeal
blood glucose levels
during the previous 2-to
3-month period)
HBAb hepatitis B antibody
HBAg hepatitis B antigen
HbAS heterozygosity for
hemoglobin A and
hemoglobin S
HBB hospital blood bank
hydroxybenzyl
benzimidazole
HbBC hemoglobin binding
capacity

HBC	high blood cholesterol
HbC	hemoglobin C
HBc	hepatitis B core
HBcAb	antibody to hepatitis B core antigen
HBcAg	hepatitis B core antigen
HbCO	carbon monoxide hemoglobin carboxyhemoglobin
HbCV	*Haemophilus b* conjugate vaccine
HBD	has been drinking hydroxybutyrate dehydrogenase (an enzyme of the oxido-reductase class)
HbD	hemoglobin D
HBDH	hydroxybutyrate dehydrogenase
HBE	His bundle electrogram
HBe	hepatitis B e
HbE	hemoglobin E
HBeAb	antibody to hepatitis B e antigen
HBeAg	hepatitis B e antigen
HBF	hepatic blood flow hypothalamic blood flow
HbF	fetal hemoglobin hemoglobin F
HBGM	home blood glucose monitoring
HbH	hemoglobin H
Hb/Hct	hemoglobin/hematocrit
HBI	high serum-bound iron
HBIG	hepatitis B immune globulin
HBL	hepatoblastoma
HBLA	human B-cell lymphocyte antigen
HBLV	human B-lymphotropic virus
HbMet	methemoglobin
HBMT	haploidentical bone marrow transplantation
HBO	hyperbaric oxygen (therapy)
HbO$_2$	oxyhemoglobin
HBOC	hereditary breast-ovarian cancer

HBOT	hyperbaric oxygen therapy
HBP	handlebar palsy hepatic binding protein high blood pressure *Helicobacter pylori*
HBPIC	High Blood Pressure Information Center (301) 496-1809
HBPM	home blood pressure monitoring
HbPV	*Haemophilus influenzae b* polysaccharide vaccine
HBS	hyperkinetic behavior syndrome
HbS	hemoglobin S (sickle cell hemoglobin)
HBs	hepatitis B surface
HBsAb	antibody to the hepatitis B surface antigen
HBsAg	hepatitis B surface antigen
HBSAII	hepatitis B surface antibody-immune indicator
HBSC	hematopoietic blood stem cell
HbSC	sickle cell hemoglobin C
HbSS	hemoglobin SS sickle cell anemia
HBT	homologous blood transfusion human breast tumor hydrogen breath test
HBV	hepatitis B vaccine hepatitis B virus
HBW	high birth weight
HbZ	hemoglobin Z
HC	hair cell hairy cell handicapped hanging cast hard cancer (scirrhous carcinoma) hardcopy head circumference (fetal) head compression Heart Card heart catheterization heart cycle heavy chain

hemoglobin concentration
heparin cofactor
hepatic candidiasis
hepatic catalase
hepatic coma
hepatocellular
hereditary coproporphyria
histamine challenge
hot compress
house call
Huntington's chorea
hyaline cast
hydatid cyst
hydrocarbon
hydrocephalus
hydrocortisone
hydroxycorticoid
hypercalcemia
hypercalciuria
hysterical convulsions

H & C hepatitis and cirrhosis
hot and cold
hypoventilation and
  cyanosis

Hc hydrocolloid

HCA health care aide
hepatocellular adenomas
home care aide
hydrocortisone acetate

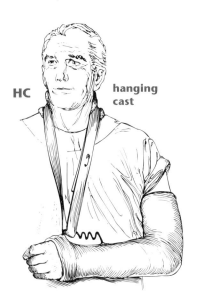

HC   **hanging cast**

hyperchloremic acidosis
hypoplastic congenital
  anemia

HCAP handicapped

H-CAP hexamethylmelamine
  (altretamine) +
  cyclophosphamide +
  Adriamycin
  (doxorubicin) + Platinol
  (cisplatin) (combination
  chemotherapy)

H. capsulatum
Histoplasma capsulatum
(fungus)

H.capsulatum

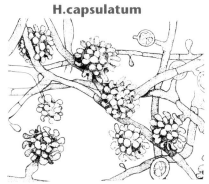

Histoplasma capsulatum

HCB hexachlorobenzene

HCBS hot cross bun skull
  (rickets)

HCC hepatocellular carcinoma
Hurthle cell cancer
husband-coached
  childbirth
25-hydroxycholecalciferol
  (active metabolite of
  vitamin D_3)

25HCC 25-hydroxycholecalciferol
  (active metabolite of
  vitamin D_3)

HCCH hexachlorocyclohexane
  (Lidane)

HCD heavy chain deposition
heavy chain disease
herniated cervical disk
high-calorie diet
high-carbohydrate diet

HCDJ	hyperostosis corticalis deformans juvenilis (juvenile Paget disease)		health care proxy (health care power of attorney)
HCF	hereditary capillary fragility		hepatocatalase peroxidase
			hereditary coproporphyria
HCFA	Health Care Financing Administration		histiocyte cytophagic panniculitis
HCFC	hydrochlorofluorocarbon		hypochondroplasia
hCFSH	human chorionic follicle-stimulating hormone	**HCPA**	health-care power of attorney
		HCR	host cell reactivation
HCG	human chorionic gonadotropin	**HCRF**	hypercarbic respiratory failure
hCG	human chorionic gonadotropin	**hCRH**	human corticotropin-releasing hormone
	hyperostosis corticalis generalisata (van Buchem's disease)	**HCS**	human chorionic somatomammotropin
			human (umbilical) cord serum
HCGR	heavy chain gene rearrangement	**17HCS**	17-hydroxycorticosteroids
HCH	hexachlorocyclohexane (benzene hexachloride)	**hCS**	human chorionic somatomammotropin
HCHO	formaldehyde	**hCSM**	human chorionic somatomammotropin
HCHP	Harvard Community Health Plan	**HCSS**	hypersensitive carotid sinus syndrome
HCHS	hydrocortisone hemisuccinate	**HCT**	heat coagulation test
HCIN	hydrocarbon-induced neoplasm		homocytotrophic
			hematopoietic cell transplantation
HCL	hairy-cell leukemia		human chorionic thyrotropin
	hard contact lens		hydrochlorothiazide (a thiazide diuretic)
	hilar cell tumor		hydrocortisone
HCLF	high carbohydrate, low fiber (diet)	**Hct**	hematocrit
HCl	hydrochloric acid	**hCT**	human calcitonin
HCM	health care maintenance		human chorionic thyrotropin
	hostile cervical mucus	**HCTU**	home cervical traction unit
	hypertrophic cardiomyopathy	**HCTZ**	hydrochlorothiazide (a thiazide diuretic)
HCMM	hereditary cutaneous malignant melanoma	**HCU**	homocystinuria
hCMV	human cytomegalovirus	**HCU-I**	homocystinuria, type I
HCN	hereditary chronic nephritis	**HCU-II**	homocystinuria, type II
	hydrogen cyanide	**HCV**	hepatitis C virus (non-A, non-B hepatitis)
	hypercalcemic nephropathy	**hCV**	human coronavirus
HCO$_3^-$	bicarbonate radical	**HCVD**	hypertensive cardiovascular disease
HCP	handicapped		
	health care provider		

HCW health care worker

Hcy homocysteine

HD Haglund deformity

Hank's dilator

Hansen's disease (leprosy)

Hartnup disease

head

hearing distance

heart disease

heloma durum
(a hard corn)

hematologic disorder

hemodialysis

hemolytic disease

hepatic disease

herniated (intervertebral)
disk

high dose

hip disarticulation

hip dislocation

Hirschsprung's disease
(congenital megacolon)

Hodgkin's disease (a form
of malignant lymphoma)

hormone-dependent

hospital day

house dust

Huntington's disease
(Huntington's chorea;
degenerative chorea)

Hurler's disease (dysotosis
multiplex)

hydroxydopamine

h.d. *heloma durum* [Latin]
hard corn
hora decubitus [Latin]
at bedtime

HD ARA C

high-dose ARA C
(cytarabine)

HDC hemoglobin dissociation
curve

high-dose chemotherapy

histidine decarboxylase

human diploid cell vaccine
(produced from rabies
virus grown in cultures of
human diploid embryo
lung cells)

hyperdistention of colon

HD CPA high-dose
cyclophosphamide

HDCV human diploid cell vaccine

HDD high-dopa dyskinesias

HDF Hereditary Disease
Foundation
(213) 458-4183
human diploid fibroblast

HDG Huntington disease gene

HDH heart disease history

HDI hemorrhagic disease of
infants
high definition imaging

HDL hepatoduodenal ligament
high-density
lipoprotein (densities of
1.063–1.21 g/ml)

HDL-C high-density lipoprotein
cholesterol

HDM host defense mechanism

HDMs house dust mites

HD MTX high-dose methotrexate
(chemotherapy)

HDN hemolytic disease of the
newborn
high-density nebulizer

hDNA hybrid deoxyribonucleic
acid (DNA)

HDP hydroxydimethylpyrimidine

HDPAA heparin-dependent
platelet-associated
antibody

HDPE high-density polyethylene

HDRA histoculture drug response
assay (detects certain
cancers)

HDRS Hamilton Depression
Rating Scale

HDRV human diploid cell rabies
vaccine

HDS health delivery system
herniated disk syndrome

HDT half disappearance time

HDU hemodialysis unit

H.ducreyi *Hemophilus ducreyi* (the
cause of soft chancres on
the genitals)
hepatic encephalopathy

HDV	hepatitis D (Delta) virus
HDZ	hydralazine (antihypertensive)
HE	hard exudates
	heat exhaustion
	hemoglobin electrophoresis
	hepatic encephalopathy
	hereditary elliptocytosis
	heterologous
H & E	hematoxylin and eosin (stain)
	heredity and environment
He	helium (an inert gaseous element present in small amounts in the atmosphere)
hEA	human erythrocyte antigen
hEAT	human erythrocyte agglutination test
HEC	human endothelial cell
	hydroxyergocalciferol
hEC	human epithelial cell
HED	*haut-einheits dosis* [German] unit of roentgen-ray dosage
	hereditary ectodermal dysplasia
HEDTA	hydroxyethylene-diamine-triacetic acid
HEENT	head, eyes, ears, nose and throat
HEEP	health effects of environmental pollutants
HEF	Hoffman external fixation (external skeletal fixation)
HEIR	high-energy ionizing radiation
HEL	hen egg-white lysozyme
	hyoepiglottic ligament
HeLa	Helen Lake (name of patient from whom cervical carcinoma cells were isolated in 1951)
HELLP	hemolysis, elevated liver enzymes, low platelets (syndrome)
hem	hemorrhage

	hemorrhoid
HEMAT	hematology
HEMB	hemophilia B
HEMI	hemiplegia (hemiparalysis)
	hemisphere
HeNe laser	
	helium neon laser
HEP	heparin (has the ability to keep blood from clotting and is used chiefly in the prevention and treatment of thrombosis)
	hepatoerythropoietic porphyria
hep	heparin (has the ability to keep blood from clotting and is used chiefly in the prevention and treatment of thrombosis)
	hepatitis
HEPA	hamster egg penetration assay
	high-efficiency particulate air (filter)
Hered	hereditary
hern	hernia
HES	hydroxyethyl starch
	hypereosinophilic syndrome
	hyperprostaglandin E syndrome
het	heterozygous
HETE	hydroxyarachidonic acid
	hydroxyeicosatetraenoic acid
HETP	hexaethyltetraphosphate
HEV	hepatitis E virus
	hepato-encphalomyelitis virus
	high (walled) endo-thelial venule
	human enteric virus
HEX	hexosaminidase (enzyme that cleaves N-acetyl hexosamine residues from glycosphingolipids)
HEX A	hexosaminidase A
Hexa	hexamethylmelamine (chemotherapy)

Hexa CAF
hexamethylmelamine + cyclophosphamide + methotrexate + 5-fluorouracil (combination chemotherapy)

HEX B hexosaminidase B

HEX C hexosaminidase C

HF Hageman factor (coagulation factor)
hair follicle
hangman's fracture (bilateral pedicle fracture of the 2nd cervical vertebra)
hay fever
head of fetus
heart failure
hemofiltration
hemorrhagic fever
hepatic fibrosis
high frequency
hip fracture
Hohl fracture
hot flashes
hyperflexion

Hf hafnium

hf high frequency

hFBT human fetal brain tissue

HFC hydrofluorocarbon

HFD high fiber diet
high forceps delivery (of fetus)

FH hemifacial hyperplasia

HFHL high-frequency hearing loss

HFI hereditary fructose intolerance
hyperostosis frontalis interna (abnormality of frontal bone's inner table)

HFIF human fibroblast interferon

HFJV high-frequency jet ventilation

HF laser hydrogen fluoride laser

Hflu *Haemophilus influenzae* (the biotype I of the species is the major cause of bacterial meningitis; biotype II and III are normal inhabitants of the nasopharynx)

HFM hemifacial microsomia

HFMD hand-foot-and-mouth disease

HFMS hand-foot-mouth syndrome

HFOV high frequency oscillatory ventilation

HFP hexafluoropropylene
hypofibrinogenic plasma

HFPPV high-frequency positive pressure ventilation

Hfr high frequency

HFRS hemorrhagic fever with renal stones
hemorrhagic fever with renal syndrome

HFS hemifacial spasm

hFSH human follicle-stimulating hormone

HFT halo-femoral traction

HFU hand-foot-uterus (syndrome)
hyperflexion of uterus

HFV high frequency ventilation
human foamy virus

HG herpes genitalis
herpes gestationis
high glucose
human genome (the total genetic endowment)
human gonadotropin
hyperglycemia

Hg hemoglobin
mercury

hG human gonadotropin

HGA homogentisic acid

Hgb hemoglobin

Hgb F fetal hemoglobin

Hgb S sickle cell hemoglobin

HGC hyperglycemic coma

HGD hypersensitivity glomerular disease
hysterical gait disorder

HGDs hallucinogenic drugs

HGE	human granulocytic ehrlichiosis
hGE	human gene encoding
HGF	hepatocyte growth factor hyperglycemic-glycogenolytic factor (glucagon)
hGG	human gamma globulin hypogammaglobulinemia
hGH	human (pituitary) growth hormone
hGHr	human (pituitary) growth hormone recombinant
HGL	hemoglobin gene loci hepatogastric ligament
HGM	human gene mapping human glucose monitoring hyoglossus muscle
HGMs	human genome maps
HGN	hypoglossal nerve (12th cranial nerve)
HGO	hepatic glucose output
HGP	Human Genome Project
HGPRT	hypoxanthine-guanine phosphoribosyltransferase
HGPS	hereditary giant platelet syndrome
hGRH	human growth hormone-releasing hormone
HGS	hourglass stomach Hutchinson-Gilford syndrome hypergalactosemia hypoglycemic shock
HGSIL	high-grade squamous intraepithelial lesion
HGT	hypergonadotropinism
hgt	height
HGU	hemoglobinuria hypoglycemia unawareness (loss of warning signals that herald the onset of an episode of low blood sugar)
HH	hard of hearing hepatic hydatidosis hiatal hernia (upward protrusion of the stomach through the

esophageal opening of the diaphragm)

HH

hiatal hernia

hyperhidrosis (excessive perspiration)
hyperhydration (overhydration)
hypogonadotropic hypogonadism

H & H	hemoglobin and hematocrit
HHA	hereditary hemolytic anemia home health aid
HHAB	hip-hinge abduction brace
HHb	deoxyhemoglobin hypohemoglobinemia
HHC	hepatic hydatid cyst home health care
HHCS	high altitude hypertrophic cardiomyopathy syndrome
HHD	hatchet-head deformity hemoglobin H disease hepatic-hypoglycemic disease home hemodialysis hydraulic hand dynamometer (records hand strength) hypertensive heart disease
HHE	health hazard evaluation
HHFM	high-humidity face mask

HHG	hypertrophic hypersecretory gastropathy
HHHO	hypotonia, hypomentia, hypogonadism, and obesity (syndrome)
HHK	hypertensive hyperkalemia
HHL	*Harvard Health Letter*
HHMI	Howard Hughes Medical Institute
HHN	hand-held nebulizer
HHNC	hyperglycemic, hyperosmotic, nonketotic coma
HHNK	hyperglycemic, hyperosmotic, nonketotic (coma)
HHNS	hyperglycemic, hyperosmotic, nonketotic syndrome
HHS	hereditary hemolytic syndrome
	Home Health Services
	hypertelorism-hypospadias syndrome
	US Departmnt of Health and Human Services
HHT	head halter traction
	hereditary hemorrhagic telangiectasia (Osler-Rendu-Weber disease)
	hydroxyheptadecatrienoic acid
	hypothalamo-hypophyseal tract
hHV	human herpes virus
hHV-1	human herpes virus – 1
hHV-2	human herpes virus – 2
hHV-3	human herpes virus – 3 (varicella-zoster virus)
hHV-4	human herpes virus – 4 (Epstein-Barr virus)
hHV-5	human herpes virus – 5 (cytomegalovirus)
hHV-6	human herpes virus – 6
hHV-7	human herpes virus – 7
HI	head injury
	health insurance
	hearing impaired
	hemagglutination inhibition
	hormone insensitivity
	hydroxyindole
	hypothermic ischemia
H	high
	histamine
	histidinemethemoglobin
HIA	hemagglutination inhibition antibody
	hemagglutination inhibition assay
HIAA	Health Insurance Association of America
5-HIAA	5-hydroxyindole acetic acid
hIAP	human intracisternal A-type particle
Hib	*Haemophilus influenzae* type b
HIC	health insurance claim (number)
	hydrogen ion concentration
HICH	hypertensive intracranial hemorrhage
HID	headache, insomnia, and depression (syndrome)
	herniated intervertebral disk
	hyperkinetic impulse disorder
HIDA	hepato-iminodiacetic acid (lidofenin nuclear scan)
HIE	Health Insurance Experiment (RAND)
	human intestinal epithelium
	hypoxic ischemic encephalopathy
hIF	human interferon
hIG	human immunoglobulin
HIH	Health Information Hotline (215) 592-0550
	hypertensive intracranial hemorrhage
HIHA	high impulsiveness, high anxiety
HIL	hypoxic-ischemic lesion
HILA	high impulsiveness,

low anxiety

HIM hepatitis-infectious
mononucleosis

H. influenzae
Haemophilus influenzae

HIO hypoiodidism (deficiency
of iodide)

HIOMT hydroxyindole-o-methyl
transferase

HIP Health Insurance Plan
homograft incus prosthesis

HIPA heparin-induced platelet
activation

HIR head injury routine

HIS histidine
home incapacity scale
hyperimmune serum

His histidine

HISL heparin-induced skin
lesion

Hist histamine

HISTLINE
history of medicine online

histo histology
histoplasmin (skin test)
histoplasmosis

HIT hemagglutination
inhibition test
heparin-induced
thrombocytopenia
histamine inhalation test
home infusion therapy
home intravenous therapy
hypertrophic infiltrative
tendinitis

HiTB *Haemophilus influenzae*
type B

HIU head injury unit
hyperplasia interstitialis
uteri

HIV human immune deficiency
virus
human immunodeficiency
virus

HIV-1 human immunodeficiency
virus type 1

HIV-2 human immunodeficiency
virus type 2

HIV Ag human immunodeficiency
virus antigen

HIVAN human immunodeficiency
virus–associated
nephropathy

HIVAT home intravenous
antibiotic therapy

HIVD herniated
intervertebral disk

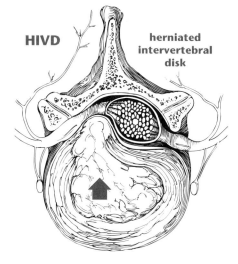

HIVD herniated
intervertebral
disk

HIVE HIV-1 encephalopathy

HIVFs hypertonic intravenous
feedings

HIV-group M
human immunodeficiency
virus, group M (strain of
virus responsible for the
worldwide AIDS
pandemic)

HIV-group O
human immunodeficiency
virus, group O (rare
strain of the HIV virus
characterized by genetic
divergence from group M
strains)

HIVIG HIV immmunoglobulin

HIV-P human immunodeficiency
virus infection with
periodontitis

HJB Howell-Jolly bodies
(remnants of nuclear
chromatin)

HJC	Henderson-Jones chondromatosis
HJR	hepatojugular reflux
HK	heat killed
	hexokinase (enzyme of the transferase class)
	hyperkeratosis
	hypokalemia
HKA	hypokalemic alkalosis
HKAFO	hip-knee-ankle-foot orthosis
HKAO	hip-knee-ankle orthosis
HKC	hypokalemic crisis
HKI	Hong Kong influenza
HKLM	heat-killed Listeria monocytogenes
HKN	hypokalemic nephropathy
HKO	hip-knee orthosis
HKRP	hinged knee replacement prosthesis
HKS	heel, knee, and shin (test)
	Heim-Kreysig sign
	hyperkinesis syndrome
HKT	heterotopic (not the normal place) kidney transplant
HL	hair line
	hairy leukemia
	hairy leukoplakia
	half-life
	hare lip (cleft lip)
	hearing level
	hearing loss
	hemilaryngectomy
	herpes labialis
	histiocytic lymphoma
	Hodgkin's lymphoma
	hyperlipidemia
	hyperlipemia
	latent hyperopia
H & L	heart and lung (bypass machine)
hl	hearing loss
	hectoliter
HLA	histocompatibility leukocyte antigen
	histocompatibility locus antigens
	homologous leukocyte antibody
	human leukocyte antigen
	human lymphocyte antigen
	human leukocyte group A antigen
HLAA	human leukocyte antigen A
HLAB	human leukocyte antigen B
HLAC	human leukocyte antigen C
HLAD	human leukocyte antigen D
HLA-SD	human lymphocyte antigen – serologically defined
HLBI	human lymphoblastoid interferon
HLD	hepatolenticular degeneration
	herniated lumbar disk
	Hippel-Lindau disease
HL/D	hemilaminectomy/discectomy
HLE	heat-labile enterotoxin
HLF	heat-labile factor
HLH	hemophagocytic lymphohistiocytosis
hLH	human luteinizing hormone
HLHS	hypoplastic left heart syndrome
HLI	human leukocyte interferon
HLK	heart, liver, kidneys
HLM	heart-lung machine
HLN	hepatic lymph node
	hilar lymph node
	hypogastric lymph node
HLP	Hunt-Lawren pouch
	hyperlipoproteinemia
HLR	heart-lung resuscitation
HLS	Hippel-Lindau syndrome
HLT	heart-lung transplantation
hLT	human lymphocyte transformation
hlth	health
HLV	herpes-like virus
HM	hand movements
	heart murmur (resulting

from turbulent
blood flow)
Heimlich maneuver
heloma molle (a soft corn)
hemifacial microsomia
Hispanic male
holosystolic murmur
humidity mask
human milk
hydatidiform mole
hypomagnesmia

Hm manifest hyperopia

HMB homatropine
methylbromide
(antispasmodic and
inhibitor of secretions)
hydroxymethylbilane

HMBA hexamethyl-bisacetamide

HMC heroin + morphine +
cocaine (mixture)
honeymoon cystitis
human mammary
carcinoma

HMD hyaline membrane disease
(idiopathic respiratory
distress of the newborn)

HME heat + massage + exercise
homatropine
methylbromide elixir
human monocytic
ehrlichiosis (tick borne
infectious disease)

HMF hydroxymethylfurfural

HMG high mobility group
hydroxy-methylglutaric
(acid)

hMG human menopausal
gonadotropin (used to
induce ovulation in the
treatment of female
infertility)

HMG-CoA hydroxy-methylglutaryl -
coenzyme A

HMI healed myocardial
infarction

HMIN hazardous materials
identification number
(e.g., trifluorochloro-
ethylene, No. 1082;

shellac, No. 1263;
mercury salicylate,
No. 1644; tetraethyl lead,
No. 1649; benzene,
No. 2971)

HMK housemaid's knee

hML human milk lysozyme

HMM hexamethylmelamine
(altretamine,
chemotherapy)

HMO Health Maintenance
Organization

HMP health maintenance
program
heavy metal poisoning
Heineke-Mikulicz
pyloroplasty
hexose monophosphate
pentose (shunt)
hexose monophosphate
pathway
hot moist packs

HMPA hexamethyl-
phosphoramide

HMR histocytic medullary
reticulosis (fatal
hereditary disorder)

H-mRNA H-chain messenger RNA
(ribonucleic acid)

HMS hexose monophosphate
shunt
horizontal mattress suture
hypermobility syndrome

HMSAS hypertrophic muscular
subaortic stenosis

hMSCs human mesenchymal
stem cells

HMSN hereditary motor and
sensory neuropathy

HMW high molecular weight

HMWC high molecular weight
component

HMWGP high molecular weight
glycoprotein

HMW-K high molecular weight
kininogen

HMX heat, massage and exercise

HN Haygarth's node
head nurse

Heberden's node (bony osteoarthritic enlargement at distal interphalangeal joint of hand)
Hensen's node
hereditary nephritis
hilar node
hydronephrosis
hypertrophic neuropathy

H & N head and neck

HNA heparin neutralizing activity

HNAD hyperosmolar nonacidotic diabetes

H. nana *Hymenolepis nana* (dwarf tapeworm)

HNB human neuroblastoma

HNI hospitalization not indicated

HNKC hyperosmolar nonketotic coma

HNL histiocytic necrotizing lymphadenitis

HNM high neonatal mortality

HNP herniated nucleus pulposus (protrusion of intervertebral disk)
human neurophysin

HNPCC hereditary non-polyposis colon cancer
hereditary non-polyposis colorectal cancer

HNPP hereditary neuropathy with liability to pressure palsies

HnRNA heterogeneous, nuclear RNA (ribonucleic acid)

hnRNA heterogeneous, nuclear RNA (ribonucleic acid)
heteronuclear RNA (ribonucleic acid)

hnRNP heterogeneous nuclear ribonucleoprotein

HNS hypernasal speech

HNSHA hereditary nonsperocytic hemolytic anemia

HNV has not voided

HO hand orthosis

high oxygen
hip orthosis
Hippocratic oath
homologous (corresponding in structure, position, development and evolutionary origin)
hyperbaric oxygen
hyperostosis

H$_2$O water

H$_2$O$_2$ hydrogen peroxide

Ho holmium (a rare-earth element)

HOA high oxygen affinity
hypertrophic osteoarthropathy

HOB head of bed

HOC human ovarian cancer
hyperosmolar coma
hydroxycorticoid

HOCM high osmolality contrast media
hypertrophic obstructive cardiomyopathy

HOE head of epididymis

HOF high output failure

HOH hard of hearing
high oxygen pressure

HOI hospital onset of infection

HOK hilum of kidney

HOM hematogenous osteomyelitis
high osmolality contrast media
high osmolar media

HOP doxorubicin (hydroxydaunomycin) + Oncovin (vincristine) + prednisone (combination chemotherapy)
high oxygen pressure

HOPA hospital-based organ procurement agency

HOPI history of present illness

hor horizontal

hor.decub.
hora decubitas [Latin] at bedtime

HORF high output renal failure

hor. som. *hora somni* [Latin] at bedtime

HOS Holt-Oram syndrome (cardiomelic syndrome)

HOSP hospital

HOT hyperbaric oxygen therapy

Hot hypotropia (a constant downward deviation of one eye not controlled by fixational efforts)

HOTS hypercalcemia-osteolysis T-cell syndrome

Ho:YAG holmium: yttrium-aluminum-garnet

HP handicapped person
hard palate
Harvard pump
Helicobacter pylori (a species causing active chronic type B gastritis; found in more than 90% of patients with duodenal ulcers and believed to play a central role in development of this condition)
hemiparkinsonism
hemiplegia
high potency
high protein
hip prosthesis
horizontal plane
Histoplasma capsulatum polysaccharide antigen
hot pack
house physician
human pituitary
humeroscapular periarthritis
hydrogen peroxide
hyperperistalsis
hyperplasia
hypersensitivity pneumonitis (extrinsic allergic alveolitis)
hypopharynx

H & P history and physical (examination)

Hp haptoglobin
Helicobacter pylori (a species causing active chronic type B gastritis; found in more than 90% of patients with duodenal ulcers and believed to play a central role in development of this condition)

hp horse power

HPA human papillomavirus
hypothalamic-pituitary-adrenal (axis)
hypothalamic-pituitary axis

HPA-23 heteropolyanion-23

HPAA hydroxyphenylacetic acid
hypothalamus-pituitary (hypophysis)-adrenal axis

Hpb haptoglobin

HPCC High-Performance Computing and Communications

HPCHA high red cell phosphatidylcholine anemia

HPD hematoporphyrin derivative
high protein diet
histrionic (hysterical) personality disorder
home peritoneal dialysis
hypothalamic-pituitary dysfunction

HPE history and physical exam
hydrostatic permeability edema

HPET *Helicobacter pylori* eradication therapy

HPETE 12-hydroperoxy-arachidonic acid (hydroperoxy-eicosatetraenoic acid)

HPF hemorrhagic peritoneal fluid
high-power field
hypocaloric protein feeding

HPFH hereditary persistence of

fetal hemoglobin

hPFSH human pituitary follicle-stimulating hormone

HPG human pituitary gonadotropin

hPG human pituitary gonadotropin

hpGRF human pancreatic growth hormone-releasing factor

HPI history of present illness

human proinsulin

HPL human parotid lysozyme

human placental lactogen

hPL human placental lactogen

human platelet lactogen

HPLA hydroxyphenyllactic acid

HPLC high-performance (pressure) liquid chromatography

high-pressure liquid chromatography

HPM hemiplegic migraine

high-pitched murmur

HPMPA hydroxy-phosphonylmethoxy-propyl-adenine (potent, broad-spectrum antiviral agent)

HPN home parenteral nutrition

hpn hypertension

HPO high-pressure oxygenation

hydroperoxide

hypertrophic pulmonary osteoarthropathy

HPP hereditary pyropoikilocytosis

hinged penile prosthesis

human pancreatic polypeptide

hyperplastic polyps

hypokalemic periodic paralysis

hPP human pancreatic polypeptide

HPPA hydroxyphenylpyruvic acid

1HPPBS 1-hour postprandial blood sugar

2HPPBS 2-hour postprandial blood sugar

HPPO high partial pressure of oxygen

HPR hypophosphatemic rickets

hPR human prolactin

hPRP human platelet-rich plasma

HPRT hypoxanthine phosphoribosyl-transferase

HPS hantavirus pulmonary syndrome

heel pain syndrome

hepatoportal sclerosis

high protein supplement

His-Purkinje system

human platelet suspension

hypertrophic pyloric stenosis

HPSC hematopoietic stem cell

His-Purkinje system conduction

HPT halo-pelvic traction

hemopneumothorax (effusion of blood accompanying accumulation of air in the chest cavity)

home pregnancy test

hyperparathyroidism

hypoparathyroidism

hPT human placental thyrotropin

hPTH human parathyroid hormone

hPTHrP human parathyroid hormone-related protein

HPTM home prothrombin time monitoring

HPV *Haemophilus pertussis* vaccine

human papillomavirus

human papilloma virus

human parvovirus

hypoxic pulmonary vasoconstriction (reflex)

HPVC hypoxic pulmonary vasoconstriction

HPVD hypertensive pulmonary vascular disease

HPVG hepatic portal venous gas

HPVI human papillomavirus

infection

Hpx hemopexin

H. pylori *Helicobacter pylori* (a species causing active chronic type B gastritis; found in more than 90% of patients with duodenal ulcers and believed to play a central role in development of this condition)

HR hallux rigidus (stiff toe; painful flexion of the big toe due to stiffness in the metatarso-phalangeal joint)
heart rate
heat rash
hemorrhagic retinopathy
high resolution
hormone receptor
hospital report
hyperimmune reaction

H & R hysterectomy and radiation
hysteria and repression

Hr blood type factor

hr hour

HRA health risk appraisal
histamine releasing activity

HRBs high-risk babies

HRC Herpes Resource Center
(415) 328-7710
high-resolution chromatography
hormone receptor complex

HRCT high-resolution computed tomography

HRE hepatic reticuloendothelial (cell)
hormone receptor enzyme

HRF histamine releasing factor
homologous restriction factor
hypothalamic releasing factors

HRI high-risk individual

hRIG human rabies immune globulin (vaccine)

HRL (fetal) head rotated left

hRLA human reovirus-like agent

hRNA heterogeneous RNA (ribonucleic acid)

HRP high-risk pregnancy
horseradish peroxidase

HRPI high-risk premature infant

HRQL health-related quality of life

HRQOL health-related quality of life

HRR (fetal) head rotated right

HRS Hamilton Rating Scale (for depression)
Hamman-Rich syndrome
hepatorenal syndrome
hormone receptor site

HRs hormone receptors

HRSEM high-resolution scanning electron microscopy

HRSS Holmes Rahe Scale of Stress

HRT heart rate
hormone replacement therapy

HRV human reovirus
human rotavirus

HS half-strength
hamstring
haversian system
hazardous substance
head sling
health screening
heart sounds
heat-stable
heat stroke
heavy smoker
Hegar's sign (softening of uterine isthmus due to pregnancy)
Heimlich sign (the characteristic sudden gesture of distress of a person with an obstruction of the airway)
heme synthetase
hemorrhagic stroke
hereditary spherocytosis
herpes simplex

Horner's syndrome
homologous serum
homosexual
Horner's syndrome
hours of sleep
house surgeon
Hunter's syndrome
  (mucopoly-
  saccharidosis II)
Hurler's syndrome
  (mucopoly-
  saccharidosis I-H)
hypersensitivity
hypersomnia
hypospadias

H & S hearing and speech
hemorrhage and shock
hypocalcemia and seizures
hysterectomy and
  sterilization

h.s. *hora somni* [Latin] at hour
  of sleep; at bedtime

HSA Hazardous Substances Act
health scientist
  administrator
Health Security Act
Health Systems Agency
heat stable antigen
hereditary sideroblastic
  anemia
horseshoe abscess
human serum albumin
hypersomnia-sleep apnea

HSAN hereditary sensory and
  autonomic neuropathy

HSAP heat-stable alkaline
  phosphatase

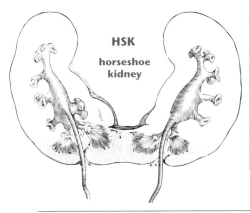

HSK

**horseshoe
kidney**

HSAS hypertrophic subaortic
  stenosis

HSC Hand-Schuller-Christian
  (syndrome)
hematopoietic stem cell
hemopoietic stem cell
hereditary spherocytosis
herpes simplex cellulitis

HSCA Health Sciences
  Communications
  Association

HSCD Hand-Schüller-Christian
  disease

HS-CoA reduced coenzyme A

HSCS Hand-Schüller-Christian
  syndrome

HSD honest significant
  difference

HSDB hazardous substances data
  bank

HSE heat-stable enterotoxin
herpes simplex
  encephalitis

Hse homoserine

HSES homorrhagic shock-
  encephalopathy
  syndrome

HSF hepatocyte-stimulating
  factor
heterosexual female
hickory-stick fracture
histamine-sensitizing factor
hypothalamic secretory
  factor

HSG herpes simplex genitalis
hysterosalpingogram
hysterosalpingography

hSGF human skeletal
  growth factor

HSH hydrogenated starch
  hydrolysates

HSI heat stress index
hypotonic saline infusion

HSK herpes simplex keratitis
horseshoe kidney

HSL herpes simplex labialis
hormone-sensitive lipase

HSLC high-speed liquid
  chromatography

HSM hepatosplenomegaly
heterosexual male
holosystolic murmur
HSN heart sounds normal
hereditary sensory
neuropathy
HSNHL hereditary sensorineural
hearing loss
H₂SO₄ sulfuric acid
hSOD human superoxide
dismutase
h. som. *hora somni* [Latin]
at bedtime
HSOR hydroxysteroid
oxidoreductase
HSP Henoch-Schönlein
purpura (anaphylactoid
purpura)
hereditary spastic
paraparesis
human serum protein
hypersensitivity
pneumonitis
HSPH Harvard School of Public
Health
HSPN Henoch-Schonlein
purpura nephritis
HSR health system reform
heated serum reagin
homogeneously staining
region
HSRC human subjects review
committee
HSS Hallermann-Streiff
syndrome
Henoch-Schönlein
syndrome
hypertrophic subaortic
stenosis
HSSE high soap suds enema
HST histplasmin skin test
HSTAT health services/technology
assessment text (free,
electronic resource that
provides access to the
full-text of documents
useful in health care
decision making)

H substance
histamine-like capillary
vasodilator
HSV herpes simplex virus

herpes simplex virus

highly selective vagotomy
HSV-1 herpes simplex virus type 1
HSV-2 herpes simplex virus type 2
HSVE herpes simplex virus
encephalitis
HT halo test
hammertoe
Hashimoto's thyroiditis
(lymphadenoid goiter)
hearing test
heart
heart transplant
heat therapy
height
hemagglutination titer
hematologic toxin
hemothorax
high temperature
high tracheostomy
home treatment
Hubbard tank
hydrotherapy
hypertension
hyperthermia
hyperthyroidism
(Graves' disease)
hypertropia
hypothalamus
hypothyroidism
3HT 3-hydroxytyramine
(dopamine)

5HT	5-hydroxytryptamine (serotonin)
Ht	heart
	height
	hot
	total hyperopia (the sum of the latent and the manifest hyperopia)
ht	height
5-HTA	5-hydroxytryptamine (serotonin)
HTACS	human thyroid adenylate cyclase stimulators
HTAT	human tetanus antitoxin
HTB	hot tub bath
HTC	hepatoma tissue culture
	homozygous typing cells
	hypertensive crisis
	hypertrophic cicatrix (hypertrophic scars)
HTCVD	hypertensive cardiovascular disease
HTE	hypothenar eminence
HTF	heterothyrotropic factor
HTG	hypertriglyceridemia
HTGL	hepatic triglyceride lipase
HTH	hypothalamus
HTHD	hypertensive heart disease

HT

hyperthyroidism

HTIG	human tetanus immune globulin
HTL	hearing threshold level
	hot tub lung
	human T-cell leukemia
	human thymic leukemia
HTLV-I	human T cell leukemia virus-type I
	human T cell lymphotropic virus-type I
HTLV-II	human T cell leukemia virus-type II
	human T cell lymphotropic virus-type II
HTLV-III	human T cell lymphotropic virus-type III
HTLVs	human T cell leukemia viruses
	human T cell lymphoma viruses
HTLV-V	human T cell lymphotropic virus-type V
HTML	Hyper Text Markup Language
HTN	hypertension
	hypertensive nephropathy
HTO	heterotopic ossification
	hospital transfer order
HTP	house-tree-person (psychological test)
	hydroxytryptophan
HTPN	home total parenteral nutrition
HTR	hemolytic transfusion reaction
HTS	head traumatic syndrome
	human thyroid stimulator
hTSAb	human thyroid-stimulating antibody
hTSH	human thyroid-stimulating hormone
hTSS	human toxic shock syndrome
HTST	high temperature, short time
HTT	high touch therapy
HTTP	Hyper Text Transport Protocol

HTV herpes-type virus
HTVD hypertensive vascular
disease
HTX hemothorax
HU hemolytic unit
human urine
hydroureter

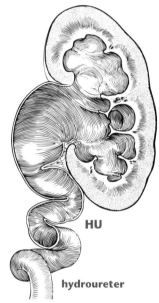

HU

hydroureter

hydroxyurea
(chemotherapy)
hyperemia unit
Hu human
HUC hypouricemia
HUD hypertonic uterine
dysfunction
hypotonic uterine
dysfunction
HuEPO human erythropoietin
HUF hot urologic forceps
(Thermajaw)
HUGH human growth hormone
HUGO Human Genome
Organization
HuIFN human interferon
Hum humerus
HUM 50/50
Humulin (half Regular,
half NPH)
HUM L Humulin Lente (insulin)

HUM N Humulin NPH (insulin)
HUM R Humulin Regular (insulin)
HUN hyperuricemic
nephropathy
HUR hydroxyurea
(chemotherapy)
HUS hemolytic-uremic
syndrome
HuSA human serum albumin
huTHAS human thymus antiserum
HV hallux valgus

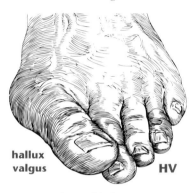

hallux valgus **HV**

has voided
hepatic vein
herpes virus
hyperventilation
(characterized by
abnormally prolonged,
rapid, deep breathing)
H & V hemigastrectomy and
vagotomy
HVA homovanillic acid
hypervitamintosis A
HVC high vocal center
HVD hypertensive vascular
disease
HVE high-voltage
electrophoresis
HVECoA high-voltage electrocortical
activity
HVEM high-voltage electron
microscopy
HVES high-voltage electrical
stimulation
HVGR host-versus-graft reaction
HVGS high-voltage
galvanic stimulation

HVH	*Herpes virus hominis*
HVIDHP	hepatic venous isolation by direct hemoperfusion
HVL	half-value layer (material that reduces radiation intensity by one half)
HVO	hallux valgus orthosis
HVPE	high-voltage paper electrophoresis
HVPG	hepatic venous pressure gradient
HVPS	hantavirus pulmonary syndrome
HVR	hypoxia ventilation response
HVS	herpes virus sensitivity
	hirsutism-virilizing syndromes
	hypovolemic shock
HVSs	hyperventilation syndromes
HVT	half-value thickness
HW	healing well
	herpetic whitlow
	hookworm (*Necator americanus, Ancylostoma duodenale*)
	housewife
HWB	hot water bottle
HWP	hot wet pack
Hx	hexyl (the isomeric forms of the organic radical C_6H_{13}-)
	history
	hospitalization
	hypoxanthine (a precursor of xanthine)
HXIS	hard x-ray imaging spectrometry
HY	hysteria
Hy	hypermetropia
	hyperopia
	hypophysis
	hysteria
HYD	hydration
hydro	hydrotherapy
Hyg	hygiene
Hyl	hydroxylysine
Hyp	4-hydroxyproline
	hypnosis
	hypothalamus
hyper al	hyperalimentation
hyper T&A	hypertrophy of tonsils and adenoids
hypno	hypnosis
hypo	hypodermic syringe
HypRF	hypothalamic releasing factor
hyst	hysterectomy
HZ	herpes zoster (shingles)
Hz	hertz (unit of frequency; 1 cycle per second = 1 hertz)
HZAN	herpes zoster acute neuralgia
HZI	hemizona assay index
	herpes zoster infection
HZL	herpes zoster lesion
HZO	herpes zoster ophthalmicus
HZV	herpes zoster virus

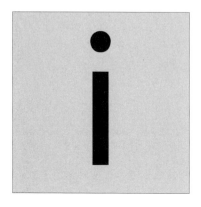

I	I-band
	ibuprofen (Advil)
	implantation
	incision
	incisor (permanent tooth)
	index
	inertia
	inhalation
	inion (a craniometric point; the most prominent point of the external occipital protuberance of the back of the skull)
	inosine
	insoluble
	inspiration
	insulin
	intensity of electric current
	intensity of magnetism
	intermittent
	internist
	intestine
	iodine
	iris
	ischium
	isoleucine
	isotope (one of two or more chemical elements in which all atoms have the same atomic number but varying atomic weights)
I	electric current

^{125}I	radioactive iodine (with relative atomic mass 125)
^{131}I	radioactive iodine (with relative atomic mass 131)
i	incisor (deciduous tooth)
IA	image amplification
	immunoadsorbent
	impedance angle
	impedance audiometry
	Impotence Anonymous
	incidental appendectomy
	incurred accidently
	indolic acid
	infantile apnea
	infantile arteritis
	infantile autism
	infected area
	infectious arthritis
	inhalation anesthesia
	initiating agent
	intra-alveolar
	intra-amniotic
	intra-aortic
I & A	irrigation and aspiration
i A	influenza A
IAA	iliac artery aneurysm
	indolylacetic acid
	infra-abdominal abscess
	insulin autoantibody
	iodoacetic acid
IAAI	intra-articular anesthetic injection
IAB	induced abortion
	intra-aortic balloon
IABC	intra-aortic balloon catheter
	intra-aortic balloon counterpulsation
IABD	ischemic-anoxic brain damage
IABM	idiopathic aplastic bone marrow
IABP	intra-aortic balloon pump
IAC	image analysis computer
	inpatient acute care
	internal auditory (acoustic) canal
	intra-arterial catheter
	intra-arterial

chemotherapy

IACD implantable automatic
cardioverter-defibrillator

IACG intermittent angle-closure
glaucoma

IACP intra-aortic
counterpulsation

IACR International Association
of Cancer Registries

IADH inappropriate antidiuretic
hormone

IADHS inappropriate antidiuretic
hormone syndrome

IADL instrumental activities of
daily living

IAF inhibiting activity factor

IAG International Association
of Gerontology

IAGT indirect antiglobulin test

IAH idiopathic adrenal
hyperplasia
implantable artificial heart
isonicotinic acid hydrazide

IAHA immune adherence
hemagglutination assay

IAHD idiopathic acquired
hemolytic disease

IAHS infection-associated
hemophagocytic
syndrome

IAI idiopathic autonomic
insufficiency
intra-abdominal infection

IAIS insulin autoimmune
syndrome

IAJ immobilization of
ankle joint

IAM internal auditory
(acoustic) meatus

IAMSSD Institute of Arthritis and
Musculoskeletal and Skin
Diseases

IAN idiopathic aseptic necrosis

IANC International Anatomical
Nomenclature
Committee

IAO immediately after onset

IAP intermittent acute
porphyria

intra-abdominal pressure

IAPB International Association
for Prevention of
Blindness

IAPP insulinoma amyloid
polypeptide
islet amyloid polypeptide

IAQ indoor air quality

IAR immediate asthma reaction

IARC International Agency for
Research on Cancer

IARF ischemic acute renal
failure

IAS idiopathic ankylosing
spondylitis
infant apnea syndrome
infantile arteriosclerosis
insulin autoimmune
syndrome
interatrial septum
internal anal sphincter
intra-amniotic saline
(infusion)

IASD interatrial septal defect

IASM intermittent air-splint
massage

IAT impedance audiometry test
indirect antiglobulin test
intraoperative autologous
transfusion
iodine-azide test

IATV interactive television

IAV influenza A viruses
intermittent assisted
ventilation

IAW Institute of Antibiotics,
Warsaw

IB inclusion body
infant botulism
infectious bronchitis
irritable bowel
Ivyblock

i B influenza B

ib. *ibidem* [Latin] in the
same place

IBA immunoblot assay
Industrial Biotechnology
Association

IBB intestinal brush border

IBC	iodine-binding capacity
	iron-binding capacity
IBCRM	impedance-based cardiorespiratory monitor
IBD	infectious bursal disease
	inflammatory bowel disease
	irritable bowel disease
IBED	inborn error of development
I. belli	*Isospora belli* (causes coccidiosis)
IBF	immunoglobulin-binding factor
IBG	iliac bone graft
	insoluble bone gelatin
IBI	intermittent bladder irrigation
ibid.	*ibidem* [Latin] in the same place
IBM	inclusion body myositis
IBNR	incurred but not reported
IBOW	intact bag of waters
IBP	iron-binding protein
IBQ	Illness Behavior Questionnaire
IBS	immunoblastic sarcoma
	irritable bowel syndrome
IBT	ink blot test
IBU	ibuprofen (Advil)
IBV	infectious bronchitis virus
	influenza B virus
IBW	ideal body weight
IC	ileocecal
	iliac crest
	immediate care
	immune complex
	immunocompromised
	immunoconjugate
	impetigo contagiosa
	incompetent cervix
	indwelling catheter
	infarctoid cardiopathy
	infection control
	inferior colliculus
	inferior concha
	inferiority complex
	informed consent

	inspiratory capacity
	institutional care
	intensive care
	intercarpal (joint)
	intercostal
	interdigitating cell
	intermediate care
	intermittent catheterization
	intermittent claudication
	internal capsule
	internal conjugate
	interstitial cystitis
	intimal cell (intimacyte)
	intracarotid
	intracellular
	intracerebral
	intracoronary
	intracranial
	intravascular coagulation
	invasive cancer
	iris coloboma
	irritable colon
	islet cells (of the pancreas)
i C	influenza C
i.c.	*inter cibos* [Latin] between meals
ICA	ileocolic artery

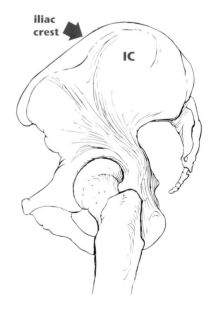

iliac crest

IC

internal carotid artery

intracranial aneurysm

islet cell adenoma

islet cell autoantigen

ICAA internal carotid artery
aneurysm

ICAb islet cell antibody

ICAM intercellular adhesion
molecule

ICAO internal carotid
artery occlusion

ICB intercostal (nerve) block

ICBF inner cortical blood flow

ICBG iliac crest bone graft

ICBN intercostobrachial nerve

ICC idiopathic calcinosis cutis

immunocompetent cells

International Consensus
Committee

intensive coronary care

intracavitary chemotherapy

intracranial cyst

islet cell carcinoma

ICCE intracapsular cataract
extraction

ICCK immunoreactive
cholecystokinin

ICCM idiopathic congestive
cardiomyopathy

ICCT intracavitary chemotherapy

ICCU intensive coronary
care unit

ICD I-cell disease

ileal conduit diversion

immune complex disease

implantable cardiac
defibrillator

impulse control disorder

infantile celiac disease

inner canthal distance

instantaneous cardiac
death

intercanthal distance

internal cardioverter
defibrillator

*International Classification of
Diseases*

intrauterine contraceptive
device

irritant contact dermatitis

ischemic coronary disease

isocitrate dehydrogenase

ICDC implantable cardioverter
defibrillator catheter

ICD10CM *International Classification of
Diseases, Tenth Revision,
Clinical Modification*
(World Health
Organization)

ICDH isocitrate dehydrogenase

ICE ice, compression and
elevation

ifosfamide + carboplatin +
etoposide (combination
chemotherapy)

intracochlear electrodes

ICEA International Childbirth
Education Association

ICEDA intracranial epidural
abscess

I cells inspiratory neurons

intercalated cells

ICES ice, compression, elevation
and splinting

ICEUS intracaval endovascular
ultrasonography

ICF immediate care facility

intermediate care facility

intracellular fluid

ICFA induced complement-
fixing antigen

ICFS intracellular fluid spaces

ICG intercritical gout

isotope cisternography

ICGN immune-complex
glomerulonephritis

ICGS intercapillary
glomerulosclerosis

ICH infantile cortical
hyperostosis
(Coffey's disease)

intracerebral hemorrhage

intracortical hemorrhage

intracranial hemorrhage

intracranial hypertension

ICI intracardiac infection

intracavitary irradiation

ICIDH International Classification

of Impairments,
Disabilities, and
Handicaps

ICL idiopathic CD4+T
lymphocytopenia

ICLE intracapsular lens
extraction

ICLN infracardiac lymph node
infraclavicular lymph node
intercostal lymph nodes

ICM inner cell mass
intercostal margin
intercostal muscle
ion conductance
modulator

ICMA intracranial
microaneurysm

ICMP inferior constrictor muscle
of pharynx

ICMVP interstitial CMV
pneumonia

ICN immune complex nephritis
intensive care nursery
International Council of
Nurses

ICNs intercostal nerves

ICNSH idiopathic central nervous
system hypersomnia

ICNV International Committee
on Nomenclature of
Viruses

ICO intracartilaginous
ossification

ICODG intracranial
oligodendroglioma

ICOH International Commission
on Occupational Health

ICP immunocompromised
patient
incubation period
infectious cell protein
intermittent
catheterization protocol
intracranial pressure
intraperitoneal cis-
platinum
ischemic cardiac pain

ICPB International Collection of
Phytopathogenic Bacteria

ICPM intracranial pressure
monitoring

ICPP intubated continuous
positive pressure

ICR intracavitary radium

ICRF immunoreactive
corticotropin-releasing
factor

ICRP International Commission
on Radiological
Protection

ICRU International Commission
on Radiological Units
and Measurements

ICS ileocecal sphincter

ICS

**ileocecal
sphincter**

immotile cilia syndrome
intercellular space
intercostal space
International College of
Surgeons
irritable colon syndrome

ICSA islet-cell surface antibody

ICSD *International Classification of
Sleep Disorders*

ICSD:DCM

*International Classification of
Sleep Disorders: Diagnostic
and Coding Manual*

ICSH International Committee
for Standardization in
Hematology
interstitial cell-stimulating
hormone

ICSI intracytoplasmic sperm
injection

ICSO intermittent coronary
sinus occlusion

ICT   icterus (jaundice)
      impaired glucose tolerance
      indirect Coombs' test
      inflammation of
        connective tissue
      insulin coma therapy
      intensive conventional
        therapy
      intermittent cervical
        traction
      interstitial cell tumor
      intracranial tumor

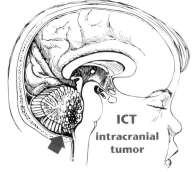

ICT
intracranial tumor

      islet cell tumor
      intracranial tumor
ICTC inferior cornu of thyroid
        cartilage
ICTS idiopathic carpal tunnel
        syndrome
ICU   immunologic contact
        urticaria
      intensive care unit
ICV   ileocecal valve
      intracellular volume
ICVH ischemic cerebrovascular
        headache
ICVS intracranial venous sinus
ICW intracellular water
ID   identification
      idiotype
      immunodeficiency
      immunodiffusion
      inappropriate disability
      inclusion disease
      infant deaths
      infectious disease
      infective dose

      initial diagnosis
      initial dose
      inside diameter
      interstitial disease
      intradermal
      Iselin disease
ID50 median infective dose
I & D incision and drainage
      irrigation and drainage
id   inside diameter
id.   *idem* [Latin] the same
IDA   iminodiacetic acid
      iron deficiency anemia
id.ac *idem ac* [Latin] the
        same as
IDAM infant of drug-abusing
        mother
      infant of drug-addicted
        mother
IDBC infiltrating ductal breast
        cancer
IDBS infantile diffuse brain
        sclerosis
IDBT immune dot-blot test
IDC   immunophilin-drug
        complex
      intervertebral disk collapse
IDCF immunodiffusion
        complement fixation
IDCP *Infectious Diseases in*
        Clinical Practice
IDCs interdigitating cells
IDCT indirect Coombs' test
IDD   insulin-dependent diabetes
      iodotyrosine deiodinase
        deficiency
IDDF investigational drug
        data form
IDDM insulin-dependent diabetes
        mellitus (type 1)
IDDS implantable drug delivery
        system
IDF   idiopathic diffuse fibrosis
      Immune Deficiency
        Foundation
      infantile digital fibroma
IDFA International Dairy Foods
        Association
IDG   interdisciplinary group

IDI immunologically
detectable insulin
implantable defibrillator
insertion
induction-delivery interval
intradiskal injection

IDIPF idiopathic diffuse
interstitial pulmonary
fibrosis

IDIS intraoperative digital
subtraction

IDISA intraoperative digital
subtraction angiography

IDK internal derangement of
the knee (joint)

IDL intermediate-density
lipoprotein (densities of
1.019–1.063 g/ml)

IDM indirect method
infant of diabetic mother

IDP inflammatory
demyelinating
polyneuropathy
initial dose period
inosine diphosphate (a
nucleotide that
participates in high-
energy phosphate
transfer)
intraductal papilloma
idiopathic pulmonary
hemosiderosis

IDR iatrogenic drug reaction
intradermal reaction

IDS immune deficiency
syndrome
immunity deficiency state
inhibitor of DNA synthesis

IDSA Infectious Diseases Society
of America
intravenous digital
subtraction angiography
(a fluoroscopic x-ray
imaging technique)

IDT immune diffusion test
indicator dilution
technique

IDTs intestine-dwelling
trematodes (*Fasciolopsis*

buski)

IDU idoxuridine (an antiviral
agent that inhibits viral
DNA synthesis)
injecting-drug user
intravenous drug use
iododeoxyuridine

IDV intermittent demand
ventilation

IDVC indwelling venous catheter

IE immunoelectrophoresis
impacted embolism
infective endocarditis
inflammatory exudate
inner ear

I.E. *immunitats einheit*
[German] immunizing
unit

I & E inspiratory and expiratory

i.e. *id est* [Latin] that is

IEA immunoelectroadsorption
immunoelectrophoretic
analysis
inferior epigastric artery

IEC infectious endocarditis
infective endocarditis
intraepithelial carcinoma

IECa intraepitheiial carcinoma

IECC intraembryonic celomic
cavity

IED individual effective dose
intraepithelial dyskeratosis
intraepithelial dysplasia

IEF inverse epicanthal fold
isoelectric focusing

IEKD intestinal enterokinase
deficiency

IEL intraepithelial lymphocyte

IEM inborn error of
metabolism

IEMG integrated
electromyography

IEN intraepithelial neoplasia

IEOAM inborn errors of organic
acid metabolism

IEP immunoelectrophoresis
intravascular endothelial
proliferation
(PEH is preferred)

isoelectric precipitation

IEPT intermediate end point
of therapy

I/E ratio inspiratory/expiratory
ratio

IES ineffective erythropoiesis
syndrome
inferior esophageal
sphincter

IEST implanted electrode
stimulation therapy

IETF Internet Engineering
Task Force

IF ictal fear
iliac fossa
immunofixation
immunofluorescence
implant failure
inferior facet
infrapatellar fat
inhibiting factor
interferon (thought to
inhibit oncogenic viral
growth)
internal fixation
interstitial fluid
intrinsic factor
involved field

IF1 interferon 1

IFA idiopathic fibrosing
alveolitis
immunofluorescence assay
immunofluorescent
antibody
indirect fluorescent
antibody (test)
indirect
immunofluorescence
assay
International Fertility
Association

I-FABP intestinal fatty acid-binding
protein

IFAT indirect fluorescent
antibody technique (test)

IFD iodoform dressing (iodine
impregnated gauze strip
dressing)

IFE immunofixation

electrophoresis

IFET ischemic forearm
exercise test

IFGO International Federation
of Gynecology and
Obstetrics

IFM immunofluorescence
microscopy
internal fetal monitoring
intrafusal muscle

IFN interferon (thought to
inhibit oncogenic
viral growth)

IFN-alpha interferon-alpha

IFN-beta interferon-beta

IFN-gamma
interferon-gamma

IFP inferior phrenic plexus
inflammatory fibroid
polyps
infrapellar fat pad
isiopathic facial paralysis

IFR infrared (the
electromagnetic radiation
beyond the red end of
the spectrum with
wavelengths too long to
be seen)
inspiratory flow rate

IFRA indirect fluorescent rabies
antibody (test)

IFSE internal fetal scalp
electrode

IFT immunofluorescence test
intrafallopian transfer

IFU interferon unit

IFV intracellular fluid volume

IG immune globulin
immunoglobulin
infantile glaucoma
inflammatory glaucoma
intestinal gas
irritable gut

Ig immune globulin
immunoglobulin

IGA infantile genetic
agranulocytosis

IgA immunoglobulin A
(gamma A globulin)

IgAD	immunoglobulin A deficiency	**IgMN**	immunoglobulin M nephropathy
IgAGN	immunoglobulin A glomerulonephritis	**IGP**	intestinal glycoprotein
IgAN	immunoglobulin A nephropathy	**IGR**	intrauterine growth retardation
IGB	ischiogluteal bursa ischiogluteal bursitis	**IGS**	inappropriate gonadotropin secretion
IgBF	immunoglobulin binding factor	**Igs**	immunoglobulins
IgD	immunoglobulin D (gamma D globulin)	**IgSC**	immunoglobulin-secreting cell
IGDM	infant of gestational diabetic mother	**IGT**	impaired glucose tolerance
		IGTN	ingrown toenail
IgE	immunoglobulin E (gamma E globulin)	**IGTT**	intravenous glucose tolerance test
IGF	insulin-like growth factor	**IGU**	iminoglycinuria (Joseph's syndrome)
IGF-I	insulin-like growth factor-type one (active in embryonic development)	**IGV**	intrathoracic gas volume
		IH	idiopathic hirsutism immediate hypersensitivity imperforate hymen incisional hernia incompletely healed indirect hemagglutination industrial hygiene infectious hepatitis inguinal hernia internal hemorrhoids intracranial hematome iris hamartomas (Lisch nodules) iron hematoxylin
IGF-II	insulin-like growth factor-type two (active postnatally; formerly called somatomedins)		
IGF-R	insulin-like growth factor receptor		
IgG	immunoglobulin G (gamma G globulin)		
IGH	immunoreactive growth hormone		
Igh-C	immunoglobulin heavy chain-constant	**IHA**	idiopathic hyperaldosteronism immunohemolytic anemia indirect hemagglutination (test)
IGHD	isolated growth hormone deficiency		
Igh-D	immunoglobulin heavy chain-diversity		
Igh-J	immunoglobulin heavy chain-joining	**IHB**	incomplete heart block intermittent heartburn
Igh-V	immunoglobulin heavy chain-variable	**IHC**	idiopathic hypercalciuria immunohistochemistry inner hair cell intrahepatic cholestasis
IgIM	immunoglobulin intramuscular		
IgIV	immunoglobulin intravenous	**IHD**	ischemic heart disease
IGM	Internet Grateful Med (program for assisted searching of MEDLINE)	**IHES**	idiopathic hypereosinophilic syndrome
		IHH	infectious human hepatitis
IgM	immunoglobulin M (gamma M globulin)	**IHM**	ictal hemimacropsia infrahyoid muscle

	in-hospital mortality
IHN	iliohypogastric nerve
IHO	idiopathic hypertrophic osteoarthropathy
IHP	idiopathic hypoparathyroidism
IHPC	intrahepatic cholestasis
IHPH	intrahepatic portal hypertension
IHR	intrinsic heart rate
IHS	idiopathic headache score
	iron-hematoxylin stain
IHSA	iodinated human serum albumin
IHSS	idiopathic hypertrophic subaortic stenosis
IHU	impaired hepatic uptake
IHW	inner heel wedge
II	image intensifier
	impaired intellect
	incapacitating illness
	incapacitating injury
	inhalation injury
	intellectual impairment
	intentional injury
	intestinal ischemia
I & I	illness and injuries
IICA	intracranial internal carotid artery
IICP	increased intracranial pressure
IICU	infant intensive care unit
	intermediate intensive care unit
IIDM	insulin-independent diabetes mellitus
IIF	immune interferon
	indirect immunofluorescence
IIFA	indirect immunofluorescence assay
IIH	insulin-induced hypoglycemia
	indirect inguinal hernia
IIN	ilioinguinal nerve
	inhibitory interneuron
IIOD	infrainguinal occlusive disease

IIP	idiopathic interstitial pneumonitis
	increased intracranial pressure
	integrated image processing
II-para	secundipara
IIS	intensive immunosuppression
IIT	ineffective iron turnover
	injectable impotence treatment
	intravenous infusion therapy
IJ	ileojejunal (parts of small intestine)
	internal jugular (vein)
IJD	inflammatory joint disease
IJO	idiopathic juvenile osteoporosis
IJP	inhibitory junction potential
	internal jugular pressure
IJV	internal jugular vein
IK	immobilized knee
	interstitial keratitis
IL	ileum
	iliolumbar
	inguinal ligament (Poupart's ligament)
	interleukin
	isoleucrine
IL-1	interleukin-1
IL-2	interleukin-2
IL-3	interleukin-3
IL-4	interleukin-4
IL-5	interleukin-5
IL-6	interleukin-6
IL-7	interleukin-7
IL-8	interleukin-8
IL-9	interleukin-9
IL-10	interleukin-10
ILA	insulin-like activity
	intestinal lymphangiectasia
ILAE	International League Against Epilepsy
ILBBB	incomplete left bundle branch block
ILBW	infant low birth weight

ILC   intermediate longitudinal crease (of hand)

ILC

intermediate longitudinal crease (of hand)

ILD   inflammatory lung disease
interstitial lung disease
ischemic limb (leg) disease

ILE   infantile lobar emphysema (congenital lobar emphysema)

Ile   isoleucine (amino acid)

ILF   indicated low forceps

ILGF I   insulin-like growth factor I (somatomedin C)

ILH   immunoreactive luteinizing hormone

ILI   influenza-like illness

ILL   iliolumbar ligament
intermediate lymphocytic lymphoma

ILM   iliocostal-longissimus muscle(s)
internal limiting membrane (innermost layer of the retina)

ILN   inguinal lymph node

ILP   interstitial laser photocoagulation
interstitial lymphocytic pneumonia

IL-1 RA   interleukin-1-receptor antagonist

IL-1ra   interleukin-1-receptor-antagonist

ILS   infrared liver scan

ILSS   integrated life support system

ILT   iliotibial tract

ILVs   inferior labial veins

IM   iatrogenic menopause
immunologic memory
Index Medicus
inferior mediastinum
infectious mononucleosis
innocent murmur
internal medicine
internal monitor
intramuscular
invasive mole
ionized magnesium

im   intramuscular

IMA   incudomalleal articulation
inferior mesenteric artery

IMB   intermenstrual bleeding

IMBC   indirect maximal breathing capacity

IMC   intermittent catheterization
interstitial myocarditis
intestinal mast cell

IMCI   induced myocardial ischemia

IMD   immunologically mediated disease
inherited metabolic disease

ImD0   median immunizing dose

IMDD   idiopathic midline destructive disease

IME   independent medical examiner
isometric exercise

IMF   idiopathic myelofibrosis
immobilization
mandibular fracture
immunofluorescence
intermaxillary fixation

IMG   international medical graduate

IMGU   insulin-mediated glucose uptake

IMI	inferior myocardial infarction
	intramuscular injection
	isolated meconium ileus
IMIG	intramuscular immune globulin
IMIg	intramuscular immunoglobulin
IMH	idiopathic myocardial hypertrophy
IMHT	indirect microhemagglutination test
IMI	impending myocardial infarction
Imi	imipramine (antidepressant)
	inferior myocardial infarction
	intramuscular injection
IMLN	internal mammary lymph node
IMM	immunization
immun	immunity
	immunization
IMN	idiopathic membranous nephropathy
	infectious mononucleosis
	initial malignant neoplasm
IMNs	internal mammary nodes (lymph nodes)
IMO	intramembranous ossification
IMP	idiopathic myeloid proliferation
	impression (opinion)
	inosine monophosphate
	intermenstrual pain
	ischemic muscle pain
imp	impacted
	impression (tentative diagnosis)
IMPA	incisal mandibular plane angle
IMPACC	intestinal multiple polyposis and colorectal cancer
ImPx	immunoperoxidase
IMR	individual medical record

	infant mortality rate
IMS	infertile male syndrome
IMSG	International Medical School graduate
IMV	inferior mesenteric vein
	intermittent mandatory ventilation
	intestinal microvilli
IMVP	idiopathic mitral valve prolapse
IN	impetigo neonatorum
	industrial nurse
	insulin neuritis
	interneuron
	internist
	interstitial nephritis
	intranasal
	inverted nipples
In	index
	indium (a metallic element)
	inion
	insulin
	inulin (a fructose polysaccharide found in roots of some underground stems; used in kidney function tests)
INA	Institute for New Antibiotics (Moscow)
INAD	infantile neuroaxonal dystrophy
	in no apparent distress
INAH	interstitial nuclei of anterior hypothalamus
	isonicotinic acid hydrazide
INB	ischemic necrosis of bone
inbr	inbreeding
INC	incision
	incomplete
	incontinence
	inferior nasal concha
INCA	infant nasal cannulae assembly
IncB	inclusion body
incr	increased
	increasing
incur	incurable
IND	investigational new drug

in d.	*in dies* [Latin] daily
INDA	investigational new drug application
indig	indigestion
INDO	indomethacin (nonsteroidal anti-inflammatory agent)
IndMed	*Index Medicus*
INE	infantile necrotizing encephalomyelopathy
inex	inexperienced
INF	infant
	infarction
	infection
	inferior
	infirmary
	interferon
	intravenous nutritional feeding
inf	infant
	infection
	inferior
INFH	ischemic necrosis of femoral head
infl	inflammation
inf mono	infectious mononucleosis
ING	inguinal
INH	isoniazid
	isonicotinic acid hydrazide
inhib	inhibitor
inj	injection
	injury
inj.	*injectio* [Latin] injection
INMT	imidazole-N-methyltransferase
INN	International Nonproprietary Names
INO	internuclear ophthalmoplegia
Ino	inosine
inoc	inoculation
inop	inoperable
IN-PT	inpatient
INPV	intermittent negative-pressure assisted ventilation
INR	International Normalized Ratio (reporting method)
INS	idiopathic nephrotic syndrome
	idiopathic neurologic syndrome
	illuminated nasal speculum
	insulin
	insurance
Ins	insulin
	insurance
insol	insoluble
InsP3	inositol triphosphate
inspr	inspiration
	inspiratory
INST	instrumental (delivery)
instab	instability
insuff	insufficient
	insufflation
INT	intermittent
	internal
	internist
int	internal
int. cib.	*intercibos* [Latin] between meals
intest	intestine
int. noct.	*inter noctem* [Latin] during the night
int obst	intestinal obstruction
intol	intolerance
intox	intoxication
int rot	internal rotation
INTRP	Negative Thoughts in Response to Pain (questionnaire)
Int trx	intermittent traction
Intub	intubation
invest	investigation
invol	involuntary
IO	infantile ovary
	intestinal obstruction
	intraocular
Io	ionium (obsolete term for the radioactive isotope of thorium, ^{230}Th)
	intestinal obstruction
	intraocular (pressure)
I & O	intake and output
IOAL	intraoperative abdominal lavage
IOB	implantation of blastocyst
IOC	intern on call

intraoperative cholangiogram

IOCG intraoperative cholecystogram
IOD integrated optical density
I/OD input/output device
IODAM infant of drug-addicted mother
IODM infant of diabetic mother
IOF infraorbital foramen
intraocular fluid
intraorbital foramen
IOFB intraocular foreign body
IOH idiopathic orthostatic hypotension
infundibulum of hypophysis
IOI intraocular implant
IOL induction of labor
intraocular lens
iron overload
islet of Langerhans

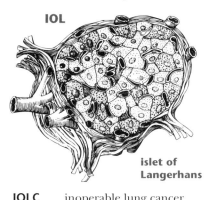

IOL

islet of Langerhans

IOLC inoperable lung cancer
IOLI intraocular lens implantation
IOM Institute of Medicine (of the National Academy of Sciences)
IOMF interosseous membrane of forearm
IOML interosseous membrane of leg
ION infraorbital nerve
ischemic optic neuropathy
IOP idiopathic osteoporosis
intraocular pressure

IOPA independent organ procurement agency
IORT intraoperative radiation therapy
IOS idiopathic oligospermia
IOT intraocular tension
intraocular tumor

IOT
intraocular tumor

ipsilateral optic tectum
IOV initial office visit
IOW infected open wound
IP icterus praecox
idiopathic parkinsonism
inactivated pepsin
incompetent patient
incubation period
infection prevention
infusion pump
inosine phosphorylase
inpatient
intellectual property
interphalangeal (joint)
interpupillary
interstitial pneumonia
intestinal polyp
intraperitoneal
intrapulmonary
invasive procedure
iron poisoning
IP-I intestinal polyposis, type I
IP-II intestinal polyposis, type II
IP-III intestinal polyposis, type III
IP3 inositol triphosphate
IPA immunoperoxidase assay
incontinentia pigmenti achromians (hypomelanosis of Ito)
individual practice association
inferior pelvic aperture
Injury Prevention Act

invasion plasmid antigens

invasive pulmonary
   aspergillosis

isopropyl alcohol

I-para   primipara

IPAs   independent practice
   associations

IPC   indirect platelet count

intraperitoneal
   chemotherapy

ion pair chromatography

ischemic preconditioning

IPCD   infantile polycystic disease

IPCP   interstitial plasma cell
   pneumonia (pneumo-
   cystis pneumonia)

IPCS   intrauterine progesterone
   contraception system

IPCT   intraperitoneal
   chemotherapy

IPD   immediate pigment
   darkening

incurable problem drinker

infantile polycystic disease

inflammatory
   pelvic disease

invasive
   pneumococcal disease

intermittent
   peritoneal dialysis

intermittent pigment
   darkening

interpubic disk

interpupillary distance

intravenous pulse dosc

IPDAS   intestinal protective drug
   absorption system

IPE   interstitial pulmonary
   emphysema

IPEH   intravascular papillary
   endothelial hyperplasia

IPEUS   intraportal endovascular
   ultrasonography

IPF   interstitial pulmonary
   fibrosis

IPFD   intrapartum fetal distress

IPFP   infrapatella fat pad

IPG   impedance
   plethysmography

implantable pulse
   generator

intestinal pteroylglutamate

IPH   idiopathic hirsutism

idiopathic portal
   hypertension

idiopathic pulmonary
   hemosiderosis

intraparenchymal
   hemorrhage

IPHP   intraperitoneal
   hyperthermic perfusion

IPHR   inverted polypoid
   hamartoma of the rectum

IPIE   intrapulmonary interstitial
   emphysema

IPIS   incomplete pulmonary
   infarction

IPJ   interphalangeal joint

IPK   indurated plantar
   keratoma

intractable plantar
   keratosis

IPKD   infantile polycystic kidney
   disease

IPL   inner plexiform layer
   (of the retina)

isolated perfused lung

IPM   immediate pigment
   darkening

infectious polymyositis

IPN   infantile periarteritis
   nodosa

infected pancreatic
   necrosis

interstitial pneumonitis

IPNA   isopropyl noradrenalin

IPOF   immediate postoperative fitting

IPOH   idiopathic orthostatic
   hypotension

IPOM   intraperitoneal onlay mesh

IPOP   immediate postoperative
   prosthesis

IPP   inferior point of pubis

inflatable penile prosthesis

intermittent positive
   pressure

intractable pelvic pain

intrapleural pressure

IPPA inspection, palpation, percussion, and auscultation

IPPB intermittent positive pressure breathing

IPPO intermittent positive pressure inflation with oxygen

IPPR intermittent positive pressure respiration

IPPV intermittent positive pressure ventilation

IPR insulin production rate

iPr isopropyl (univalent radical)

iPrA isopropyl alcohol

iPrM isopropyl myristate

iPrRA isopropyl rubbing alcohol

iPrTG isopropyl thiogalactose

IPS idiopathic postprandial syndrome

inferior petrosal sinus

infundibular pulmonary stenosis

initial prognostic score

International Psychogeriatric Society

intrapartum stillbirth

ischiopubic synchondrosis

IPSF immediate postsurgical fitting

IPSID immunoproliferative small intestinal disease

IPSP inhibitory postsynaptic potential

I-PSS International Prostate Symptom Score

IPT immunologic pregnancy test

intermittent pelvic traction

interpersonal therapy

iPTH immunoreactive parathyroid hormone

IPTX intermittent pelvic traction

IPV inactivated polio vaccine

inactivated poliovirus (vaccine)

inactivated poliovirus

vaccine

infectious peritonitis virus

infectious pustular vaginitis

internal pudendal vein

IPW ice-pick wound

IPZ insulin protamine zinc

IQ intelligence quotient

i.q. *idem quod* [Latin] the same as

IR immune response

immunoreactive

incidence rate

inferior rectus (eye muscle)

information retrieval

infrared (the electromagnetic radiation beyond the red end of the spectrum that is invisible)

inspiratory reserve

insulin reaction

insulin resistance (the state in which a given amount of insulin does not produce the expected amount of glucose transported into body cells)

insulin resistant

internal reduction

ionizing radiation (x-rays plus alpha, beta and gamma radiation)

Ir iridium (the chemical element with the greatest resistance to corrosion)

IRA immunoradioassay

implant resection arthroplasty

intravenous regional anesthesia (Bier block)

IR-ACTH immunoreactive adrenocorticotropic hormone

IR-AVP immunoreactive arginine vasopressin

IRB institutional review board

IRBBB incomplete right bundle

branch block

IRBC immature red blood cell
(erythroblast)

IRC immunoreactive calcitonin
indirect radionuclide
cystography
inspiratory reserve capacity
International Red Cross
intrastromal corneal ring

IRD infantile Refsum's
syndrome
infrared detector

IRDM insulin-resistent diabetes
mellitus

IRDS idiopathic respiratory
distress syndrome
infant respiratory distress
syndrome

IRE internal rotation
in extension

IRF idiopathic retroperitoneal
fibrosis
internal rotation in flexion

IRG immune response genes
immunoreactive glucagon
initial review group

IRGH immunoreactive growth
hormone

IRGI immunoreactive glucagon

IRH idiopathic renal hematuria
intraretinal hemorrhage

IRhGH immunoreactive human
growth hormone

IRI immunoreactive insulin
insulin resistance index

IRIA indirect radioimmunoassay

IRIg insulin-reactive
immunoglobulin

IRIC International Research
Information Center

IRIS Integrated Risk
Information System
(online database)
interleukin regulation of
immune system

IRM immune response modifier

IRMA immunoradiometric assay
intraretinal
microangiopathy

intraretinal microvascular
abnormalities

iRNA informational RNA
(ribonucleic acid)

IRP insulin-releasing
polypeptide
interstitial radiation
pneumonitis

IRPGN idiopathic rapidly
progressive
glomerulonephritis

IRR intrarenal reflux

Irr irradiation

irreg irregular

irrig irrigation

IRS infrared
spectrophotometry
irritant respiratory
syndrome

IRT intermediate renal tubule
(ascending and
descending thin limbs of
nephron)

IRTR impaired renal tubular
reabsorption

IRU interferon reference unit

IRV inspiratory reserve volume
inverse ratio ventilation

IS ichthyosis simplex
immediate sensitivity
immune serum
immunosuppressive
inguinal syndrome
incentive spirometer
infectious spondylitis
information system
insight response
in situ [Latin] in place
intercostal space
interrupted suture
intestinal stenosis
intraspinal
iris scan (personal
identification
technology)
ischial spine
isometric strength
isotonic strength

ISA incudostapedial
articulation

intrinsic sympathomimetic
activity

iodinated serum albumin

ISADH inappropriate secretion of
antidiuretic hormone

ISB incentive spirometry
breathing

ISBI International Society for
Burn Injuries

ISBN International Standard
Book Number

ISC insoluble collagen

International Society of
Chemotherapy

interstitial cell

isolette servo-control

I. scampularis

Ixodes scampularis (black-
legged tick capable of
inflicting a painful bite)

ISCF interstitial cell fluid

Iscom immunostimulating
complex

ISCR intrastromal corneal ring

ISCs immunoglobulin-
secreting cells

irreversible sickle cells

ISD immune-suppression drug

immunosuppressive drug

inhibited sexual desire

interventricular
septal defect

intractable seizure disorder

intrinsic sleep disorder

iron-storage disease

isosorbide dinitrate
(vasodilator)

ISDN isosorbide dinitrate
(vasodilator)

ISE ion-selective electrode

ISEM immunosorbent electron
microscopy

ISF interstitial fluid

ISG immune serum globulin

ISH icteric serum hepatitis

idiopathic stabbing
headache

in situ hybridization

isolated systolic

hypertension

ISHLT International Society for
Heart and Lung
Transplantation

ISH icteric serum hepatitis

ISI infarct size index

injury severity index

Institute for Scientific
Information

insulin sensitivity index

intestinal sucrase-
isomaltase

ISIS integrated shape
imaging system

ISJ iliosacral joint

ISL interspinous ligament
(connects the adjacent
spinous processes of
vertebrae)

inverse square law

ISMA infantile spinal muscular
atrophy

ISMN isosorbide mononitrate

ISMP Institute for Safe
Medication Practices

ISO International Standards
Organization

isolette

isoproterenol (synthetic
adrenergic derived from
norepinephrine)

ISOs isoenzymes

ISP interspace

interspinal

interspinous plane

interstitial pneumonia
(chronic fibrous
pneumonia)

isosexual precocity

ISPCAN International Society for
Prevention of Child
Abuse and Neglect

i.s.q. *in status quo* [Latin]
unchanged

ISR information storage and
retrieval

insulin secretion rate

ISRM International Society of
Reproductive Medicine

ISS	inferior sagittal sinus
	injury severity score
	International Staging System
	irritable stomach syndrome
ISSVD	International Society for the Study of Vulvar Disease
IST	immunosuppressive therapy
	insulin sensitivity test
	insulin shock therapy
	inversion stress test
I-sub	inhibitor substance
ISW	interstitial water
IT	iliotibial
	immunity test
	immunotherapy (hyposensitization)
	impacted tooth
	implantation test
	individual therapy
	infective thrombosis
	infective thrombus
	inferior turbinate
	inhalation test
	inhalation therapy
	inspiratory time
	insulin therapy
	intensive therapy
	intention tremor
	intermittent traction
	intradermal test
	intrathecal
	intrathoracic
	intratracheal tube
	ischial tuberosity
	isomeric transition
ITA	influenza type A
	internal thoracic artery (internal mammary artery)
ITB	iliotibial band (tractus iliotibialis)
	influenza type B
ITBS	iliotibial band syndrome
ITCP	idiopathic thrombocytopenic purpura

ITCVD	ischemic thrombotic cerebrovascular disease
ITD	immune thyroid disease
	intensely transfused dialysis
	iodide transport defect
ITE	insufficient therapeutic effect
ITF	infratemporal fossa
	interferon (thought to inhibit oncogenic viral growth)
ITFDE	International Task Force for Disease Eradication
ITFR	inferior transverse fold of rectum
ITFS	incomplete testicular feminization syndrome
ITG	intrathoracic goiter

ITG

intra-thoracic goiter

	isthmus of thyroid gland
ITI	intertragic incisure
ITL	intrathoracic tuberculous lymphadenopathy
ITLC	instant thin-layer chromatography
ITM	impacted third molar
ITN	infratrochlear nerve
	ingrown toenail

intertragus notch

ITO intertrochanteric
osteotomy

ITP idiopathic
thrombocytopenic
purpura
inosine triphosphate
islet-cell tumor of pancreas

ITPA inosine triphosphatase

ITS inhaled tobacco smoke
(principal carcinogenic
agent in the atmosphere)

ITT iliotibial tract
insulin tolerance test
internal tibial torsion

ITU intensive therapy unit

IU immunizing unit
International Units
intrauterine
in utero [Latin] within
the uterus

IUA intrauterine adhesions

IUC idiopathic ulcerative colitis

IUCD intrauterine contraceptive
device

IUD incoordinate uterine
dysfunction
intrauterine death
intrauterine
(contraceptive) device

IUFB intrauterine foreign body

IUFD intrauterine fetal demise

IUFT intrauterine fetal
transfusion

IUG intrauterine growth
intravenous urography

IUGR intrauterine growth
retardation

IUI intrauterine insemination

IU/L international units per liter

IUM internal urethral meatus

IUP intrauterine pregnancy

IUPC intrauterine pressure
catheter

IUT infundibulum of
uterine tube
intrauterine transfusion

IUTD immunizations updated

IV influenza vaccination

initial visit
interventricular
intervertebral
interview
intravaginal
intravascular
intervenous
intraventricular
intravertebral

iv intravenous

i.v. *in vitro* [Latin] within glass
in vivo [Latin] within a
living body

IVAs intravenous anesthetics

IVB intraventricular block

IVC inferior vena cava

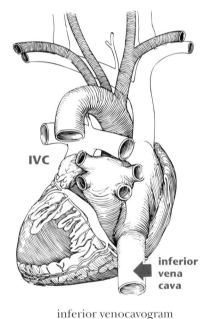

IVC

**inferior
vena
cava**

inferior venocavogram
inspiratory vital capacity
interventional cardiology
intravascular catheter
intravascular coagulation
intravenous
cholangiography
intraventricular catheter

IVCC intravascular comsumptive
coagulopathy

IVCD intraventricular
conduction delay/defect

IVCH	intravenous cholangiography
IVCP	inferior vena cava pressure
IVCT	inferior vena cava thrombosis
IVCV	inferior venacavography
IVD	induced vestibular dysfunction
	intervertebral disk

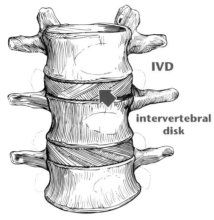

IVD

intervertebral disk

	intravenous drip
	intraventricular delay
	ischemic vascular disease
IVDA	intravenous drug abuse
	intravenous drug abuser
IVDD	intervertebral disk disease
	intervertebral disk displacement
IVDU	intravenous drug user
IVF	interventricular foramen
	intervertebral foramen
	intravenous feeding
	intravenous fluid
	in vitro fertilization
IVFA	intravenous fluorescein angiogram
IVF-ET	*in vitro* fertilization with embryo transfer
IVFT	intravenous fluid therapy
IVGG	intravenous gamma globulin
IV-GTT	intravenous glucose tolerance test
IVH	intravenous

	hyperalimentation
	intraventricular hemorrhage
IVIG	intravenous immune globulin
	intravenous immunoglobulin
IVIg	intravenous immunoglobulin
	intraventricular hemorrhage
IVIT	intravenous infusion theapy
IVJ	intervertebral joint
IVJC	intervertebral joint complex
IVL	intravenous leiomyomatosis
IVLBW	infant of very low birth weight
IVM	intervertebral muscle
	intravascular mass
	involuntary muscle
IVN	inferior vertebral notch
	intravenous nutrition
IVOX	intravascular oxygenation
IVP	increased vascular permeability
	influenza virus pneumonia
	intravenous pyelogram (urogram)
	intravenous pyelography
	intraventricular pressure
IVPF	isovolume pressure flow
IVR	idioventricular rhythm
IVRA	intravenous regional anesthesia
IVRP	isovolumic relaxation period
IVRT	isovolumic relaxation time
IVS	inappropriate vasopressin secretion
	intervening segments
	interventricular septum
	intervillous space
	irritable voiding syndrome
IVSD	interventricular septal defect
IVT	intravenous transfusion

IVU	intravenous urography
IVUS	interventional ultrasonography
	intravascular ultrasound
IVV	influenza virus vaccine
	intravenous vasopressin
IVWLs	intracapsular volar wrist ligaments
IWF	iliac wing fracture
IWI	inferior wall infarct
IWL	insensible water loss
IWMI	inferior wall myocardial infarction
IWS	index of work satisfaction
IWT	impacted wisdom (3rd molar) tooth
IZ	infarction zone
IZS	insulin zinc suspension

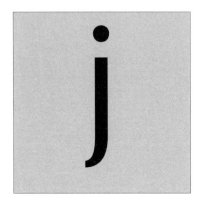

J	joint
	joule (SI unit of energy)
	journal
	juice
	juvenile
	magnetic polarization
JA	judgment analysis
	juvenile arthritis
	juvenile atrophy
JAGS	*Journal of the American Geriatric Society*
JAMA	*Journal of the American Medical Association*
JAMG	juvenile autoimmune myasthenia gravis
jaund	jaundice
JBE	Japanese B encephalitis
JC	jacket crown
	Jakob-Creutzfeldt (disease)
	joint contracture
	juvenile cataract
jc	juice
JCA	juvenile chronic arthritis
JCAH	Joint Commission on Accreditation of Hospitals
JCAHO	Joint Commission on Accreditation of Healthcare Organizations
JCAI	Joint Council of Allergy and Immunology
JCD	Jakob-Creutzfeldt disease (Creutzfeldt-Jakob disease)
JCF	juvenile calcaneal fracture
JCMHC	Joint Commission on Mental Health of Children
JCML	juvenile chronic myelocytic leukemia
JCP	juvenile chronic polyarthritis
jct	junction
JCV	JC virus (human papovavirus)
JD	jaundice
	jet douche
	juvenile delinquent
	juvenile diabetes
JDC	Joslin Diabetes Center (617) 732-2400
JDF	Juvenile Diabetes Foundation
JDFIH	Juvenile Diabetes Foundation International Hotline (800) 223-1138
JDLN	jugulodigastric lymph node
JDM	juvenile-onset diabetes mellitus
JDMS	juvenile dermatomyositis
JE	Japanese encephalitis
	jacksonian epilepsy
	junctional escape (rhythm)
JEB	junctional escape beat
jej	jejunum
JEM	*Journal of Experimental Medicine*
JER	junctional escape rhythm
JET	high frequency ventilation
JEV	Japanese encephaltis virus
JF	Jefferson fracture
	joint fluid
	Jones fracture
	jugular foramen
JFS	jugular foramen syndrome
JG	juxtaglomerular
JGA	juxtaglomerular apparatus
JGB	juxtaglomerular body
JGC	juxtaglomerular complex
j-g complex	
	juxtaglomerular complex
JGCs	juxtaglomerular cells
JGCT	juxtaglomerular cell tumor
J gene	joining gene

JH	jogger's heel
J-HR	Jarisch-Herxheimer reaction
JI	jejunoileitis
JIBP	jejuno-ilial bypass (for treating morbid obesity)
JIS	jujunoileal shunt
	juvenile idiopathic scoliosis
JJ	jaw jerk (jaw reflex)
JK	jumper's knee
Jk	Kidd blood group
JLP	juvenile laryngeal papilloma
	juvenile macular degeneration
JLS	jet lag syndrome
JME	juvenile myoclonic epilepsy (impulsive petit mal)
JMRO	Joint Medical Regulating Office
JN	junctional nevus
JNC V	Joint National Committee on Detection, Evaluation, and Treatment of High Blood Pressure (5th report)
JND	just noticeable difference
jnt	joint
JOD	juvenile-onset diabetes
JODM	juvenile-onset diabetes mellitus (type 1 diabetes mellitus)
JOLN	jugulo-omohyoid lymph node
Jour	journal
JP	Jackson-Pratt (catheter; drain)

JGA

juxtaglomerular apparatus

	joint pain
	juvenile periodontitis
	juvenile polyposis
JPA	juvenile psoriatic arthritis
JPB	junctional premature beat
JPC	Jackson-Pratt catheter
	junctional premature contraction
JPD	juvenile plantar dermatosis
JPMN	juvenile polymorphonuclear leukocyte (band cell)
JPS	juvenile polyposis syndrome
JR	junctional rhythm
JRA	juvenile rheumatoid arthritis
JROM	Joint range of motion
JS	Jaccoud syndrome (chronic arthritis following recurring episodes of rheumatic fever)
	Jacksonian seizure
	Jackson syndrome (paralysis of cranial nerves X, XI, and XII)
	jejunal syndrome (dumping syndrome)
	Jeune's syndrome (asphyxiating thoracic dystrophy)
	Job syndrome (autosomal recessive disorder of neutrophils)
	joint stiffness
	jugular foramen syndrome (Vernet's syndrome)
J seg	joining segment (of DNA encoding immunoglobulins)
JSV	Jerry-Slough virus
JT	jejunostomy tube
Jt	joint
JTE	javelin thrower's elbow
JTPS	juvenile tropical pancreatitis syndrome
Jts	joints
JTT	Jackson tracheostomy tube

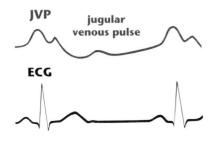

J tube   jejunostomy tube
jug   jugular
junct   junction

juv	juvenile
juxt.	*juxta* [Latin] near
JV	jugular vein
JVC	jugular venous catheter
JVD	jugular venous distention
JVP	jugular venous pressure
	jugular venous pulse
JVPT	jugular venous pulse tracing
JVS	Jamaican vomiting sickness
Jx	joint
	junction
JXG	juvenile xanthogranuloma

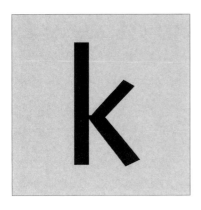

K cathode
constant
electrostatic capacity
equilibrium constant
Kell blood system
keloid
Kelvin (preferred
  temperature scale)
keratometry
kidney
killer (cell)
kilobyte
kilocalorie
kilodalton
kilogram
Klebsiella (frequent cause of
  wound infections)
knee
lysine (betaine)
potassium (*kalium*)
K equilibrium constant
17K 17-ketosteroids
k constant
kilo (prefix denoting
  decimal factor 10^3)
kilo-ohm
reaction rate
k fractional disappearance
  rate
KA keep abreast
ketoacanthoma
ketoacidosis
keto acids
ketoaciduria

kA kiloampere
ka cathode
KAF conglutinogen activating
  factor
KAFO knee-ankle-foot orthosis
KAO knee-ankle orthosis
KAT kanamycin
  acetyltransferase
kat katal (measure of
  enzymatic activity)
KB ketone bodies
knee-bearing
knee brace
kb kilobase
kilobyte
KBr potassium bromide
KC kangaroo care (to treat
  premature infants)
keratoconjunctivitis
keratoconus
killer cells (cytotoxic cells)
knee cap (patella)
Krebs cycle (tricarboxylic
  acid cycle)
Kupffer cells (phagocytic
  cells that line the walls of
  the liver sinusoids)

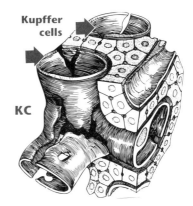

**Kupffer
cells**

KC

Kc Krebs cycle
kc kilocycle
Kcal kilocalorie (1000 calories)
KCC Kulchitsky cell carcinoma
KCCT kaolin-cephalin
  clotting time
K cell killer cell (cytotoxic cell)
kCi kilocurie

KCl	potassium chloride
KCP	knee-chest position
kc/ps	kilocycles per second
KCS	keratoconjunctivitis sicca
K cycle	Krebs cycle
KD	Kawasaki's disease (mucocutaneous lymph node syndrome)
	kidney donor
	Kohler disease
kD	kilodalton (unit of molecular mass)
kDa	kilodalton (unit of molecular mass)
KDA	known drug allergies
KDU	kidney dialysis unit
KE	Kagel exercises
	kinetic energy
KE	exchangeable body potassium
KEB	Krause's end-bulb
Keq	equilibrium constant
Kera	keratitis
17 Keto	17 ketosteroids
keV	kiloelectron-volt
KF	keloid formation
	Kerckring's folds
	Kocher fracture
Kf	glomerular ultrafiltration coefficient
KFAb	kidney-fixing antibody
KFD	Kyasanur Forest disease (a severe hemorrhagic fever seen primarily in India)
KFR	Kayser-Fleischer ring (a circular brownish discoloration of the cornea seen in some liver disorders)
KFS	Klinefelter syndrome (47XXY); most frequent major abnormality of sexual differentiation
	Klippel-Feil syndrome
KFT	kidney function test
KG	keratoglobus
	ketoglutarate
Kg	kilogauss
	kilogram(s) (1000 grams)

kG	kilogauss
kg	kilogram
kg-cal	kilocalorie
KGA	ketoglutaric acid
KGF	keratinocyte growth factor
kg/l	kilograms per liter
Kgn	kininogen (kinin precursor)
KGS	ketogenic steroid
KHb	potassium hemoglobinate
KHD	kinky-hair disease
KHM	keratoderma hereditaria mutilans
KHN	Knoop hardness number
KHS	keyhole surgery (minimally invasive laparoscopic surgery)
	kinky-hair syndrome (Menkes' disease)
kHz	kilohertz
KI	karyotype index
	potassium iodide
KIC	keto isocaproic acid
KID	keratitis, ichthyosis and deafness (syndrome)
KIDS	kids in integrated day care settings
kilo	kilogram
KIMG	Kulturensammlung am Institut für Mikrobiologie (West Germany)
KISS	kids in safety seats
	potassium iodide saturated solution
KJ	kilojoule
	knee jerk (quadriceps jerk; reflex test))
KJR	knee-jerk reflex
KK	knee kick (knee jerk)
	knock-knee (genu valgum)
kl	kiloliter
KITA	Kitasato Institute for Infectious Diseases (Tokyo)
KL	Kidner lesion
KLB	Klebs-Loeffler bacillus (*Corynebacterium diphtheriae*)
kl	kiloliter

Kleb	*Klebsiella* (frequent cause of wound infections)
KLH	keyhole limpet hemocyanin
KLPC	krypton laser photocoagulation
KLS	kidneys, liver, and spleen
	Kleine-Levin syndrome (episodic periods of excessive sleep and overeating)
KLWT	Kirsch laser welding technique
KM	kneading massage
km	kilometer
KMnO$_4$	potassium manganate (VII) (the old name for which was potassium permanganate
KMS	Kasabach-Merritt syndrome
KMV	killed measles (virus) vaccine
Kn	knee
K nail	Kuntscher nail
KNO	keep needle open
KO	keep open
	killed organism
	knee orthosis
KOH	potassium hydroxide
kΩ	kilo-ohm
KP	keratic punctata
kp	kilopound
KPA	kidney plasminogen activator (prourokinase)
	kissing pseudarthrosis
KPB	ketophenylbutazone
KPE	Kelman pharmacoemulsification
KPI	karyopyknotic index
KPM	kilopond meters
K. pneumoniae	
	Klebsiella pneumoniae
KPTT	kaolin partial thromboplastin time
Kr	krypton (an inert gaseous element)
KRBB	Krebs-Ringer bicarbonate buffer

KRBS	Krebs-Ringer bicarbonate solution
KRS	Krebs-Ringer solution
KS	Kallmann's syndrome (hypogonadotropic eunuchoidism)
	Kaposi's sarcoma
	Kawasaki syndrome (mucocutaneous lymph node syndrome)
	Kehr's sign (sharp pain in the left shoulder seen in some cases of spleen rupture)
	Kernig's sign (sign of meningitis)
	ketosteroid
	kidney stone
	Klinefelter's syndrome (male genetic disorder caused by one or more extra X sex chromosomes)
	Koplik's spots (mucous membrane lesions)
	Korsakoff syndrome (amnestic syndrome)
	Kostmann's syndrome (infantile genetic agranulocytosis)
	Krackow suture
	Krause's syndrome (encephalo-ophthalmic dysplasia)
	Kunkel's syndrome (lupoid hepatitis)
	kyphoscoliosis
17-KS	17-ketosteroids
ks	kilosecond
KSHV	Kaposi's sarcoma-associated herpes virus
KS-OI	Kaposi's sarcoma with opportunistic infections
KSS	Kearns-Sayre syndrome
KT	Kaplan's test (for globulin-albumin in spinal fluid)
	Kapsinow's test (for bile pigments)
	Kashiwado's test (for

pancreatic disorder)
Katayama's test (for
carbonyl-hemoglobin)
Kelling's test (for lactic
acid in the stomach)
Kerner's test (for
creatinine)
kidney transplant
Killian's test (for
carbohydrate tolerance)
Kinberg's test (for liver
function)
Klimow's test (for blood
in urine)
Knapp's test (for glucose
in urine)
Kober test (qualitative
analysis for estrogens)
Kobert's test
(for hemoglobin)
Krokiewicz's test (for bile
pigment in urine)
Kveim test (for sarcoidosis)

KTP potassium, titanium,
phosphate
KTS Klippel-Trenaunay
syndrome
KTU kidney transplant unit
KTWS Klippel-Trenaunay-Weber
syndrome
KUB kidney ultrasound biopsy
kidney, ureter and bladder
KUF kidney ultrafiltration rate
KUS kidney, ureter and spleen
KV killed vaccine
kraurosis vulvae
kV kilovolt
kv kilovolt
KVE Kaposi's varicelliform
eruption

KVO keep vein open
KW Keith-Wagener
(retinopathy
classification)
Kimmelstiel-Wilson
syndrome (intercapillary
glomerulosclerosis)
K-wire Kirschner wire

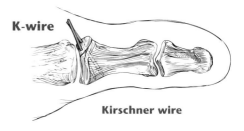

K-wire

Kirschner wire

kW kilowatt
kw kilowatt
KWB Koch-Weeks bacillus
(*Haemophilus aegyptius*)
Keith-Wagener-Barker
(classification)
KWF Kirschner wire fixation
kW-hr kilowatt-hour
KWIC keyword in context (index)
K-wire Kirschner wire
KWL Kimmelstiel-Wilson Lesion
(at periphery of
glomerular tufts)
KWOC keyword out of context
(index)
KWS Kimmelstiel-Wilson
syndrome
kx crystallography unit
Kyph kyphosis
KZ ketoconazole
(broad-spectrum
antifungal agent)

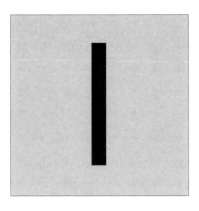

L   coefficient of induction
Lactobacillus (bacteria
  found widely in the
  human mouth, vagina,
  and intestinal tract)
lambda
lambert
latex
Latin
left
Legionella
length
lente insulin
leptin
lethal
leucine
leukocyte
lewisite
lidocaine (anesthetic,
  analgesic, sedative and
  anticonvulsant drug)
ligament
light
light chain
lingual
liter
liver
lumbar
lumbar vertebra
lumen
lung
lymph
lymphocyte
lysosome

l   left
length
lethal
ligament
liter
long
lung

L1 first lumbar spinal nerve
first lumbar vertebra

L2 second lumbar spinal
    nerve
second lumbar vertebra

L/2 lower half

L3 third lumbar spinal nerve
third lumbar vertebra

L/3 lower third

L4 fourth lumbar spinal nerve
fourth lumbar vertebra

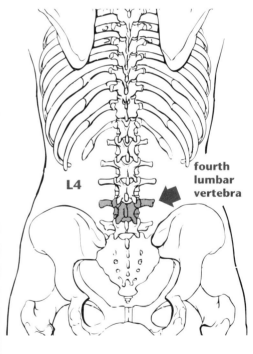

L/4 lower fourth

L5 fifth lumbar spinal nerve
fifth lumbar vertebra

L/5 lower fifth

l. *ligamentum* [Latin]
ligament

LA	lactic acid
	lactic acidosis
	laryngeal atresia
	late antigen
	latex agglutination (test)
	latex allergy
	left arm
	left atrium
	left auricle
	Legionella antigens
	lenticular astigmatism (astigmatism due to irregularity of lens)
	leucinamide
	leukemia antigen
	levator ani (muscle)
	linea alba
	linea aspera
	linoleic acid
	linolenic acid
	Lisfranc amputation
	lobar pneumonia
	local anesthesia
	locomotor ataxia
	long acting
	low anxiety
	Ludwig's angina
	lunula
	lupus anticoagulant
	Lyme arthritis (Lyme disease; recurrent multisystemic disorder caused by the spirochete *Borrella burgdorferi*, transmitted by the tick *Ixodes dammini*)
	lymphadenectomy (lymph node excision)
L & A	light and accommodation (reaction of the pupil)
	living and active
LA50	lethal area (area of the body burned resulting in 50% of patient death)
La	lanthanum (rare metallic element)
LAA	leukemia-associated antigen

	lupus anticoagulant antigen
	lymphocyte activating antigens
LAAM	levo-alpha-acetylmethadol (Orlaam, a long-acting methadone)
LAAO	L-amino acid oxidase
LAB	lower airway burns
lab	laboratory
LAC	laceration
	lactic acid
	lactose (milk sugar)
	long-arm cast (extends from wrist to axilla)
	lung adenocarcinoma cell
	lupus anticoagulant
Lac	lactose (milk sugar)
lac	laceration
LACN	lateral antebrachial cutaneous nerve
lacr	lacrimal
lact	lactate
LAD	lactic acid dehydrogenase
	language acquisition device
	left anterior descending (branch of left coronary artery)
	leukocyte adhesion deficiency
	look-alike drugs
	lymphocyte-activating determinant
LADA	left anterior descending (coronary) artery
LADCA	left anterior descending coronary artery
LADH	lactic acid dehydrogenase
LAE	left atrial enlargement
laev.	*laevus* [Latin] left
LAF	leukocyte-activating factor
	lymphocyte-activating factor
LAG	lymphangiogram
LAH	lactalbumin hydrolysate
	left atrial hypertrophy
	lithium, aluminum, hydroxide

LAHB   left anterior hemiblock
LAHV   leukocyte-associated herpes
           virus
LAISK laser-assisted *in situ*
           keratomileusis (corneal
           procedure for vision
           correction)
LAIT   latex agglutination-
           inhibition test
LAK   lymphocyte-activated
           killer (cells)
           lymphokine-activated
           killer (cells)
LAK cells lymphokine-activated
           killer cells
LAL   left axillary line
           lysosomal acid lipase
LAM   late ambulatory
           monitoring
           left atrial myxoma
           levator ani muscle
           lymphangio
           leiomyomatosis
Lam   laminectomy
           laminogram
LAMA   laser-assisted
           microanastomosis
LAMB syndrome
           lentigines, atrial myxoma,
           mucocutaneous myxomas
           and blue nevi syndrome
LAMI   laminectomy
           laminotomy
LAMMA laser microprobe
           mass analyzer
LA MYX left atrial myxoma
LANC   long-arm navicular cast
LAO   left anterior oblique (view)
LAOF   longitudinal arch of foot
LAP   laparoscopy
           laparotomy
           left atrial pressure
           leucine aminopeptidase
           leukocyte adhesion
           stimulator
           leukocyte alkaline
           phosphatase
           low atmospheric pressure
           lyophilized anterior

           pituitary tissue
Lap Chole
           laparoscopic
           cholecystectomy
LAPMS long arm posterior
           molded splint
LAPSE long-term ambulatory
           physiologic surveillance
LAR   laryngology
           late asthma reaction
lar   larynx
laryn laryngitis
LAS   lateral amyotrophic sclerosis
           laxative abuse syndrome
           leucine acetylsalicylate
           lysine acetylsalicylate
           long-arm splint
           low Apgar score
           lower abdominal surgery
           lupus anticoagulant
           syndrome
           lymphadenopathy
           syndrome
LASE   laser-assisted spinal
           endoscopy
LASER light amplifiction by
           stimulated emission
           of radiation
LASH   left anterosuperior
           hemiblock
LASIK laser-assisted *in situ*
           keratomileusis (a corneal
           procedure for vision
           correction)
L-ASP L-asparaginase
           (chemotherapy)
LASS   labile aggregating-
           stimulating substance
LAT   latex agglutination test
           (fixation test)
           left atrial thrombus
lat   latent
           lateral
           latex
lat men lateral meniscectomy
LATS   long-acting thyroid
           stimulator
LATS-P long-acting thyroid
           stimulator-protector

LAUP	laser-assisted uvulopalatoplasty (to help alleviate snoring)
LAV	AIDS virus [French] lymphadenopathy-associated virus
LAVV	left atrioventricular valve
lax	laxative
LB	large bowel
	left breast
	left buttock
	lipid body
	live birth
	liver biopsy
	lung biopsy
lb.	*libra* [Latin] pound
LBA	left brachial artery
	linebacker's arm
LBAT	leukocyte bactericidal assay test
LBB	left breast biopsy
	left bundle branch
LBBB	left bundle branch block
LBC	large-bore catheter
LBCD	left border of cardiac dullness
LBCV	left brachiocephalic vein
LBD	lamellar body density (count)
	large bile duct
LBH	length, breadth and height
LBI	live-born infant
	low back injury
	low serum-bound iron
LBL	lymphoblastic lymphoma
LBM	lean body mass
	loose bowel movement
LBO	large bowel obstruction
LBP	low back pain
	low blood pressure
LBPS	low back pain syndrome
LBR	labor room
LBRF	louse-borne relapsing fever
LBS	low back syndrome
LBT	low back tenderness
L. bulgaricus	*Lactobacillus bulgaricus* (the homofermentative

	bacteria that produces Bulgarian milk)
LBV	left brachial vein
LBW	low birth weight (infant)
LBWI	low birth weight infant
LC	Laënnec's cirrhosis (atrophic cirrhosis of the liver with scarring)
	lamina cribrosa
	laparoscopic cholecystectomy
	lateral canthus
	leg cramp
	leukocyte count
	Leydig cell
	Library of Congress
	lidocaine (an anesthetic, analgesic, anticonvulsant, sedative and cardiac depressant drug)
	Lieberkühn's crypt
	life care
	light chain
	lipid cytosomes
	lipocalins
	liquid chromatography
	liver cancer
	liver cirrhosis
	living child
	living children
	low calorie
	lung cancer
L & C	laxatives and cathartics
LC₅₀ LC_{50}	median lethal concentration
LCA	lacrimal canaliculus atresia
	laser coronary angioplasty
	left coronary artery
	leukocyte common antigen
	lymphocyte chemotactic activity
LCa	lung cancer
LCAR	late cutaneous anaphylactic reaction
LCAT	latex cryptococcal agglutination test
	lecithin-cholesterol acyltransferase
LCC	laparoscpic

cholecystectomy
large cell carcinoma
life-care community
liver cell carcinoma

LCCA left circumflex
coronary artery
left common carotid artery

LCCN Library of Congress card
number

LCCS low cervical cesarean
section

LCD left crus of diaphragm
light-chain deposition
liquid crystal diode
liquid crystal display
liquor carbonis dertergens
(coal tar solution)
lobster-claw deformity
(abnormal cleft
between the central
metacarpal bones)
low calorie diet

LCDD light-chain deposition
disease

LCE legal counsel for
the elderly

LCF left circumflex (branch
of left coronary artery)

LCFA long-chain fatty acids

LCFU leukocyte colony-
forming unit

LCG Langerhans cell
granulomatosis

LCGL large-cell granulocytic

LCA

left
coronary
artery

leukemia

LCGU lesser curve gastric ulcer
local cerebral glucose
utilization

LCH Langerhans cell histiocytosis

L chain light chain

LCI local cerebral ischemia

LCIS lobular carcinoma *in situ*

LCL large cell carcinoma
lateral capsular ligament
lateral (fibular)
collateral ligament
lumbocostal ligament
lymphocytic leukemia
lymphocytic
lymphosarcoma

LCLC large cell lung carcinoma

LCM large coloboma of macula
latent cardiomyopathy
left costal margin
lymphocytic
choriomeningitis (virus)

LCMG long-chain monoglyceride

LCMv lymphocytic
choriomeningitis virus

LCO kow cardiac output

LCP leukocytopoiesis
long-chain polyunsaturated
(fatty acid)

LCPD Legg-Calvé-Perthes disease

LCR late cutaneous reaction
ligase chain reaction

LCS lateral crural steal
liquid chemical
sterilization
low continuous suction

LCSFP low cerebrospinal
fluid pressure

LCSW licensed clinical
social worker

LCT Leydig cell tumor
liquid crystal thermogram
long-chain triglyceride
lymphocytotoxin

LCTA lymphocytotoxic antibody

LCV leucovorin (folinic acid)
leukocytoclastic vasculitis

LCX left circumflex
(coronary) artery

LD	labyrinthine dysfunction
	lactase deficiency
	lactate dehydrogenase
	lactic dehydrogenase
	last dose
	learning disability
	learning disorder
	Legionnaires' disease (a life-threatening disease caused by the gram-negative bacillus *Legionella pneumophila*)
	Leigh's disease (subacute necrotizing encephalomyelopathy)
	lethal dose
	leukodystrophy
	levodopa
	linguodistal (tooth surfaces)
	lipodystrophy
	Lisfranc dislocation
	living donor
	loading dose
	low density
	low dosage
	Lyme disease (Lyme arthritis; recurrent multisystemic disorder caused by the spirochete *Borrella burgdorferi*, transmitted by the tick *Ixodes dammini*)

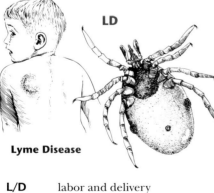

Lyme Disease

L/D	labor and delivery
L & D	labor and delivery
LD50	median lethal dose (dose

	required to kill half of subject animals)
LD100	invariably lethal dose (dose required to kill all of the subject animals)
LDA	left dorso-anterior (fetal position)
	lymphocyte-dependent antibody
LDAC	low-dose cytosine arabinoside
LDAR	latex direct agglutination reaction
LDAT	low dosage antimicrobial therapy
LDB	Legionnaire's disease bacteria
LD & B	Lyme disease and babesiosis
LDC	lysine decarboxylase
LDCI	low-dose continuous infusion
LDD	lactate dehydrogenase deficiency
	laser disk decompression
	low-dopa dyskinesias
	lumbar disk disease
LDDST	low-dose dexamethasone test
LDE	low-dose estrogen
	low-dose exposure
LDE & P	low-dose estrogen and progesterone
LDF	laser Doppler fluxometry
LDG	lingual developmental groove
LDH	lactate dehydrogenase deficiency (type XI glycogenosis)
LDH A	lactic dehydrogenase A
LDH B	lactic dehydrogenase B
LDH C	lactic dehydrogenase C
LDHK	lactic dehydrogenase K
	lactic acid dehydrogenase
	lactic dehydrogenase
	low-dose hydrochlorothiazide
	lumbar disk herniation
LDIH	left direct inguinal hernia

LDIR	low-dose ionizing radiation
LDL	loudness discomfort level
	low-density lipoprotein
	(densities of
	1.006–1.019 g/ml)
LDL-C	low-density lipoprotein
	cholesterol
LDLP	low-density lipoprotein
LDM	latissimus dorsi muscle
L. donovani	
	Leishmania donovani
	(causes kala azar)
L-dopa	L-dihydroxyphenylalanine
	levodopa
LDP	left dorsoposterior
	(fetal position)
LDR	labor, delivery, and
	recovery (room)
LDS	late dumping syndrome
	Lucey-Driscoll syndrome
LDT	left dorsotransverse
	(fetal position)
LDTs	liver-dwelling trematodes
	(*Fasciola hepatica*)
	lung-dwelling trematodes
	(*Paragonimus westermani*)
LDUB	long double upright brace
LDV	lactic dehydrogenase virus
	laser Doppler velocimeter
	laser Doppler velocimetry
LE	laryngeal edema
	lazy eye (amblyopia; poor
	vision in an eye that did
	not develop normal sight
	during early childhood)
	left ear
	left eye
	leukocyte esterase
	life expectancy
	lower extremity
	low exposure
	lupus erythematosus
	lysosomal enzyme
LE-I	lymphedema, type I
LE-II	lymphedema, type II
LEA	lower extremity
	amputation
	lumbar epidural anesthesia
LEAP	lower extremity

	amputation protocol
LEC	lateral epicondyle
	lateral epicondylitis
	(tennis elbow)
	leukoencephalitis
LECCE	left extracapsular cataract
	extraction
LE cell	lupus erythematosus cell
LECH	lateral epicondyle
	of humerus
LED	lupus erythematosus
	disseminatus
LEDs	light-emitting diodes
LEE	last eye examination
LEEP	left end-expiratory
	pressure
	loop electrosurgical
	excision procedure
LEF	lupus erythematosus factor
LEH	liposome-encapsulated
	hemoglobin
LeIF	leukocyte interferon
leio	leiomyoma
LEL	lowest effect level
LEM	light emission microscopy

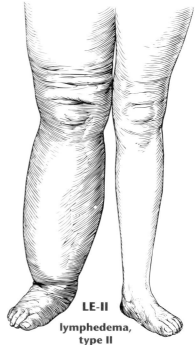

LE-II
**lymphedema,
type II**

LEMS   Lambert-Eaton myasthenic
             syndrome
lenit.   *leniter* [Latin] gently
LEOPARD
             lentigines, ECG
             abnormalities, ocular
             hypertelorism,
             pulmonary stenosis,
             abnormalities of
             genitalia, retarded
             growth, and
             sensorineural deafness
             (syndrome)
LEP   lipoprotein electrophoresis
LER   lysozomal enzyme release
LES   Lambert-Eaton syndrome
             lower esophageal sphincter
             lupus erythematosus
             systemic
les   lesion
LESP   lower esophageal sphincter
             pressure
LET   linear energy transfer
LETD   lowest effective toxic dose
LETS   large extenal
             transformation-sensitivity
LEU   leukocyte equivalent unit
Leu   leucine (an essential
             amino acid)
leuk   leukemia
levit.   *leviter* [Latin] lightly
l/ex   lower extremity
LF   lactoferrin (iron
             binding protein)
             laryngofissure
             Lassa fever
             lethal factor
             leukotactic factor
             ligamenta flava
             Lisfranc fracture
             liver fluke (*Fasciola
             hepatica*)
             low fat (diet)
             low forceps
             low frequency
             lung fluke (*Paragonimus
             westermani*)
lf   low frequency
LFA   lavage fluid analysis

left femoral artery
left frontoanterior
  (fetal position)
leukotactic factor activity
Lupus Foundation of
  America
low friction arthroplasty
lymphocyte function-
  associated antigen
LFA-1   leukocyte function-
             associated antigen 1
LFA-2   leukocyte function-
             associated antigen 2
LFA-3   leukocyte function-
             associated antigen 3
LFC   lateral femoral condyle
             left flexure of colon
             low fat and cholesterol
             (diet)
LFD   lactose-free diet
             lateral facial dysplasia
             least fatal dose of a toxin
             low fat diet
             low fiber diet
             low forceps delivery
LFF   LeFort fracture
LFH   left femoral hernia
LFJ   lumbar facet joints
LFL   left frontolateral
             (fetal position)
LFN   lactoferrin (iron-binding
             protein)
LFP   left frontoposterior
             (fetal position)
LFPPV   low frequency positive-
             pressure ventilation
LFR   lymphoid follicular
             reticulosis
LFS   lateral facet syndrome
             Li-Fraumeni syndrome
             Lignac-Fanconi syndrome
             long face syndrome
LFT   latex fixation test
             latex flocculation test
             left frontotransverse
             (fetal position)
             liver-function test
LFV   Lassa fever virus
LFx   linear fracture

LG	large	**LHBV**	left heart blood volume
	laryngectomy	**LHC**	Langerhans cell
	lateral geniculate		histiocytosis
	(nucleus)		left heart catheterization
	linguogingival		left hypochondrium
	(tooth surfaces)	**LHE**	lateral humeral
lg	large		epicondylitis
LGA	large for gestational age		(tennis elbow)
	left gastric artery		lateral humeral
LGB	lateral geniculate body		epicondylalgia
LGC	laboratory-grown cartilage	**LHF**	left heart failure
LGCSP	lateral gray column of		luteinizing hormone-
	spinal cord		releasing factor
LGD	Lou Gehrig disease	**LHL**	left hepatic lobe
	(amyotrophic lateral	**LHON**	Leber's hereditary optic
	sclerosis)		neuropathy
LDG	low-grade disease	**LHP**	left hemiparesis
LGF	low-grade fever	**LHPT**	loculated
LGH	lactogenic hormone		hydropneumothorax
LGI	large glucagon	**LHR**	leukocyte histamine
	immunoreactivity		release (test)
	lower gastrointestinal	**LHRF**	luteinizing hormone-
LGL	large granular leukocyte		releasing factor
	large granular lymphocyte		(gonadorelin)
	(null cells)	**LH-RH**	luteinizing hormone-
	Lown-Ganong-Levine		releasing hormone
	(syndrome)	**LHSC**	lateral horn of spinal cord
LGM	lymphogranuloma	**LHSV**	laparoscopic highly
LGMD	limb-girdle muscular		selective vagotomy
	dystrophy	**LHT**	left hypertropia
LGN	lobular glomerulonephritis	**LHV**	lymphotropic human
	(membranoproliferative		herpes virus
	glomerulonephritis)	**LI**	labeling index
LGT	late generalized tuberculosis		lactose intolerance
lgth	length		large intestine
LGV	large granular vesicle		laser iridotomy
	lymphogranuloma		linguoincisal
	venereum		(tooth surfaces)
LgX	lymphogranulomatosis X		liver infarct
LH	lanugo hair		low impulsiveness
	laparoscopic	**Li**	lithium (metallic element)
	herniorrhaphy	**LIA**	Laser Institute of America
	left hand		leukemia-associated
	left hemisphere (of brain)		inhibiting activity
	left hyperphoria		lymphocyte-induced
	lidocaine hydrochloride		angiogenesis
	(Xylocaine)	**LIB**	left in bottle
	luteinizing hormone	**LIBC**	latent iron-binding
L & H	laxity and hypermobility		capacity

LIC   left iliac crest
left internal carotid
(artery)
limiting isorrheic
concentration
LICA   left internal carotid artery
LICCE   left intracapsular cataract
extraction
LICH   lobar intracranial
hemorrhage
LICM   left intercostal margin
LICS   left intercostal space
ID   lymphocytic infiltrative
disease
Lido   lidocaine (an anesthetic,
analgesic, sedative, and
anticonvulsant drug)
LIF   laser induced fluorescence
left iliac fossa
left index finger
leukemic-inhibiting factor
leukocyte-inhibiting factor
leukocytosis-inducing
factor
LIFT   lymphocyte
immunofluorescence test
LIG   ligament
lig   ligation
lig.   *ligamentum* [Latin]
ligament
ligg   ligature
LIH   left inguinal hernia
leucine-induced
hypoglycemia
leukocyte inhibiting factor
LIHA   low impulsiveness,
high anxiety
LIJ   left internal jugular (vein)
LILA   low impulsiveness,
low anxiety
LIMA   left internal mammary
artery (left internal
thoracic artery)
LINUS   Local Independently
Nucleated Units of
Structure (to honor
Linus Pauling)
LIO   laser indirect
ophthalmoscope

left interior oblique
(radiologic view)
LIP   lithium-induced polydipsia
lymphocytic interstitial
pneumonia
lymphocytic interstitial
pneumonitis
lymphoid interstitial
pneumonia
LIQ   lower inner quadrant
liq   liquid
liq pt   liquid pint
LIS   left intercostal space
locked-in syndrome
low intermittent suction
(during surgery)
LITH   lithotomy
Lith   lithium
litho   lithotripsy
liv   live
LivB   live birth
LJ   lockjaw (tetanus)
LJM   limited joint mobility
LJP   localized juvenile
periodontitis
LK   left kidney
lymphokine (a hormone-
like factor produced by
sensitized lymphocytes
when they come in
contact with the antigen
to which they were
sensitized)
LKC   latch key child
latch key children
Lkc   leukocyte
Lkcs   leukocytes
LKM   liver-kidney microsomes
LK   lamellar keratoplasty
LKS   liver, kidneys and spleen
LL   large lymphocyte
lateral lemniscus
left leg
left lung
lepromatous leprosy
long leg (brace)
lower lid (of eye)
lower limb
lower lip

lower lobe
lymphoblastic lymphoma
lymphoid leukemia
lysolecithin

I. I. *lapus linguae* [Latin] slip of the tongue

LLB long-leg brace

LLC laparoscopic laser cholecystectomy
long leg cast (extends from upper thigh to toes)

LLCC long-leg cylinder cast

LLB long leg brace

LLD late-life depression
leg length discrepancy
lipid-lowering drug

LLE left lower extremity
Little League elbow

LLES lower limb extensor spasticity

LLETZ large loop excision of transitional zone

LLF lower limb fracture

LLL left liver lobe
left long leg (brace)
left lower leg
left lower lid (of eye)
left lower limb
left lower lobe (of lung)

LLLE low-level lead exposure

LLMS longitudinal layer of muscles of stomach

LLN lower limit of normal

LLOs Legionella-like organisms

LLP late luteal phase

LLR left lateral rectus (eye muscle)

LLRW low-level radioactive waste

LLQ left lower quadrant (of abdomen)

LLS later-life sexuality
lazy leukocyte syndrome
Little League shoulder
long-leg splint

LLSB lower left sternal border

LLT lipid-lowering therapy
lysolecithin (seen in trace amounts in the pancreas)

LLTG left lobe of thyroid gland

LLV lymphatic leukemia virus

LLWC long-leg walking cast (extends from upper thigh to toes with a rubber sole walker)

LLX left lower extremity

LM labia majora
labia minora
Lamaze method
laryngeal mucosa
lateral malleolus
lateral meniscus
left mental
legal medicine
lentigo maligna
licentiate in widwifery
light microscopy
linguomesial (tooth surfaces)
loud murmur

l/min liters per minute

LMA left mentoanterior (fetal position)

L. mactans *Latrodectus mactans* (black widow spider)

LMB left main bronchus
leiomyoblastoma

LMC lipomeningocele
lymphocyte-mediated cytotoxicity

LMCA left middle cerebral artery

LMCL left midclavicular line

LMD local medical doctor

LME left mediolateral episiotomy

LMF leukocyte mobilizing factor
limited motor function
lymphocyte mitogenic factor

LMI leukocyte migration inhibition

LMIF leukocyte migration inhibition factor

L/min liters per minute

LMKJ left meniscus of knee joint

LMLE left medial lateral episiotomy

LMM lentigo maligna melanoma
lumbar motion monitor

LMN	lower motor neuron
LMNL	lower motor neuron lesion
L monocytogenes	
	Listeria monocytogenes
LMP	last menstrual period
	latent membrane protein
	left mentoposterior (fetal position)
	low malignant potential (tumor)
	lumbar puncture
LMR	localized magnetic resonance
	lymphocytic meningoradiculitis
LMS	lateral medullary syndrome
	Laurence-Moon syndrome
	leiomyosarcoma (common sarcoma of the uterus)
	levator muscle of scapula
	levator muscle syndrome
LMT	lateral meniscus tear
	left mentotransverse (fetal position)
LMV	larva migrans visceralis
LMW	low molecular weight
lmwd	low molecular weight dextran
LMW NOD	
	low molecular weight nonoligomeric drug
LN	left nostril
	leukonychia
	lipoid nephrosis
	lobular neoplasia
	low necrosis
	lupus nephritis
	lymph node
LN$_2$	liquid nitrogen
LNB	lumbar nerve block
	lymph node biopsy
LNC	lateral nasal cartilage
LND	lymph node dissection (lymph node excision)
LNE	lymph node enlargement
	lymph node excision
LNKS	low natural killer syndrome
LNM	lymph node metastases

LNMP	last normal menstrual period
LNN	lower nephron nephrosis
LNPF	lymph node permeability factor
LNS	Lesch–Nyhan syndrome (a disorder of purine metabolism and excess uric acid with death usually occurring during childhood due to kidney damage)
LO	lateral oblique (radiologic view)
	left occipital
	linguo-occlusal (tooth surfaces)
Lo	low
LOA	lateral osseous ampulla
	leave of absence
	Leber's optic atrophy
	left anterior oblique (radiologic view)
	left occipito-anterior (fetal position)
	left occiput anterior (fetal position)
	lysis of adhesions
LOB	loss of balance
LOC	laxative of choice
	level of care
	level of consciousness
	local
	loss of consciousness
LOCD	late-onset Alzheimer's disease
loc. dol.	*loco dolenti* [Latin] to the painful spot
lo chol	low cholesterol
LOCM	low osmolality contrast medium
LOF	low output failure
LOFD	low outlet forceps delivery
LOG	lipoxygenase (converts arachidonic acid to HPETE and HETE)
log	logarithm to any base
log$_{10}$	logarithm to base 10
LOH	loop of Henle

loss of heterozygosity
LOHF late-onset hepatic failure
LOI level of injury
limit of impurities
LOL left occipital lateral
(fetal position)
left occipitolateral
(fetal position)
LOM left otitis media
limitation of motion
limitation of movement
low osmolality
contrast media
low osmolar media
LoNa low sodium
long longitudinal
LOP lactosuria of pregnancy
left occipitoposterior
(fetal position)
left occiput posterior
(fetal position)
level of pain
LOPS length of patient stay
LOQ lower outer quadrant
LOR loss of righting (reflex)
Lord lordosis
LOS length of stay
level of significance
lumen of stomach
LOT left occipitotransverse
(fetal position)
left occiput transverse
(fetal position)
lot. *lotio* [Latin] lotion
LOV loss of vision
LOZ lozenge
LP labor pain
lactic peroxidase
laryngopharyngeal
laser printer
latency period
latent period
lead poisoning
lichen planus
light perception
lipid pneumonia
lipoid proteinosis
lipoprotein
loss of privileges

low power
lumbar plexus
lumbar puncture
lung parenchyma
lymphoid plasma
lymphomatoid papulosis
L/P lactate/pyruvate (ratio)
lymphocyte/PMN (ratio)
lymph/plasma (ratio)
Lp lipoprotein
Lp III intermediate lipoproteins
LPA lateral periodontal abscess
latex particle agglutination
(test)
left pulmonary artery
Little People of America
LpA lipoprotein A
L-PAM L-phenylalanine mustard
(melphalan)
LPB lipoprotein B
LPC laser photocoagulation
LPD Legg-Perthes disease
low protein diet
luteal phase defect
lymphoproliferative
disorder
LPDA left posterior descending
(coronary)artery
LPE lipoprotein electrophoresis
LPF lead pipe fracture
lesser palatine foramen
leukocytosis-promoting
factor
localized plaque formation
lower palpebral furrow
low-power field
lymphocytosis-
promoting factor
LPG lipophosphoglycan
LPH left posterior hemiblock
lipotropic hormone
(lipotropin)
low-pressure
hydrocephalus
lumbar puncture headache
(postpuncture headache)
LPHB left posterior hemiblock
LPHS loin pain hematuria
syndrome

LPI   laser peripheral iridectomy
     long process of incus
LPK   liver pyruvate kinase
LPL   lipoprotein lipase
LPM   lateral pterygoid muscle
LPN   licensed practical nurse
LPNA   leucine-p-nitroanilide
L. pneumophilia
     Legionella pneumophilia
      (the causative agent of
      legionnaires' disease)
LPO   left posterior oblique
      (fetal position)
     light perception only
LPP   lateral pterygoid plate
LPPH   late postpartum
      hemorrhage
LPR   late phase reaction
L proj   light projection
LPS   last Papanicolaor smear
     levator pelpebrae
      superior (muscle)
     lipopolysaccharide
      (endotoxin)
LPT   licensed physical therapist
     lipotropin (precursor
      molecule of endorphins,
      enkephalins and
      melanocyte-stimulating
      hormones)
LPV   left pulmonary veins
     lymphotropic papovavirus
Lp-X   lipoprotein X
LQ   longevity quotient
     lowcr quadrant
lq   liquid
LQTS   long (prolonged) QT
      syndrome
LR   laboratory report
     labor room
     lacrimation reflex
     lactated Ringer's (solution)
     latency reaction
     light reaction
     light reflex
     low renin
L & R   left and right
Lr   lawrencium
      (chemical element)

LRA   left radial artery
     left renal artery
     life resuscitation
      ambulance
LRD   living-related donor
     living-renal donor
     low-residue diet
LRDT   living-related donor
      transplant
LRE   least restrictive
      environment
     lymphoreticuloendoth-
      eliosis
L. redusa *Loxesceles redusa* (brown
      recluse spider)
LRF   liver residue factor
     luteinizing hormone
      releasing factor
LRH   luteinizing hormone-
      releasing hormone
LRI   lower respiratory infection
LRM   left radical mastectomy
LRMP   last regular menstrual
      period
LRN   lateral reticular nucleus
LRP   LDL receptor-related
      protein
     long-range planning
LRQ   lower right quadrant
LRR   labor room
     labyrinthine righting reflex
LRS   lactated Ringer's solution
LRs   likelihood ratios
LRSB   low right sternal border
LRT   local radiation thcrapy
     lower respiratory tract
     lymphoreticular tissue
LRTD   living relative
      transplant donor
LRTI   lower respiratory
      tract infection
LRV   left renal vein
LS   lactiferous sinus
     Ladin's sign
     Laënnec's sign
     Landry's syndrome (acute
      febrile polyneuritis)
     Langoria's sign
     laparoscopic

Larcher's sign
laser surgery
latent syphilis
late syphilis
Laugier's sign
lecithin supplements
left sacral
left side
Leichtenstern's sign
leiomyosarcoma
length of stay
Lennox syndrome
Lenz's syndrome
leopard syndrome
Leredde's syndrome
Leriche's syndrome
Lermoyez's syndrome
Levasseur's sign
levator syndrome
Libman's sign
lichen sclerosis
lichen simplex
Liddle's syndrome
ligature sign
light sleep
limbic system
liver scan
Livierato's sign
Löeffler's syndrome
Lombardi's sign
low salt
low sodium
Lucas' sign
Ludloff's sign
lumbar spine
lumbosacral
Lutembacher's syndrome
lymphosarcoma

L/S lecithin/sphingomyelin
(amniotic fluid ratio)

LSA left sacroanterior
(fetal position)
left subclavian artery
Leukemia Society of
America
lichen sclerosus atrophicus
low serum albumin
lumbosacral agenesis
lymphosarcoma

LSANA leukocyte-specific
antinuclear antibody

LSA/RCC lymphosarcoma –
reticulum-cell carcinoma

LSB left sternal border
lumbar spinal block
lumbar sympathetic block

LS BMD lumbar spine bone
mineral density

LSC late systolic click
lichen simplex chronicus
liquid scintillation counter
liquid-solid
chromatography

LSc local scleroderma

LScA left scapuloanterior
(fetal position)

LSCC lateral (horizontal)
semicircular canal

LSCL lymphosarcoma cell
leukemia

LScP left scapuloposterior
(fetal position)

LSCS lower segment cesarean
section
left subclavian artery

LSCV left subclavian vein

LSD least significant difference
Letterer-Siwe disease
life-sustaining device
lipid storage disease
low salt diet
low sodium diet
lysergic acid diethylamide
(continued intake can
precipitate a persistent
psychotic state)
lysosomal storage disease

LSD II lysosomal storage disease
(Pompe disease)

LSE low-set ear

LSF lesser sciatic foramen
low saturated fat

LSFA low saturated fatty acid

LSG low serum globulins

LSH lutein-stimulating
hormone
lymphocyte-stimulating
hormone

LSK   liver, spleen, and kidneys
LSL   left sacrolateral
              (fetal position)
              left short leg (brace)
              lymphosarcoma leukemia
LSM   laser scanning microscopy
              late systolic murmur
              levator scapulae muscle
              lipid storage myopathy
LSN   lesser sciatic notch
LSO   left salpingo-ophorectomy
              lumbosacral orthosis
LSP   left sacroposterior
              (fetal position)
              lumbosacral plexus
LSp   life span
L-spine lumbar spine
LSR   lecithin-sphingomyelin
              ratio (in amniotic fluid)
              left superior rectus
L/S ratio lecithin/sphingomyelin
              ratio
LSRI   lumbosacral root injury
LSS   laparoscopic surgery
              lateral spinal stenosis
              limb-salvage surgery
              lumbar spinal stenosis
LSSA   lipid-soluble secondary
              antioxidant
LS spine lumbosacral spine
LST   left sacrotransverse
              (fetal position)
LSTL   laparoscopic tubal ligation
LSU   life support unit
LSV   lateral sacral vein
              left sinus of Valsalva
              left subclavian vein
LT   heat-labile
              Lamaze technique
              laser therapy
              left
              less than
              leukotridene
              Levin tube
              levothyroxine
              light therapy
              locum tenens
              long term
              low temperature

              low tracheostomy
              lung transplantation
              lumbar triangle
              (Petit's triangle)
              lymphotoxin
lt   left
LTA   leisure-time activity
              leukotriene A
              lidocaine topical spray
              lipoteichoic acid
              lymphocyte-transforming
              activity
LTA$_4$ leukotriene A$_4$
LTB   laryngotracheobronchitis
              (croup)
              lead-time bias
              length-time bias
              leukotriene B
LTB4   leukotriene B4
LTBU4u   leukotriene BU4u
LTC   leukotriene C
              long-term care
              long-term complications
              long-term consequences
              low transverse cervical
LTC4   leukotriene C$_4$
LTCF   long term care facility
LTCI   long-term care insurance
LTCS   low transverse
              Cesarean section
LTCU4u   leukotriene CU4u
LTD   leukotriene D
LTDU4u   leukotriene DU4u
LTE   leukotriene E
              long-term effect
LTF   lactotransferrin
              lymphocyte
              transforming factor
LTG   long-term goal
              low-tension glaucoma
LTH   luteotropic hormone
              (prolactin)
LTL   laparoscopic tubal
              (uterine) ligation
LTM   long-term management
              long-term memory (for an
              indefinite period of time)
LTP   lateral tibial plateau
              long-term problem

long-term potentiation
L-tryptophan
LTPA leisure-time physical activity
LTRs long terminal repeats
LTS lidocaine topical spray
long-term survivors
low-threshold spike
LTT lactose tolerance test
long-term treatment
lymphocyte transformation
test
LTTPBA late third trimester partial
birth abortion
LTUI low transverse uterine
incision
LTVC long-term venous catheter
LU left upper
left ureter
L & U lower and upper
Lu lutetium (chemical
element)
LUCE low urinary calcium
excretion
LUE left upper extremity
Lues I primary syphilis
Lues II secondary syphilis
Lues III tertiary syphilis
LUF luteinized unruptured
follicle
LUFS luteinizing unruptured
follicle syndrome
LUL left upper lid (of eye)
left upper lobe (of lung)
lumb lumbar
left ureteral orifice
LUMD lowest usual
maintenance dose
LUOQ left upper outer quadrant
LUQ left upper quadrant
(of abdomen)
LUS laparoscopic ultrasound
lower uterine segment
LUT lower urinary tract
LUTD lower urinary tract
dysfunction (commonly
caused by benign
prostatic hyperplasia)
LV laryngeal vestibule
Latino virus
lateral ventricle (of brain)

left ventricle (of heart)

leucovorin
(antitumor agent)
leukemia virus
live vaccine
live virus
lumbar vertebrae
lung volume
Lv leave
leukovorin
LVA left ventricular aneurysm
left vertebral artery
LVAD left ventricular assist device
L-VAM leuprolide acetate +
vinblastine + Adriamycin
(doxorubicin) +
mitomycin (combination
chemotherapy)
LVB lomustine + vindesine +
bleomycin sulfate
(combination
chemotherapy)
LVC laser vision correction
LVCH last value carried forward
LVCS low vertical Cesarean
section
LVD left ventricular dysfunction
LVDP left ventricular

	diastolic pressure
LVDV	left ventricular diastolic volume
LVE	left ventricular enlargement
LVED	left ventricular end-diastole
LVEDD	left ventricular end-diastolic dimension
LVEDP	left ventricular end-diastolic pressure
LVEDV	left ventricular end-diastolic volume
LVEF	left ventricular ejection fraction
LVEP	left ventricular end pressure
LVET	left ventricular ejection time
LVF	left ventricular failure
LVFP	left ventricular filling pressure
LVFU	leucovorin + fluorouracil (combination chemotherapy)
LVG	left ventriculography lesser vestibular gland
LVH	left ventricular hypertrophy
LVHWR	lateral ventricle hemispheric width ratio
LVI	left/ventricular insufficiency
LVL	left vastus lateralis (muscle)
LVM	lateral vastus muscle left ventricular mass
LVN	licensed visiting nurse licensed vocational nurse
LVOT	left ventricular outflow tract
LVOTO	left ventricular outflow tract obstruction
LVP	left ventricular pressure levator veli

	palatini (muscle)
LVPW	left ventricular posterior wall
LVS	left ventricular strain
LVSO	left ventricular systolic output
LVSP	left ventricular systolic pressure
LVSV	left ventricular stroke volume
LVV	left ventricular volume Le Veen valve
LVW	left ventricular wall left ventricular work
LVWI	left ventricular work index
LVWT	left ventricular wall thickness
LW	lacerating wound living will
L & W	living and well
LWOT	left without therapy left without treatment
LWS	lavage with saline
LX	local irradiation lower extremity
Lx	latex
lx	larynx lux (metric unit of illumination)
LXC	laxative of choice
LXT	left exotropia
LYG	lymphomatoid granulomatosis
lym	lymphocyte
lymphs	lymphocytes
Lys	lysine (essential amino acid)
lytes	electrolytes
Lx	laboratory examination
Lyx	lyxose (an aldopentose)
lzm	lysozyme (an enzyme that catalyzes the breakdown of some bacterial cell walls)

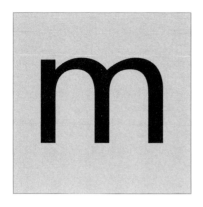

M	macerate
	macrophage
	male
	malignant
	mandible

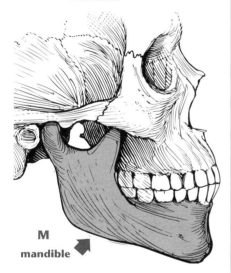

M
mandible

marijuana (cannabis)
married
masculine
mass
massage
maternal
mature
maxilla
maximum
mean
measles (rubeola)

meatus
medial
median
medical
Medicare
mega (prefix denoting decimal factor 10^6)
meiosis
membrane
memory
meningeal
mesial
metabolite
metastases
metatarsus
meter
methionine
methyl
microvillus
minimum
minute
mitochondrion
mitosis
mixture
M line
modiolus
mol
molar
molarity
mole
molecule
month
morgan
morphine
mother
mouth
mucus
multipara
murmur

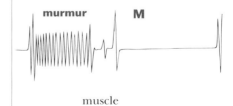

murmur   M

muscle
myopia

M.   *misce* [Latin] mix

M₁   first mitral (left
     atrioventricular)
     valve sound
     mitral valve closure
M₂   second mitral (left
     atrioventricular)
     valve sound
M-2   Oncovin (vincristine) +
     BCNU (carmustine) +
     Cytoxan
     (cyclophosphamide) +
     melphalan + prednisone
     (combination
     chemotherapy)
M²   square meter
M/3   middle third
m   married
     mass
     median
     meter(s)
     milli (prefix denoting
     decimal factor 10^{-3})
     molality
     molar
     motile
     murmur
m   mass
     molal
m.   *misce* [Latin] mix
     musculus [Latin] muscle
MA   malignant astrocytoma
     (glioblastoma)
     masseter (muscle)
     mechanical atherectomy
     medical assistant
     medical audit
     medical authorization
     megaloblastic anemia
     menstrual age
     mental age
     meta-analysis
     metabolic acidosis
     microadenoma
     microaneurysm
     milliampere
     mitochondral antibody
     moderately advanced
     monoclonal antibody
     monomorphic adenoma

     myelinated axon
Ma   male
mA   milliampere
ma   milliampere
MAA   macroaggregated albumin
     melanoma-associated
     antigen
     monoarticular arthritis
Mab   monoclonal antibody
mAb   monoclonal antibody
MABP   mean arterial blood
     pressure
Mabs   monoclonal antibodies
MAC   macrophage
     macula
     maintained anesthesia care
     maximum allowable
     concentration (of
     hazardous substance)
     maximum allowable cost
     (of program)
     membrane-attack complex
     membranous aplasia cutis
     minimum alveolar
     (anesthetic)
     concentration
     minimal antibiotic
     concentration
     monitored anesthesia care
     Mycobacterium avium complex
Mac-1   macrophage-1 glycoprotein
MACC   medical acute care clinic
     methotrexate +Adriamycin
     (doxorubicin) + cyclo-
     phosphamide + CCNU
     (lomustine)
     (combination
     chemotherapy)
MACINH   membrane attack complex
     inhibitor
MACO   mucinous adenocarcinoma
     of ovary
MACOPB   methotrexate +
     Adriamycin
     (doxorubicin) +
     cyclophosphamide +
     Oncovin (vincristine) +
     prednisone + bleomycin
     (combination

chemotherapy)

Macro macrocyte
macrocytosis
MACs mastoid air cells
MACT multiple-agent
chemotherapy
MAD maximal allowable dose
methylandrostenediol
milk-alkali disease
mind-altering drug
minimal average dose
MADA muscle adenylate
deaminase
MADD Mothers Against Drunk
Driving (817) 268-MADD
multiple acyl CoA
dehydrogenation
deficiency
MADS mixed anxiety/depression
syndrome
MADU methylaminodeoxyuridine
MAE moves all extremities
MAEQW moves all extremities
quite well
MAF macrophage-activating
factor (type II interferon)
macrophage agglutinating
factor
MAFA movement-associtated
fetal acceleration
(of heart rate)
MAG myelin-associated
glycoprotein
mag magnesium (metallic
element; its salts are
essential in nutrition)
mag cit magnesium citrate (citrate
of magnesia)
MAggF macrophage agglutination
factor
MAHA microangiopathic
hemolytic anemia
MAHH malignancy-asociated
humoral hypercalcemia
MAI *Mycobacterium avium-*
intracellular
MAID mesna + Adriamycin
(doxorubicin) +
ifosfamide + dacarbazine

(combination
chemotherapy)
MAIDS murine acquired immune
deficiency syndrome
MAL midaxillary line
malig malignant
MALS median arcuate
ligament syndrome
MALT mucosa-associated
lymphoid tissue
MALTL mucosa-associated
lymphoid tissue
lymphoma
MAM methylazomethanol
MAm myopic astigmatism
MAMC mid-arm muscle
circumference
mammo mammogram
MAN malignant acanthosis
nigricans
man. *mane* [Latin] in
the morning
mand mandible
manip manipulation
MANOVA
multivariate analysis
of variance
MAN-6-P mannose-6-phosphate
man. pr. *mane primo* [Latin] early in
the morning
MAO maximal acid output
monoamine oxidase
MAO-A monoamine oxidase,
type A
MAO-B monoamine oxidase,
type B
MAOI monoamine oxidase
inhibitor
MAP maxilla alveolar process
mean airway pressure
mean aortic pressure
mean arterial pressure
megaloblastic anemia of
pregnancy
methyl alcohol poisoning
mitomycin + Adriamycin
(doxorubicin) + Platinol
(cisplatin) (combination
chemotherapy)

monophasic action
potential
multiple antigen peptide
muscle action potential
MAPC migrating action potential
complex
mar marrow
MARKS mitogen-activated
protein kinases
MAS malabsorption syndrome
McCune-Albright
syndrome (Albright's
disease; fibrous dysplasia)
meconium aspiration
syndrome
milk-alkali syndrome
(kidney failure,alkalosis
and hypercalcemia)
Morgagni-Adams-Stokes
syndrome (Adams-Stokes
disease)
mas masculine
MASD menstrual-associated
sleep disorder
MASER microwave amplification by
stimulated emission of
radiation
MASH Mobile Army Surgical
Hospital
MASS Morgagni-Adams-Stokes
syndrome
MAST medical antishock trausers
(pneumatic antishock
garment)
military antishock trousers
(pneumatic antishock
garment)
mast mastoid
MAT maternity
mean absorption time
microagglutination test
Miller analogy test
multifocal atrial
tachycardia
multiple-agent therapy
MAU microalbuminuria
MAVR maxillary and aortic valve
replacement
max maxillary
maximum
MB mamillary body

menstrual blood
methyl bromide
methylene blue
midbrain
(mesencephalon)
Milwaukee brace

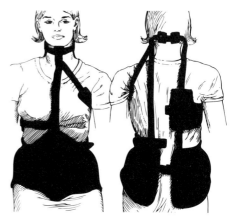

MB Milwaukee brace

mucosal barrier
mucosal bleeding
m.b. *misce bene* [Latin] mix well
Mb megabyte
myoglobin
MBA megaloblastic anemia
mBACOD
methotrexate + bleomycin
+ adriamycin +
cyclophosphamide +
Oncovin +
dexamethasone
(combination
chemoherapy)
MBAR myocardial beta adrenergic
receptor
MBC male breast cancer
maximum bladder capacity
maximum breathing
capacity
metastatic breast cancer
minimum bactericidal
concentration
MBD maple bark disease
marble bone disease

Marchiafava-Bignami
disease
Marie-Bamberger disease
metabolic bone disease
methylene blue dye
Meyer-Betz disease
minimum brain damage
minimum brain
dysfunction
Moeller-Barlow disease
MBE may be elevated
MBF myocardial blood flow
MBG mean blood glucose
MBI maximal blink index
methylene bisphenyl
isocyanate
mycobacterial infection
MBK methyl butyl ketone
MBL Marine Biological
Laboratory
(Woods Hole, MA)
menstrual blood loss
MBM mother's breast milk
MBO mesiobucco-occlusal
(converging
tooth surfaces)
MBO$_2$ oxymyoglobin
MBP major basic protein
malignant bone pain
mean blood pressure
modified Bagshawe
protocol
myelin basic protein
MBPS Münchausen-by-proxy
syndrome
MBT massive blood transfusion
MC macula coloboma
malignant carcinoid
mast cell
mature cataract
maximum concentration
medial canthus
medullary cavity
megalocornea
meibomian cyst
(chalazion)
Meissner's corpuscle
(tactile corpuscle)
melanocytoma

membranous cataract
meningocele
meningococcemia
mental confusion
menstrual cycle
mesenteric cyst
metacarpal
microcephaly
miscarriage
mixed cryoglobulinemia
molluscum contagiosum
monocyte
mucous cell
muscle cramps
myocarditis
myotonia congenita
3-MC 3-methylcholanthrene
M & C morphine and cocaine
mc millicurie
MCA methylcholanthrene
microsurgical
approximator
middle carotid artery
middle cerebral artery
monoclonal antibodies
mucinous cystadenoma
multiple congenital
abnormalities
MCAB monoclonal antibody
MCAT Medical College
Admission Test
Medical College
Aptitude Test
monoclonal antibody
therapy
M. catarrhalis
Moraxella catarrhalis
(bacteria that normally
inhabits the nasal cavity
and nasopharynx,
occasionally causing
respiratory disease and
ear aches)
mCBF mean cerebral blood flow
McB pt McBurney's point (point
on the skin that overlies
the normal position of
the appendix)
MCBR minimum concentration of

bilirubin
MCBs metacarpal bones
MCC mesenchymal cell
concentration
mesenteric chylous cysts
metacentric chromosome

MCC

**metacentric
chromosome**

midstream clean-catch
(urine sample)
mucocutaneous candidiasis
MCCI multichannel cochlear
implant
MCD mad cow disease
(bovine spongiform
encephalopathy) (human
equivalent: Creutzfeldt-
Jakob disease)
medullary collecting
duct (kidney)
medullary cystic disease
metaphyseal
chondrodysplasia
minimal cerebral
dysfunction
minimal change disease
multiple carboxylase
deficiency
MCE multiple cartilaginous
exostoses
myocardial embolism
M cell memory cell
MCES multiple cholesterol
emboli syndrome
MCF macrophage chemotactic
factor
middle cranial fossa
myocardial contraction
force
myocardial fascicles
MCFA medium-chain fatty acid
MCFP mean circulatory
filling pressure

MCFS median cleft face
syndrome
middle cranial fossa
syndrome
MCG middle cervical ganglion
monoclonal gammopathy
(plasma cell dyscrasia)
musculocutaneous graft
mcg microgram
MCGN minimal-change
glomerulonephritis
MCH maternal and child
health service
mean cell hemoglobin
mean corpuscular
hemoglobin
mineralocorticoid
hormone
muscle contraction
headache
myocardial hypertrophy
MCHB Maternal and Child
Health Bureau
MCHC mean cell hemoglobin
concentration
mean corpuscular
hemoglobin
concentration
Missing Children – Help
Centers (813) 623-5437
MCHgb mean corpuscular
hemoglobin
MCHR Medical Committee for
Human Rights
mchr millicurie-hour
(measurement used in
radiation therapy)
MCI mean cardiac index
midcarpal instability
myocardial infarct
myocardial insufficiency
myocardial ischemia
mCi millicurie
MCINS minimal change idiopathic
nephrotic syndrome
MCJ mucocutaneous junction
MCK muscle-specific creatine
kinase
MCKD multicystic kidney disease

MCL	mature corpus luteum
	maximum
	contamination level
	medial collateral ligament
	midclavicular line
MCLNS	mucocutaneous lymph
	node syndrome
MCM	meningococcal meningitis
	metastatic carcinomatous
	meningitis
MCMP	middle constrictor muscle
	of pharynx
MCN	malignant cystic neoplasm
	minimal change
	nephropathy
	musculocutaneous nerve
MCNS	minimal change nephrotic
	syndrome
MCO	multicystic ovary
MCOS	magnesium citrate
	oral solution
MCOs	managed care
	organizations
MCP	managed care physician
	managed care program
	mean carotid pressure
	melphalan +
	cyclophosphamide +
	prednisone (combination
	chemotherapy)
	membrane cofactor
	protein
	metacarpophalangeal
	(joint)
	metatastic carcinoma
	of prostate
	midclavicular plane
	mucin clot prevention
MCP-1	monocyte chemotactic
	protein
MCPA	2-methyl-4-
	chlorophenoxyacetic acid
MCPI	Medical Consumer Price
	Index
MCPJ	metacarpophalangeal joint
MCR	metabolic clearance rate
MCRC	metastatic colorectal
	cancer
MCRD	medullary cystic

	renal disease
MCRI	multifactorial cardiac
	risk index
MCS	malignant carcinoid
	syndrome
	mesocaval shunt
	metachronous seeding
	(metastases arising from a
	secondary neoplasm)
	multi-chemical sensitivity
M-CSF	macrophage colony-
	stimulating factor
	monocyte-macrophage
	colony-stimulating factor
MCSS	multiple chemical
	sensitivity syndrome
MCT	manual cervical traction
	mature cystic teratoma
	mean circulating time
	medium-chain triglyceride
	medullary carcinoma
	of thyroid
	mucin clot test
MCTB	medial calcaneal tubercle
	bursitis
MCTD	Marie-Charcot-Tooth
	disease
	mixed connective
	tissue disease
MCU	maximum care unit
MCUG	micturating
	cystourethrogram
MCV	mean cell volume
	mean clinical value
	mean corpuscular volume
	measles-containing vaccine
	meningococcus vaccine
	middle cardiac vein
	motor conduction velocity
MD	macrodontia
	macula degeneration
	macula densa
	magnesium deficiency
	maintenance dose
	major depression
	malignant disease
	manic-depressive
	maximum dose

mean deviation
Meckel's diverticulum
(an occasional
sacculation of the ileum)

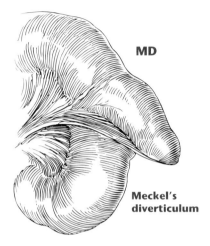

MD

Meckel's diverticulum

medical directive
(living will)
medical doctor
medium dosage
Ménierè's disease
mental deficiency
mental depression
mental disorder
Milroy disease
minimum dose
mitral disease
moderate disability
mnemonic device (scheme
for remembering and
recalling information)
Monteggia dislocation
mood disorder
Mouchet's disease
multiple dose
muscular dystrophy
myotonic dystrophy
Md mendelevium (radioactive
chemical element)
MDA malondialdehyde
mento-dextra anterior [Latin]
right mentoanterior
(fetal position)
methylene draniline

minimal deviation
adenocarcinoma
motor discriminative acuity
Muscular Dystrophy
Association
MD-BD major depression and
bipolar disorder
MDC major diagnostic category
mullerian duct cyst
MDD major depression disorder
male development
disorder
manic depressive disorder
mean daily dose
MDE major depressive episode
mammary duct ectasia
MDF myocardial depressant
factor
MDGF macrophage-derived
growth factor
MDH maleate dehydrogenase
MDI manic depressive illness
metered-dose inhaler
multiple daily injections
MDM medical decision making
mid-diastolic murmur
MDMA 3,4-methylenedioxy-
methamphetamine
(ecstasy; illicit drug)
mdn median
mDNA mitochondrial DNA
MDNB metadinitrobenzene
MDP major duodenal papilla
manic-depressive psychosis
mento-dextra posterior [Latin]
right mentoposterior
(fetal position)
methylene diphosphate
minor duodenal papilla
muramyl dipeptide
muscular dystrophy,
progressive
MDPD maximum daily
permitted dose
MDPI maximum daily
permitted intake
MDQ memory deviation quotient
MDR microbial drug resistance
minimal daily requirement

	multidrug resistance
MDRI	multidrug-resistant infection
MDRT	multidrug-resistant tuberculosis
MDR TB	multidrug-resistant tuberculosis
MDS	maternal deprivation syndrome
	milk drinker's syndrome
	myelodysplastic syndrome
	myocardial-dysplasia syndrome
MDSO	mentally disturbed sex offender
MDT	*mento-dextra transversa* [Latin] right mentotransverse (fetal position)
	multidisciplinary team
	multidrug therapy
MDTP	multidisciplinary treatment plan
MDUO	myocardial disease of unknown origin
MDV	multiple dose vial
MDY	month, date, year
MDZ	midazolam
ME	macular edema
	magnitude estimation
	male escutcheon
	manic episode
	maximal efficacy
	medial episiotomy
	mediastinal emphysema
	Medical Examiner
	medication error
	meningoencephalitis
	microelectrode
	microemboli
	microscopic examination
	middle ear
	multiple embolisms
	multiple exostoses
	myalgic encephalomyelitis
	myoepithelium
M:E	myeloid-erythroid ratio
Me	methyl
MEA	multiple endocrine

	adenomatosis
	multiple endocrine adenopathy
MEA-1	multiple endocrine adenomatosis, type I
MEA-II	multiple endocrine adenomatosis, type II
meas	measure
MEB	Medical Evaluation Board
MeB	methylene blue (methylthionine chloride)
MEC	medial epicondyle
	median effective concentration
	middle ear canal
	middle ear chamber
	mucoepidermoid carcinoma
mec	meconium (mixture of intestinal secretions and amniotic fluid found in the intestine of full term fetuses)
MeCbl	methylcobalamin
MeCCNU	methylchloroethylcyclo-hexylnitrosourea (semustine)
MECH	medial epicondyle of humerus
MECY	methotrexate + cyclophosphamide (combination chemotherapy)
MED	medical
	medication
	medicine
	medium
	minimal effective dose
	minimal erythema dose
	multiple endocrine deficiency
	multiple epiphyseal dysplasia (Fairbank's disease)
med	medial
	medication
	medicine
medic	medical corpsman in

the armed forces

MEDLARS
MEDical Literature Analysis and Retrieval System (database)

MEDLINE
MEDLARS on-Line

medmen medial meniscectomy

Med Tech
medical technologist

MEE measured energy expenditure
middle ear effusion

MEF maximal expiratory flow (respiratory rate)
middle ear fluid
midexpiratory flow

MEFR maximal expiratory flow rate

MEFV maximal expiratory flow volume

MEG magnetoencephalography
male external genitalia

Mega megakaryocyte

MegaCSF
megakaryocyte-colony - stimulating factor

MEI metastatic efficiency index
middle-ear infection

MEK methyethylketone

MEL metabolic equivalent level

mel melanoma

MELAS mitochondrial encephalomyopathy with acidosis and stroke

memb membrane

MEN meningitis
multiple endocrine neoplasia (syndrome)

MEN-I multiple endocrine neoplasia type I

MEN-II multiple endocrine neoplasia type II

men meninx
meniscus
menorrhea
menses
mental
menthol

menton (a craniometric landmark)
mentum (the chin)

MEnk met-enkephalin

MENS microamperage electrical nerve stimulation

MEO malignant external otitis
Medical Examiner's Office

MeOH methyl alcohol

MEOS microsomal ethanol-oxidizing system

MEP maximal expiratory pressure
mean effective pressure
motor end-plate
motor evoked potential

mep meperidine (a synthetic narcotic analgesic)

MEPRS medical expense and performance reporting system

mEq milliequivalent

meq milliequivalent

mEq/L milliequivalent per liter

MER mean ejection rate
medical error reduction
methanol extraction residue

M/E ratio
myeloid: erythrocyte ratio

MERB Medical Examination and Review Board

MERG macular electroretinogram

MERIT Method to Extend Research in Time

MERLIN Medical Emergency Relief International

MERP Medical Errors Reporting Program (physicians call anonymously to report errors; (800) 233-7767)

MERRF myoclonic epilepsy with ragged-red fiber (syndrome)

MES maximal electroshock
multi-endocrine syndrome

mes mesial

MESA microsurgical epididymal sperm aspiration

myoepithelial sialadenitis

Mesc mescaline (an intoxicating poisonous alkaloid that produces delusions of music and color)

MeSH medical subject headings

MesPGN mesangial glomerulonephritis

MESS mangled extremity severity score

MET metastasis

mid-expiratory time

Met methionine (an essential amino acid)

META metamyelocyte

meta metanephrine

Metf metformin (Glucophage; it sensitizes the body's tissues to the effects of insulin)

meth methyl

Met Hb methemoglobin

methyl-CCNU

semustine (antineo- plastic agent)

MetMb metmyoglobin

m. et n. *mane et nocte* [Latin] morning and night

m. et sig. *misce et signa* [Latin] mix and label

METT maximal exercise tolerance test

MEV maximal exercise ventilation

middle ear ventilation

MeV megavolt

megavoltage

million electron volts

MF Maisonneuve fracture

Malgaigne fracture

mallet finger

mallet fracture

mandibular foramen

march fracture

microfilament

midcavity forceps

Mickey Finn (chloral hydrate and alcohol)

mitogenic factor

Monteggia fracture

Montercaux fracture

Moore fracture

Muller fracture

multifactorial

multiform extrasystole

mutation frequency

mycosis fungoides

myelofibrosis (replacement of bone marrow by fibrous tissue)

myocardial fibrosis

M & F male and female

mother and father

mf microfilaria

MFA macrofollicular adenoma

MFAT multifocal atrial tachycardia

MFB metallic foreign body

MFCS Mason fracture classification system

MFD mandibulofacial dysostosis

mid-forceps delivery (of fetus)

milk-free diet

Monteggia fracture- dislocation

MFEM maximal forced expiratory maneuver

MFG magnetic field gradient

MFH malignant fibrous histiocytoma

MFM maternal-fetal medicine

MFP myofascial pain

MFR mid-forceps rotation

mean flow rate

MFS maxillofacial surgery

MFT muscle function test

MFW multiple fragment wounds

MG macroglossia

mammary gland (lactiferous gland)

medial gastrocnemius (muscle)

megaloglossia

menopausal gonadotropin

methylguanidine

micoglia

	monoglycerides myasthenia gravis (neuromuscular disorder) myoglobin (an oxygen- transporting pigment of muscle) myoglobulin (a globulin in muscle serum)
Mg	magnesium (a component of both intra- and extracellular fluids)
mg	milligram(s) (1/60 grain)
MGA	mammary gland adenoma
MgATP	magnesium adenosine triphosphate
MGB	medial geniculate body
MGC	microglial cell minimal glomerular change multinucleated giant cell
MGCE	multifocal giant cell encephalitis
MGCT	mixed germ cell tumor
MGD	maternal genetic disease maximal glucose disposal meibomian gland dysfunction mixed gonadal dysgenesis
MGE	megaloblastic erythropoiesis
MGF	macrophage growth factor multipotent growth factor Myasthenia Gravis Foundation
MGH	mammogenic hormone Massachusetts General Hospital monosodium glutamate headache
mg hr	milligram-hour (unit used in radiation therapy)
MGI	macrophage-granulocyte inducer
mg/l	milligrams per liter
Mgl	myoglobin (an oxygen- transporting protein found in muscle fibers, similar to hemoglobin)

MGN	medial geniculate nucleus membranous glomerulonephritis
Mg(OH)$_2$	magnesium hydroxide (milk of magnesia)
MGP	matrix Gla protein mucin glycoprotein
MGR	marrow graft rejection
MGS	male gonadal shield
MgSO$_4$	magnesium sulfate
MGT	multiple glomus tumors multiplex genetic testing
Mgtis	meningitis
MGTN	metastatic gestational trophoblastic neoplasia
MGUS	monoclonal gammopathy of uncertain significance monoclonal gammopathy of undetermined significance
MGW	magnesium sulfate, glycerin, and water (enema solution)
M-GXT	multistage-graded exercise test
MH	malignant histiocytosis malignant hypertension malignant hyperthermia marital history medical history menstrual history mental health mental hygiene migraine headache moist heat Morgagni hernia mylohyoid (muscle) myocardial hypertrophy
MHA	major histocompatibility antigen methemalbumin microangiopathic hemolytic anemia microhemagglutination assay middle hepatic artery multiplex heteroduplex analysis
MHA-TP	microhemagglutination

assay for antibodies to
Treponema pallidum

MHB maximum hospital benefits

MHb myohemoglobulin

MHC major histocompatibility
complex (class I and II
antigens)

mental health clinic

myosin heavy chain

MHCA minor histocompatibility
antigen

MHCC major histocompatibility
complex (class I and II
antigens)

MHD maintenance hemodialysis

mean hemolytic dose

minimum hemolytic
dilution

minimum hemolytic dose

MHDA multiplex heteroduplex
analysis

MHE malignant
hemangioendothelioma
(hemangiosarcoma)

medial humeral
epicondylitis
(golfer's elbow)

MHI malignant histiocytosis
of intestine

minor head injury

MHL mylohyoid line (a ridge on
the inner surface of the
mandible that affords
attachment to the
mylohyoid muscle)

MHM mill-house murmur

mylohyoid muscle

MHMA 3-methoxy-4-
hydroxymandelic acid

MHN massive hepatic necrosis

morbus hemolyticus
neonatorum

mylohyoid nerve

MHO medical house officer

microsomal heme
oxygenase

mho unit of conductance

MHP malignant hyperpyrexia

modified Hughes

procedure

monosymptomatic hypo-
chondriacal psychosis

MHPG 3-methoxy-4-
hydroxyphenylglycol

MHR malignant hyperthermia
resistance

maternal heart rate

methemoglobin reductase

MHS major histocompatibility
system

malignant hyperthermia
syndrome

MHT malignant hyertension

malignant hyperthermia

medical history taking

mixed hemagglutination
test

MHV magnetic heart vector

NHW medial heel wedge

M Hx medical history

MHz megahertz

MI malassezia infection
(pityriasis)

maturation index

mechanical incontinence

medical improvement

Mendelian inheritance

menstruation induction

mental illness

mercaptoimidazole

mild irritant

mitosis index

mitral (left
atrioventricular)
incompetence

mitral (left
atrioventricular)
insufficiency

monilial intertrigo

myocardial infarction

myocardial ischemia

MIAs mechanically insensitive
afferents

MIB Medical Information
Bureau

MIBG metaiodobenzyl guanidine

MIC magnesium ion
concentration

maternal and infant care

methacholine inhalation
challenge
microscope
minimal inhibitory
concentration
minimal isorrheic
concentration

MICC milia-like idiopathic
calcinosis cutia
microinvasive carcinoma
of cervix
mitogen-induced cellular
cytotoxicity

MICE mesna + ifosfamide +
carboplatin + etoposide
(combination
chemotherapy)

micro-IF microimmunofluorescence

MICU medical intensive care unit

MID median incisal diastema
minimal infecting dose
minimal infective dose
minimal inhibiting dose
minimal irradiation dose
multi-infarct dementia

mid middle

mid/3 middle third

MIDCAB minimally invasive direct
coronary artery bypass
(surgery)

MIE medical improvement
expectation

MIF macrophage inhibiting
factor
maximum inspiratory force
melanocyte inhibiting
factor
Merthiolate (thimerosal)-
iodine-formalin
microimmunofluorescence
migration-inhibiting factor
migration-inhibitory factor
mixed immuno-
fluorescence
mullerian (duct)
inhibiting factor

MIFR maximal inspiratory
flow rate

MIg measles immune globulin

MIH migraine with

interparoxysmal
headache
migraine with interval
headache

MILP mitogen-induced
lymphocyte proliferation

MIM meglumine iocarmate
myelography
mendelian inheritance
in man

MIMOL Mendelian inheritance
in man online

MIN motor interneuron

min minimal
minor
minute(s)

MINA monoisonitrosoacetone

MINE medical improvement
negative expectations
mesna + ifosfamide +
Novantrone
(mitoxantrone) +
etoposide (combination
chemotherapy)

MINT middle internodal tract
(between S-A node and A-
V node)

MIO minimal identifiable odor

MIP maximal inspiratory
pressure
mean incubation period
mean intravascular
pressure
minimal inspiratory
pressure

MIRL membrane inhibitor of
reactive lysis
minimal invasive
procedure

MIRP major iron-regulated
protein
myocardial infarction
rehabilitation program

MIRS medical improvement
review standard

MIS melanoma *in situ*
minimally invasive surgery
mitral (left
atrioventricular)

insufficiency
mullerian-inhibiting
  substance (antimullerian
  hormone)

misc   miscarriage
miscellaneous

MISG   modified immune
  serum globulin

MISO   misonidazole

mist.   *mistura* [Latin] a mixture

MIT   male impotence test
Massachusetts Institute
  of Technology
monoiodotyrosine
myocardial infarction
  triage

MITO-C   mitomycin-C
  (antineoplastic agent)

mIU   milli-International Unit

MJ   marijuana
Minerva jacket (cast
  immobilization)

MKB   megakaryoblast

MKC   megakaryocyte

MkCSF   megakaryocyte colony-
  stimulating factor

MKHS   Menkes' kinky-hair
  syndrome

MkL   megakaryoblastic leukemia

mks   meter-kilogram-second
  (system)

ML   macula lutea
malignant lymphoma
medial leminiscus
memory loss
middle lobe (of lung)
midlife
midline
milk letdown
mucolipidosis (hereditary
  lysosomal storage diseases
  in which
  mucopolysaccharides
  and lipids accumulate
  in the tissues)
myeloid leukemia

ML I   mucolipidosis I
  (lipomucopolysaccharidosis)

ML II   mucolipidosis II (I-cell

disease)

MS III   mucolipidosis III (pseudo-
  Hurler polydystrophy)

MS IV   mucolipidosis IV

mL   milliliter(s)

ml   milliliter(s)

MLA   Medical Library
  Association
mento-laeva anterior [Latin]
  left mento-anterior
  (fetal position)
monophosphoryl lipid A

MLAP   mean left atrial pressure

MLBP   mechanical low back pain

MLBW   moderately low
  birth weight

MLC   mid-life crisis
minimal lethal
  concentration (minimal
  bactericidal
  concentration)
mixed leukocyte culture
mixed lymphocyte culture
morphine-like compound
multilumen catheter
myosin light chain

MLCK   myosin light chain kinase

MLCP   myosin light chain
  phosphatase

MLCT   mixed lymphocyte
  culture test

MLD   median lethal dose
metachromatic
  leukodystrophy
microlumbar diskectomy
minimal lethal dose

MLD50   median lethal dose

MLD-I   mucolipidosis, type I

MLD-II   mucolipidosis, type II

MLD-III   mucolipidosis, type III

MLE   midline episiotomy

M. leprae   *Mycobacterium leprae* (the
  causative agent of
  leprosy)

MLF   median longitudinal
  fasciculus

MLG   midline granuloma
mitochondrial lipid
  glycogen

MLGN minimal lesion glomerulonephritis

ML H malignant lymphoma, histiocytic

ml/l milliliters per liter

MLL middle lobe of lung

MLN mediastinal lymph nodes
membranous lupus nephropathy
mesenteric lymph nodes

MLNS mucocutaneous lymph node syndrome (Kawasaki disease)

MLO mesio-linguo-occlusal (tooth surfaces)

MLP *mento-laeva posterior* [Latin] left mento-posterior (fetal position)
microsomal lipoprotein

MLR middle latency response
mixed leukocyte reaction
mixed leukocyte response
mixed lymphocyte reaction
mixed lymphocyte response

MLS Maroteaux-Lamy syndrome (mucopoly-saccharidosis VI)
mean life span
Means-Lerman scratch (pericardial friction rub)
middle lobe syndrome

MLs Mendelian laws

MLSE malformed low-set ears

MLT medical laboratory technician
medical laboratory technologist
mento-laeva transversa [Latin] left mento-transverse (fetal position)

MLTC mixed lymphocyte tumor cell

MM main memory
major medical (insurance policy)
malignant melanoma
medial malleolus
medial meniscus

medical monitoring
meningococcal meningitis
menstrual migraine
methadone maintenance
Milch maneuver
mitral murmur
mononeuropathy multiplex
mouse mite (agent of rickettsialpox)
mucormycosis
mucous membrane
multiple myeloma
murmurs
muscles
musical murmur
myeloid metaplasia
myelomeningocele

M & M Medicare and Medicaid
morbidity and mortality

mM millimole
millimolar

mm millimeter(s)
mucous membrane
muscles

mm² square millimeter

mm. *musculi* [Latin] muscles

MMA methylmalonic acid
minor motor aphasia

MMB mouth-to-mouth breathing (resuscitation)

MMC meningomyelocele

MMC
meningomyelocele

migrating myoelectric complex

mitomycin C
(antitumor agent)
mucosal mast cell
myelomeningocele

MMCB motor neuropathy with
conduction block

MMD milkmaid's dislocation
myotonic muscular
dystrophy

MMDI Minnesota Multiphasic
Personality Inventory

MME milkmaid's elbow
M-mode echocardiography

MMEF maximal midexpiratory
flow

MMF mean maximum flow

MMFR maximal midexpiratory
flow rate

MMG mean maternal glucose

mmHg millimeters of mercury

MMI macrophage migration
inhibition

MMIF macrophage migration
inhibitory factor

MMIHS megacystis-microcolon-
intestinal hypoperistalsis
syndrome

MMJ mere medical judgment

MMK Marshall-Marchetti-Krantz
(cystourethroplexy)

MMKJ medial meniscus of
knee joint

MML myelomonocytic leukemia

MMLV Moloney murine leukemia
virus (affects mice and/
or rats)

MMM mitoxantrone +
methotrexate +
mitomycin (combination
chemotherapy)
mucous membrane moist
myelofibrosis with myeloid
metaplasia
myelosclerosis with
myeloid metaplasia

mmm millimicron

MMMF man-made mineral fibers

MMMT malignant mixed
mesodermal tumor
metastatic mixed

müllerian tumor

MMN multiple mucosal neuroma

mmol millimole

MMOV malignant melanoma
of vagina

MMP multiple medical problems

MMPI matrix metalloproteinase
inhibitor
Minnesota Multiphasic
Personality Inventory
(test)

mmpp millimeters partial pressure

MMPR methylmercaptopurine
ribonucleoside

MMR maternal mortality rate
measles, mumps, rubella
(vaccine)
mild mental retardation
mobile mass x-ray
mouth-to-mouth
resuscitation

M & M rates mortality and morbidity
rates

MMS megacystis-megaureter
syndrome
methionine malabsorption
syndrome
milkman's syndrome
mini-mental status
minimum methadone
service
mixed mesodermal
sarcoma
mixed müllerian sarcoma
(most common sarcoma
of the uterus)
Mohs micrographic
surgery
myasthenic-myopathic
syndrome

MMSE mini-mental state
examination

mm/sec millimeters per second

MMT malignant mixed tumor
manual muscle testing
medial meniscus tear
methadone maintenance
treatment
methylcyclopentadienyl

manganese tricarbonyl

MMTP methadone maintenance
treatment program

mμ millimicron

mμg millimicrogram

MMV mandatory minute
ventilation

MMWR *Morbidity and Mortality
Weekly Report* (prepared
by CDC)

MN Masugi nephritis
malignant nephrosclerosis
melanocytic nevus
membranous nephropathy
mesenteric (lymph) node
midnight
mononuclear
Morton neuroma
motor neuron

M & N morning and night
mydriacyl and
neosynephrine

Mn manganese (a
metallic element that
resembles iron)

mn midnight

MNA mucositis necroticans
agranulocytica

MNB mandibular nerve block

MNBCCS multi-nevoid basal-cell
carcinoma syndrome

MNC multinucleated cell

MNCV motor nerve conduction
velocity

MND minor neurologic
dysfunction
motor neuron disease

MNES median nerve entrapment
syndrome

MNF myelinated nerve fiber

MNG multinodular goiter

mng morning

MNJ myoneural junction

MNL marked neutrophilic
leukocytosis

MNM motile (sperm) with
normal morphology

MNN median nerve neuropathy

MNP median nerve palsy

mononuclear phagocyte

MNS malignant nephrosclerosis

Mn-SOD manganese-superoxide
dismutase

MNT Morton's neuroma of toe
mouse infection
neutralization test

MNU methylnitrosourea

MNV milker's node virus
(pseudocowpox)

MO macro-orchidismomal-
occlusion
mechanical obstruction
medial oblique (x-ray view)
medical officer
medulla oblongata
mineral oil (liquid
petrolatum)
monoamine oxidase
mono-oxygenase
morbid obesity
mumps orchitis
myositis ossificans

Mo molybdenum (a metallic
essential trace element)

mo mode

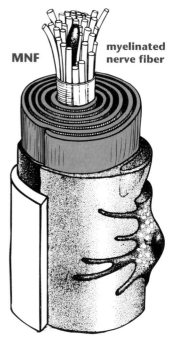

MNF myelinated
nerve fiber

month(s)
MOA mechanism of action
monoamine oxidase
MOAb monoclonal antibody
MOBP mitomycin + Oncovin
(vincristine) + bleomycin
+ Platinol (cisplatin)
(combination
chemotherapy)
MOC maximum oxygen
consumption
MOCA methotrexate + Oncovin
(vincristine) +
cyclophosphamide +
Adriamycin
(doxorubicin)
(combination
chemotherapy)
4,4'methylene-bis
(2-chloroaniline)
MOD maturity-onset diabetes
(usually type II diabetes
mellitus)
mesio-occlusodistal
(relating to tooth
surfaces)
mod moderate
modem *mod*ulate and *dem*odulate
MODM mature-onset diabetes
mellitus (usually type II
diabetes mellitus)
MODS multiple organ dysfunction
syndrome
MODY maturity-onset diabetes of
the young
maturity-onset diabetes
of youth
MOF mal-union of fracture
mature ovarian follicle
methotrexate + Oncovin
(vincristine) +
fluorouracil
(combination
chemotherapy)
multiple organ failure
(MODS is preferred)
multisystem organ failure
MOFS multiple organ
failure syndrome

mΩ milliohm
MOI monoamine oxidase
Inhibitor
multiplicity of infection
mol mole (unit of
measurement
of substance)
molecule
molc molar concentration
mol/kg moles per kilogram
mol/l moles per liter
moll. *mollis* [Latin] soft
mol mass molecular mass
mol wt molecular weight (relative
molecular mass)
MOM main outcome measure
milk of magnesia (aqueous
suspension of magnesium
hydroxide)
mucoid otitis media
MOMA methylhydroxymandelic
acid
mo/ma monocyte/macrophage
MOMP major outer
membrane protein
MOMS Mothers Offering
Maternal Support
MONAb monoclonal antibody
mono monocyte

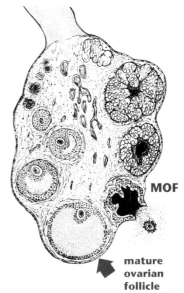

MOF

mature
ovarian
follicle

	mononucleosis (kissing disease)
monos	monocytes
MOP	medical outpatient
	multiple oocytes per disk
	myositis ossificans progressiva (fibrodysplasia ossificans progressiva)
MOPP	mechlorethamine (nitrogen mustard) + Oncovin (vincristine) + prednisone + procarbazine (combination chemotherapy)
MOPV	monovalent oral poliovirus vaccine
mor	morphine
MOR	main operating room
	morphine
	morphology
mor. dict.	*more dicto* [Latin] as directed
mor. sol.	*more solito* [Latin] in the usual manner
MOS	macula of saccule (of inner ear)
	myelofibrosis osteosclerosis
	myocardial oxygen supply
mos	months
MOSF	multiple organ system failure
mOsm	milliosmole
mOsmol	milliosmole
mot	motor
MOTT	mycobacterium other than tuberculosis
MOU	macula of utricle (of inner ear)
MOUS	many occurrences of unexplained symptoms
MOW	Meals-on-Wheels
MP	macrophage
	malpractice
	manganese poisoning
	mastoid process
	McBurney's point (surface site of appendix)

	mean pressure
	melting point
	menstrual pain
	menstrual period
	mercury poisoning
	metacarpophalangeal (joint)
	microphakia
	micturition pain
	middle phalanx
	monophosphate
	mouthpiece
	mucopolysaccharide
	mucopurulent
	mucous plug
	multiparous
	muscle pain
	mycoplasmal pneumonia
	myenteric plexus
4-MP	4-methylpyrazole
6-MP	6-mercaptopurine (used in treatment of acute leukemia)
	6-methylprednisolone
M & P	melphenal and prednisone
mp	melting point
m.p.	*modo prescripto* [Latin] in the manner prescribed
MPA	medroxyprogesterone acetate

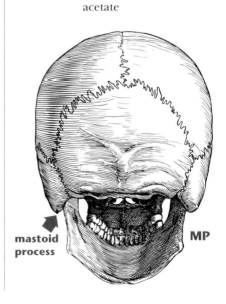

mastoid process

MP

mycoplasma pneumoniae antibody

MPAN macrosopic polyarteritis nodosa

microscopic polyarteritis nodosa

MPAP mean pulmonary artery pressure

MPAQ McGill Pain Assessment Questionnaire

MPB male-pattern baldness

meprobamate (an oral sedative for the relief of anxiety and tension)

mucopurulent bronchitis

MPC maximal permissible concentration

mean plasma concentration

meningococcal protein conjugate

midpalmar crease

mucopurulent cervicitis

multipolar cell

MPCM middle pharyngeal constrictor muscle

MPCO micropolycystic ovary (syndrome)

MPD main pancreatic duct

maximal permissible dose (within the limits of safety)

membrane potential difference

minimal perceptible difference

multiple personality disorder

muscle phosphoralase deficiency (type V glycogenosis)

myeloproliferative disorder

myofascial pain dysfunction

myophosphorylase deficiency (McArdle's disease)

MPDS mandibular pain dysfunction syndrome

myofascial pain dysfunction syndrome

MPE malignant pericardial effusion

maximal permissible exposure (within the limits of safety)

Molt periosteal elevator

MPEC multipolar electrocoagulation

MPED minimal phototoxic erythema dose

M-PFL methotrexate + Platinol (cisplatin) + fluorouracil + leucovorin (combination chemotherapy)

MPGM monophosphoglycerate mutase

MPGN membranoproliferative glomerulonephritis (lobular glomerulonephritis)

mesangial proliferative glomerulonephritis

MPGT mediastinal paraganglionic tumor

MPH male pseudohermaphroditism

mesh plug hernioplasty

MPHD multiple pituitary hormone deficiency

MPHP maximal predicted heart rate

MPI mannose phosphate isomerase

maximal permissible intake

MPJ metaphalangeal joint

MPL maximum permissible level

medial palpebral ligament

MPM malignant pepillary mesothelioma

medial papillary muscle

medial pterygoid muscle

mortality probability model

multiple primary malignancy

MPN most probable number

multiple primary neoplasm

M. pneumoniae
  Mycoplasma pneumoniae
    (Eaton agent)
MPO minimal perceptible odor
    misconduct policy officer
    myeloperoxidase
MPOA medical power of attorney
MPOD myeloperoxidase
    deficiency
MPP malleable penile prosthesis
    massive periretinal
      proliferation
    medial pterygoid plate
    medical personnel pool
    mycoplasmal pneumonia
mppcf millions of particles per
    cubic foot of air
MPPN malignant persistent
    positional nystagmus
MPQ McGill Pain Questionnaire
MPR mannose-6-phosphate
    receptor
    maximal pulse rate
    myeloproliferative reaction

M protein
    matrix protein
MPS mean prognostic score
    meconium plug syndrome
    melanin pigmentation
      system
    mononuclear
      phagocyte system
    mucopolysaccharide
    mucopolysaccharidosis
    myocardial perfusion
      scintigraphy
    myofacial pain syndrome
MPSI midpalmar space infection
MPS I mucopolysaccharidosis
    type I (Hurler syndrome)
MPS II mucopolysaccharidosis
    type II (Hunter
      syndrome)
MPS III mucopolysaccharidosis
    type III (Sanfilippo
      syndrome)
MPS IV mucopolysaccharidosis
    type IV (Morquio
      syndrome)

MPS V-S mucopolysaccharidosis
    type V (Scheie syndrome)
MPS VI mucopolysaccharidosis
    type VI (Maroteaux-Lamy
      syndrome)
MPS VII mucopolysaccharidosis
    type VII (beta-
      glucuronidase deficiency)
MPSS methylprednisolone
    sodium succinate
MPSV myeloproliferative sarcoma
    virus
MPTP 1-methyl-4-phenyl-1,2,5,6-
    tetrahydropyridine
MPU malposition of uterus

malposition of uterus

MPU

    multiparous uterus
MPV mean platelet volume
    metatarsus primus varus
    mitral (left
      atrioventricular) valve
      prolapse
MQ memory quotient
MR magnetic resonance
    may repeat
    medical record
    medical release
    medical resident
    megaroentgen
    mental retardation
    metabolic rate
    mitral (left atrioventricular
      valve) regurgitation
    Moro's reflex
    mortality rate
    multiple regression
    muscle relaxant
M & R measure and record

mR	milliroentgen
MRA	magnetic resonance angiography
mrad	millirad
MRAP	mean right atrial pressure
MRBF	mean renal blood flow
MRC	major renal calix
	Medical Research Council
	minor renal calix
MRD	Medical Records Department
	metabolic renal disease
	minimal reactive dose
	minimal renal disease
MRE	maximal resistive exercise
	meals ready to eat
mrem	millirem
MRF	moderate renal failure
	müllerian regression factor
mRF	monoclonal rheumatoid factor
MRFIT	Multiple Risk Factor Intervention Trial
MRH	melanocyte-stimulating hormone-releasing hormone
MRI	magnetic resonance imaging (nuclear magnetic resonance)

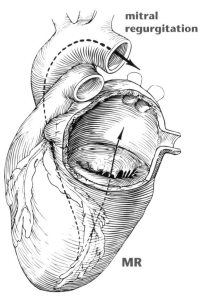

mitral regurgitation

MR

	moderate renal insufficiency
MRKHS	Mayer-Rokitansky-Küster-Hauser syndrome (a rudimentary uterus with congenital absence of the vagina)
MRL	medical records librarian
	minimal response level
MRM	modified radical mastectomy
	modified Ritgen maneuver
	multiple residue method
MRN	malignant renal neoplasm
mRNA	messenger ribonucleic acid
MRO	Medical Review Officer
	minimal recognizable odor
MRPS	midline retroperitoneal syndrome
MRS	magnetic resonance spectroscopy
	male reproductive system
MRSA	methicillin-resistant *Staphylococcus aureus*
MRT	median reaction time
	median relapse time
MRV	mixed respiratory vaccine
MRVI	multi-viral respiratory infection
MRVP	mean right ventricular pressure
MRx	manifest refraction
MS	Maffucci's syndrome
	malabsorption syndrome
	malignant Schwannoma (neurosarcoma)
	Malin's syndrome (autoerythrophagocytosis)
	Marfan's syndrome
	Maric-Strumpell (syndrome)
	Marinesco-Sjögren's (syndrome)
	Martorell's syndrome (pulseless disease)
	maxillary sinus
	Meckel's syndrome (dysencephalia splanchnocystica)

medical student
megalosperm
Meigs' syndrome (ascites + hydrothorax associated with a pelvic tumor)
Mengert's shock (syndrome)
Ménière's syndrome (recurrent episodes of severe vertigo associated with hearing loss and tinnitis)
Menkes' syndrome (kinky-hair syndrome)
menopausal syndrome
microstomia
Mikulicz's syndrome (painless enlargement of the salivary and lacrimal glands, accompanied by decreased lacrimation and dryness of the mouth)
Milkman's syndrome (Looser-Milkman syndrome)
milk sugar
mitral stenosis
Möbius' syndrome (congenital oculofacial paralysis)
Mohs' surgery
Mohs' syndrome (oral-facial-digital syndrome, type II)
Mönckeberg sclerosis
Morel syndrome (hyperostosis frontalis interna)
morning sickness
morning stiffness
morphine sulfate
Morquio's syndrome (mucopoly-saccharidosis IV)
motion sickness
Moynahan syndrome (progressive cardiomyopathic lentiginosis)

multiple sclerosis (frequent cause of neurologic disability)
Münchausen's syndrome (chronic factitious disorder with physical symptoms)
muscle spasm
musculoskeletal
myelosclerosis
myocardial scintigraphy
myosarcoma

MS I   a first-year medical student (freshman)

MS II   a second-year medical student (sophomore)

MS III   a third-year medical student (junior)

MS IV   a fourth year medical student (senior)

Ms   manuscript
murmurs

ms   manuscript
millisecond

MSA   major serologic antigen
medical savings accounts
middle sacral artery
multi-system atrophy

MSAF   meconium-stained amnionic fluid

MS AFP   maternal serum alpha-fetoprotein

MSAP   mean systemic arterial pressure

MSAS   muscular subaortic stenosis

MSB   mid-small bowel

MSBC   maximal specific binding capacity

MSCDs   membranous semicircular ducts (of inner ear)

MSCRP   Mississippi scale for combat-related post-traumatic stress disorder

MSD   maple-syrup disease
Marie-Strümpell disease (rheumatoid spondylitis)
mean square deviation
microsurgical discectomy
mild sickle cell disease

mule spinner's disease

MSDS material safety data sheets

MSDI Martin suicide depression inventory

MSE mental status examination

muscle strengthening exercise

msec millisecond

MSER mean systolic ejection rate

MSF macrophage slowing factor

Mediterranean spotted fever

megakaryocyte stimulating factor

MSFC multiple sort flow cytometry

MSG merocrine sweat gland

MSG

merocrine sweat gland

monosodium glutamate

MSH medical self-help

melanocyte-stimulating hormone (intermedin)

MSHRH melanocyte-stimulating hormone-releasing hormone

MSHSE multiple self-healing squamous epithelioma

MSI magnetic source imaging

multiple subcutaneous injections

MSK medullary sponge kidney

MSKCC Memorial Sloan-Kettering Cancer Center

MSL midsternal line

multiple symmetric lipomatosis

MSLT multiple sleep latency test (test to assess excessive sleepiness)

MSM mid-systolic murmur

MSMP mainstream medical practice

MSN mildly subnormal

MSO mentally stable and oriented

MSOF multisystems organ failure

MSP major sperm protein

maxillary sinus pain

Münchausen syndrome by proxy

musculoskeletal pain

MSPGN mesangial proliferative glomerulonephritis

MSPS musculoskeletal pain syndrome

myocardial stress perfusion scintigraphy

MSR muscle stretch reflexes

MSRP maximal static respiratory pressure

MSRS multisegmental root syndrome

MSS Marie-Sainton syndrome

Marie-Strümpell spondylitis

marital satisfaction scale

massage

minor surgery suite

motion sickness susceptibility

musculoskeletal stress (physical stress)

musculoskeletal system

mucus-stimulating substance

multiple sclerosis susceptibility

MSs muscle spindles

MST maxillary sinus tumor

McCarthy screening test

mean survival time

median sulcus of tongue

MSTI many soft tissue injuries

MSTS MindSet toe splint (splint worn inside a regular shoe)

Musculoskeletal Tumor Society

MSU maple syrup urine

midstream urine

monosodium urate

MSUD   maple syrup urine disease
(alpha-keto-acid
decarboxylase
enzyme defect)

MSV   maximal sustained level
of ventilation

     murine sarcoma virus

MSW   multiple stab wounds

MT   malignant teratoma

     mammary tumor

     Mantoux test
(intracutaneous
tuberculin test)

     marathoner's toe

     medical technologist

     medical transcriptionist

     melatonin (hormone
synthesized by the pineal
body in the brain)

     metatarsal

     methoxytyramine

     methyltestosterone

     microtome

     microtubule

     middle turbinate

     more than

     Morton toe

     multiple tics

     muscle testing

     muscle trauma

M & T   muscles and tendons

MTA   malignant teratoma,
anaplastic

     metatarsus adductus

     myoclonic twitch activity

MT bar   metatarsal bar

MTBE   meningeal tick-borne
encephalitis

MTC   maximal toxic
concentration

     medullary thyroid
carcinoma

     mitomycin-C
(chemotherapy)

MTD   maximal tolerated dose

     metastatic trophoblastic
disease

     monotropic thyrotropin
deficiency

     multiple tic disorder

MTDDA   Minnesota Test for
Differential Diagnosis
of Aphasia

mtDNA   mitochondrial
deoxyribonucleic
acid (DNA)

MTE   multiple trace elements

MTET   modified treadmill
exercise test

MTF   mild thyroid failure

     modulation transfer
function

     murine typhus fever

MTFR   middle transverse fold
of rectum

MTHL   medial thyrohyoid
ligament

MTHS   middle turbinate headache
syndrome

MTI   malignant teratoma,
intermediate

MTJ   metatarsophalangeal joint

     midtarsal joint

MTLP   metabolic toxemia of late
pregnancy

MTP   maximum tolerated
pressure

     medial tibial plateau

     medical termination
of pregnancy

     metatarsal pads

     metatarsophalangeal
(joint)

     microtubule protein

     musculotendinous pain

MTPJ   metatarsophalangeal joint

MTPJI   metatarsophalangeal
joint injury

MTQ   methaqualone (a hypnotic
and sedative)

MTSS   medial tibial stress
syndrome

MTST   maximal treadmill
stress test

MTT   malignant teratoma,
trophoblastic

     mean transit time

MTU   malignant teratoma,

undifferentiated
methylthiouracil

M. tuberculosis
Mycobacterium tuberculosis
(the causative agent of
tuberculosis)

MTV   mammary tumor virus
metatarsus varus

MTX   methotrexate

MTZ   mitoxantrone

MU   membranous urethra
micturation urgency
million units
motor unit

mU   milliunit

mu   million units
mouse unit

μ   mu [Greek letter]
micro (prefix denoting
decimal factor 10^{-6})
micrometer
micron

μA   microampere

MUA   middle uterine artery

MUAC   middle upper arm
circumference

MUAP   motor unit action potential

MUC   maximum urinary
concentration
moniliasis of uterine cervix
multiparous uterine cervix

muc   mucus

μc   microcurie

MUD   matched unrelated donor
minimum urticarial dose

MUDDLES
miosis, urination, diarrhea,
defecation, lacrimation,
excitation and salivation

MUE   medication use evaluated

μg   microgram

MUGA   multigated blood pool
analysis
multigated acquisition
analysis
multigated angiogram
multiple gated acquisition
multi-unit gated
acquisition

μg/l   micrograms per liter

MUL   median umbilical ligament

μL   microliter

mult   multiple

multi-CSH
multipotential colony-
stimulating factor

multip   multiparous

MuLV   murine leukemia virus

μM   micromolar

μm   micrometer

μmg   micromilligram
(nanogram)

μmm   micromillimeter
(nanometer)

μmol   micromole

μμg   micromicrogram
(picogram)

MUO   myocardiopathy of
unknown origin

μΩ   micro-ohm

MUP   maximal urethral pressure
motor unit potential

MUPS   metastases with unknown
primary site

MURC   measurable undesirable
respiratory contaminants

MUS   midstream urine specimen

4MUS   4-methylumbelliferyl
sulfate

musc   muscle
muscular

MUUF   Mobin-Uddin umbrella
filter

MV   measles virus
mechanical ventilation
megavolt
microvilli
minute ventilation
minute volume
mitral (left
atrioventricular) valve
multivesicular

mV   millivolt

MVA   malignant ventricular
arrhythmias
mechanical ventilatory
assistance
microvascular angina

	mitral (left atrioventricular) valve atresia
	motor vehicle accident
	multivariable analysis
mV-A	millivolt-ampere
M-VAC	methotrexate + vinblastine + Adriamycin (doxorubicin) + and cyclo-phosphamide (combination chemotherapy)
MVB	microventricular bolt (catheter with transducer on the end)
	mixed venous blood
	multivesicular bodies
MVC	maximum vital capacity
	maximal voluntary contraction
	mitral (left atrioventricular)- valve cusps
	myocardial vascular capacity
MVD	Doctor of Veterinary Medicine
	microvascular decompression
	mitral (left atrioventricular)- valve disease
	multivalvular disease
MVE	mitral (left atrioventricular)- valve embolism
	mitral (left atrioventricular)- valve endocarditis
MVFL	macrovesicular fatty liver
MVH	major vessel hemorrhage
	massive vitreous hemorrhage
MVI	mitral (left atrioventricular)- valve insufficiency
	multiple vitamin infusion
MVL	mitral (left atrioventricular) valve leaflet

MVO	mitral (left atrioventricular) valve orifice
MVO$_2$	mixed venous oxygen content (saturation)
MVP	mean venous pressure
	mitral (left atrioventricular) valve prolapse (floppy-valve syndrome)
	mitral (left atrioventricular) valvuloplasty
MVPP	mechlorethamine + vinblastine + procarbazine + prednisone (combination chemotherapy)
MVPS	Medicare volume performance standard
	mitral (left atrioventricular) valve prolapse syndrome
MVR	mitral (left atrioventricular) valve regurgitation
	mitral (left atrioventricular) valve replacement
MVRI	mixed vaccine, respiratory infections
MVRT	multivoltage radiation therapy
MVS	mature vesicular follicle
	mesenteric venous system
	midvoid stream (urine specimen)
	mitral valve stenosis
MVT	maximal ventilation time
	megavitamin therapy
	mesenteric venous thrombosis
	multivitamin
mvt	movement
MVV	maximal voluntary ventilation
MW	mean weight
	megawatt (one million watts)

	microwave
	midwife
	molecular weight (former name for relative molecular mass)
	mosaic wart
	multiple warts
mW	milliwatt (one-thousandth of a watt)
MWD	microwave diathermy
MWG	maternal weight gain
MWP	mean wedge pressure
MWR	microwave radiation
MWS	Mallory-Weiss syndrome
	Muckle-Wells syndrome
MWT	maintenance of wakefulness test (test to assess degree of daytime sleepiness)
	myocardial wall thickness
Mx	computer statistical software program for the type of modeling used in genetic studies
	maxilla
My	myopia
Mycol	mycology
MyD	myotonic dystrophy
myel	myelinated

MW

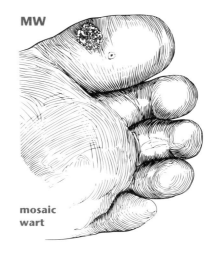

mosaic wart

Myelo	myelocytes
MyG	myasthenia gravis
MyMD	myotonic muscular dystrophy
Myop	myopia
MYS	myasthenic syndrome
MYX	myxedema
	myxoma
MZ	monozygotic (twins)
MZT	monozygotic twins (developed from one zygote)

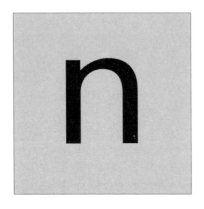

N asparagine (a nonessential
amino acid)
nasal
nasion
negative
nerve
neuroglia
neutron number
nevus (birthmark)
newton
nitrogen
node
nodule
normal
normal concentration
normality (of a solution)
notified
nucleoside
nucleus
number

N normal (solution)
population size

N₂ nitrogen

n nano-(prefix denoting
decimal factor 10^{-9})
nasal
nerve
neutron
refractive index
sample size

n. *naris* [Latin] nostril
nervus [Latin] nerve

n chromosome number
(haploid)

NA Narcotics Anonymous
(818) 780-3951
nasal allergy
Native American
needle aspiration
neuraminidase
neutrophil antibody
nicotine addiction
nicotinic acid (niacin is
preferred)
nodulus aranti
Nomina Anatomica (official
anatomic terminology)
nonadherent
not admitted
not applicable
not available
nuclear antigen
nucleic acid
nucleus ambiguus
numerical aperture (light
gathering power of an
optical fiber or lens)
nurse anesthetist
nurse's aid

N & A nipple and areola

N/A not applicable

Na *Necator americanus*
(hookworm that attaches
to small bowel mucosa)
natrium [Latin] sodium

NAA N-acetyl aspartate
neutrophil aggregation
activity
no apparent abnormalities

NAAC no apparent anesthesia
complication

NAAF National Alopecia Areata
Foundation

NAANAD
National Association of
Anorexia Nervosa and
Associated Disorders
(708) 83103438

NAAQS National Ambient Air
Quality Standard

NAB nitric acid burns
North American
blastomycosis
not at bedside

Nab	neutralizing antibodies
NaBi	sodium bicarbonate
NABS	normoactive bowel sounds
NABX	needle aspiration biopsy
NAC	N-acetylcysteine
	National Asthma Center
	(800) 222-5864
	no acute changes
NACC	National Association of
	Childbearing Centers
NACE	National Association of
	Childbirth Education
NaCl	sodium chloride (salt)
NACOA	National Association for
	Children of Alcoholics
	(714) 499-3889
NACOR	National Advisory
	Committee on Radiation
NACT	neoadjuvant chemotherapy
NAD	National Association of
	the Deaf
	nicotinamide adenine
	dinucleotide
	(coenzyme 1)
	nicotinic acid
	dehydrogenase
	no active disease
	no acute distress
	no apparent distress
	no appreciable disease
	nothing abnormal
	detected
NAD+	nicotinamide-adenine
	dinucleotide (oxidized
	form) (DPN)
NaD	sodium dialysate
NADA	new animal drug
	application
NADD	National Association for
	the Dually Diagnosed
NADG	nicotinamide adenine
	dinucleotide
	glycohydrolase
NADH	nicotinamide-adenine
	dinucleotide (reduced
	form) (DPNH)
NADP	nicotinamide-adenine
	dinucleotide
	phosphate (TPN)

NADP+	nicotinamide-adenine
	dinucleotide phosphate
	(oxidized fom)
NADPH	nicotinamide-adenine
	dinucleotide phosphate
	(reduced form) (TPNH)
NADS	National Association for
	Down's Syndrome
NAEMT	National Association of
	Emergency Medical
	Technicians
NAF	nafcillin (a semisynthetic
	penicillinase-resistant
	penicillin)
	National Ataxia
	Foundation
NaF	sodium fluoride
NAG	narrow angle glaucoma
NAH	National AIDS Hotline
	(800) 342-2437
NAHMOR	
	National Association of
	Health Maintenance
	Organization Regulators
NAHSAL	National Association for
	Hearing and Speech
	Action Line
	(800) 638-8255
NAI	no acute inflammation
	non-accidental injury
NAIC	National Association of
	Insurance Commissioners
Na/K ratio	
	sodium/potassium ratio
NAL	North American
	Loxoscelism
NALD	neonatal
	adrenokeukodystrophy
NAM	natural actomyosins
	normal adult male
NAME	National Association of
	Medical Examiners
	nevi, atrial myxoma,
	myxoid neurofibroma
	and ephilides (syndrome)
NAN	N-acetylneuraminic (acid)
NANA	N-acetylneuraminic acid
NANB	non-A, non-B (hepatitis)
	(hepatitis C)

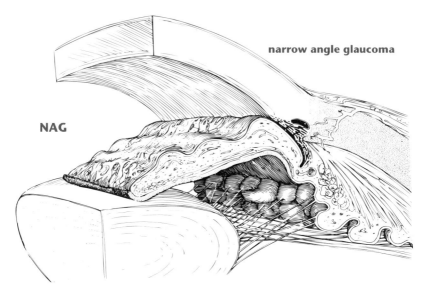

narrow angle glaucoma

NAG

NANBH non-A, non-B hepatitis
(hepatitis C)
NANC nonadrenergic,
noncholinergic
NANDA North American Nursing
Diagnosis Association
NANs negative axillary nodes
NAOO National Association of
Optometrists and
Opticians
NAP nerve action potential
nucleic acid phosphatase
NAPA *N*-acetyl-*p*-aminophenol
N-acetylprocainamide
NAPAP National Acid Precipitation
Assessment Program
NAPARE National Association for
Prenatal Addiction
Research and Education
(312) 329-2512
NAPCA National Air Pollution
Control Administration
Na Pent Sodium Pentothal
(thiopental sodium)
NAPHT National Association of
Patients on Hemodialysis
and Transplantation
NAPM National Association of
Pharmaceutical
Manufacturers

NAR no action required
no adverse reaction
not at risk
NARA Narcotic Addict
Rehabilitation Act
National Association of
Recovered Alcoholics
Nar Anon Narcotics Anonymous
Narc narcotic
narcotics officer
Narco narcolepsy
narcotic
NARD nonarticular rheumatic
disorder
NARIC National Rehabilitation
Information Center
(800) 346-2742
NARS National Acupuncture
Research Society
NAS nasal
National Academy of
Sciences
neonatal abstinence
syndrome
no abnormality seen
no added salt
NASA National Aeronautics and
Space Administration
NAT N-acetyltransferase
no action taken

NATA	Narcotic Addict Treatment Act
NAVH	National Association for Visually Handicapped
NB	nailbed
	needle biopsy
	nephroblastoma (Wilms' tumor)
	neuroblastoma
	nerve block
	newborn

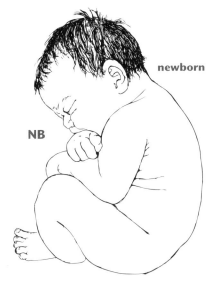

newborn

NB

	night blindness
	nosebleed
	nutrient broth
Nb	niobium (former name columbium)
n. b.	*nota bene* [Latin] note well
NBC	nasobiliary catheter
	nursing bottle caries
NBCCS	nevoid basal cell carcinoma syndrome
NBD	neurogenic bladder dysfunction
	no brain damage
NBE	nonbacterial endocarditis
NBF	no breast feeding
	not breast fed
NBFs	nucleotide-binding folds
NBI	no bone injury

NBICU	newborn intensive care unit
NBL	Naval Biological Laboratory (Oakland)
NBM	no bowel movement
	normal bone marrow
	nothing by mouth
NBME	National Board of Medical Examiners
	normal bone marrow extract
NBN	newborn nursery
NBP	needle biopsy of prostate (under ultrascan)
	nonbacterial prostatitis
NBS	National Bureau of Standards
	no bacteria seen
	normal blood serum
	normal bowel sounds
	normal brainstem
NBT	nitroblue tetrazolium (test)
	normal breast tissue
NBTE	nonbacterial thrombotic endocarditis
NBTNF	newborn, term, normal, female
NBTNM	newborn, term, normal, male
NBTS	National Blood Transfusion Service
NBTT	nitroblue tetrazolium test
NBW	normal birth weight
NC	nasal cannula
	nasal catheter
	natural childbirth
	neonatal cholestasis
	nephrocalcinosis
	neural crest
	night call
	nitrocellulose
	no caffeine
	no change
	no charge
	no complaints
	non-cirrhotic
	non-compliance
	noncontributory

nose clip
not completed
nurse counseling
N/C no complaints
nc nanocurie
nasal cannula
n/c no change
NCA National Council on Aging
National Council on
Alcoholism (800)
NCA-CALL
neurocirculatory asthenia
neutrophil chemotactic
activity
no congenital
abnormalities
Noise Control Act
nuclear cerebral
angiogram
NCADD National Council on
Alcoholism and Drug
Dependency
(800) 622-2255
NCADI National Clearinghouse for
Alcohol & Drug
Information
(301) 443-6500
NCADV National Coalition Against
Domestic Violence
NCAE National Council for
Alcohol Education
NCAH National Child Abuse
Hotline (800) 422-4453
NCAM neuronal cell adhesion
molecule
NcAMP nephrogenous cyclic AMP
NCAP nasal continuous
airway pressure
NCB natural childbirth
NCBE nonciliated bronchiolar
epithelium (Clara cell)
NCBI National Center for
Biotechnology
Information
NCC neurocysticercosis
non-coronary cusp
NC & C normal coitus and climax
NCCDC National Center for
Chronic Disease Control

NCCEA Neurosensory Center
Comprehensive
Examination for Aphasia
NCCF National Cancer Care
Foundation
NCCHR National Commission on
the Confidentiality of
Health Records
NCCLS National Committee for
Clinical Laboratory
Standards
NCD National Council on Drugs
neurocirculatory dystonia
normal childhood
disorders
not considered disabling
NCDA National Council on
Drug Abuse
NCE Naughton cardiac exercise
negative contrast
echocardiography
neurologic clinical
examination
nonconvulsive epilepsy
NCEF Non-Circumcision
Educational Foundation
NCEP National Cholesterol
Education Program
NCF neutrophil chemotactic
factor
NCFB National Collection of
Food Bacteria
NCG nicotine chewing gum
NCH National Cocaine Hotline
(800) COCAINE
NCHCA National Commission
for Health Certifying
Agencies
NCHGR National Center for
Human Genome
Research
NCHS National Center for Health
Statistics
NCHSR National Center for Health
Services Research
(at NIH)
NCI National Cancer Institute
(at NIH)
negative chemical
ionization

Netherlands Cancer
Institute
nosocomial infection
(cross infection)
nCi nanocurie
NCIM National Commission on
Infant Mortality
NCJ needle catheter
jejunostomy
NCL neuronal ceroid
lipofuscinosis
NCLD National Center for
Learning Disabilities
(212) 687-7211
NCMEC National Center for
Missing and Exploited
Children
NCMHI National Clearinghouse
for Mental Health
Information
NCN nasociliary nerve
NCNCA normochromic,
normocytic anemia
NCNR National Center for
Nursing Research
(at NIH)
NCPA National Committee for
the Prevention of
Alcoholism and other
Drug Dependencies
nCPAP nasal continuous positive
airway pressure
NCPCA National Committee
for Prevention of
Child Abuse
NCPPA National Coalition for
Promoting Physical
Activity
NCPR National Center for
Patients' Rights
no cardiopulmonary
resuscitation
NCPSIDS National Center for
Prevention of Sudden
Infant Death Syndrome
NCQA National Committee for
Quality Assurance
NCRC non-child-resistant
container

NCRP National Council for
Radiation Protection
NCRPO National Consortium
of Resident Physician
Organizations
NCRR National Center for
Research Resources
(at NIH)
NCRV National Committee for
Radiation Victims
NCS nystagmus compensation
syndrome
NCSA National Center for
Supercomputer
Applications
NCSCC National Child Safety
Council Childwatch
(800) 222-1464
NCSE nonconvulsive status
epilepticus
NCT nerve conduction time
neural crest tumor
noncontact tonometry
nursing care technician
NCTC National Cancer
Tissue Culture
National Collection of
Type Cultures (London)
NCV nerve conduction velocity
NCVIA National Childhood
Vaccine Injury Act
ND nasal deformity
natural death
neonatal death
neoplastic disease
neurologic demyelination
neurotic depression
Newcastle disease
new drug
nil disease
no data
no disease
noise dosimetry
nondetectable
nondiabetic
nondisabling
nondistended
normal delivery
normal development

nose drops
not determined
not diagnosed
not done
nothing done
notifiable disease
nutritionally deprived
nutrition disorder

N& D nodular and diffuse

N/D no defects
normally developed
not done

Nd neodymium
(a rare element)

NDA new drug application
new drug approval
no data available
no detectable antibody

NDC National Drug Code
nondifferentiated cell

NDCD *National Drug Code Directory*

NDD no dialysis days

NDDIC National Digestive Diseases
Information
Clearinghouse
(301) 654-3810

NDE near death experience

NDF new dosage form
no disease found

NDI nephrogenic diabetes
insipidus

NDIR nondispersive infrared
analyzer

NDMDA National Depressive and
Manic Depressive
Association

NDMREA
National Diabetes
Mellitus Research and
Education Act

nDNA native deoxyribonucleic
acid (DNA)

NDP net dietary protein

NDR neonatal death rate
normal detrusor reflex

NDS new drug submission

NDSC National Down
Syndrome Congress

NDSSH National Down Syndrome

Society Hotline
(800) 221-4602

NDT noise detection threshold

NDTI National Disease and
Therapeutic Index

NDV Newcastle disease virus

Nd:YAG neodymium: yttrium-
aluminum-garnet (laser)

Nd:YLF neodymium: yttrium-
lithium fluoride (laser)

NE necrotic enteritis
nerve ending
nervous exhaustion
neuroepithelium
neurologic examination
nocturnal emission
no effect
no exposure
nonendogenous
norepinephrine
not examined
not exposed
nuclear envelope

Ne neon (an inert
gaseous element)

NEA no evidence of abnormality

NEAA nonessential amino acids

NEB nebulizer
neuroepithelial bodies

nebul. *nebula* [Latin] spray

NEC necrotizing enterocolitis
no essential changes
nonesterified cholesterol

NED no evidence of disease
no expiration date

NEE needle electrode
examination

NEEP negative end-expiratory
pressure

NEFA Narcotic Educational
Foundation of America
(213) 663-5171
nonesterified fatty acid
(free fatty acids)

NEFG normal external female
genitalia

NEG negative
nonenzymatic glycosylation

NEGL neglect

NEI	National Eye Institute (at NIH)
NEISS	National Electronic Injury Surveillance System
NEJ	neuroeffector junction
NEJM	*New England Journal of Medicine*
NEM	N-ethylmaleimide
	no evidence of malignancy
nema	nematode (roundworm)
NEMD	nonspecific esophageal motility disorder
N Engl J Med	
	New England Journal of Medicine
NENU	N-ethyl-N-nitrosourea
NEO	neomycin (a broad-spectrum antibacterial antibiotic)
	neonatology
NEOM	no evidence of malignancy
NEOP	no evidence of pathology
NEP	negative expiratory pressure
	no evidence of pathology
Neph	nephrology
NER	no evidence of recurrence
NERD	no evidence of recurrent disease
NERO	non-invasive evaluation of radiation output
NESHAP	National Emission Standards for Hazardous Air Pollutants
NESS	National Easter Seal Society (800) 221-6827
NET	nasoendotracheal tube
	nerve excitability test
	neuroendocrine transducer
NETF	nasoenteric tube feeding
n. et m.	*nocte et mane* [Latin] night and day
neuro	neuroanatomy
	neurologic
neut	neutrophil
NF	nafcillin (a semisynthetic penicillinase-resistant penicillin)

	National Formulary (an official publication of the American Pharmaceutical Association that provides authoritative information on drugs)
	necrotizing fasciitis
	neurofibroma
	neurofibromatosis
	nevus flammeus
	noise factor
	not found
NF I	neurofibromatosis type I (von Recklinghausen's disease)
NF II	neurofibromatosis type II
NFAIS	National Federation of Abstracting and Indexing Services
NFAR	no further action required
NF-AT	nuclear factor of activated T cells
NFB	National Foundation for the Blind
	negative feedback
NFC	National Fertility Center
NFD	neurofibrillary degeneration
	no family doctor
	non-familial disease
NFDI	National Foundation for Depressive Illness
NFH	nonfamilial hematuria
NFI	no-fault insurance
NFID	National Foundation for Infectious Diseases
NFMH	negative family medical history
NFMM	nonfamilial malignant melanoma
NFN	nodular fat necrosis
NFND	National Foundation for Neuromuscular Diseases
NFNID	National Foundation for Non-Invasive Diagnostics
NFP	not for publication
NFPDFY	
	National Federation of Parents for Drug-Free

Youth (417) 836-3709
NFT neurofibrillary tangle
no further treatment
NFTD normal full-term delivery
NFTs neurofibrillary tangles
NFTSD normal full-term
spontaneous delivery
NFTT nonorganic failure
to thrive
NFUO nosocomial fever of
unknown origin
NFW nursed fairly well
NG nasogastric (tube)
new growth
nitroglycerin
nodose
(sympathetic) ganglion
nodular goiter
norgestrel
(a potent progestin)
normoglycemia
nomogram (for calculating
body surface area)
not given
not good
ng nanogram
nasogastric
NGB neurogenic bladder
NGC neurogenic claudication
nucleus reticularis
gigantocellularis
NGF nerve growth factor
NGFR nerve growth
factor receptor
NGHDC non-growth hormone
deficient child
NGI nasogastric intubation
ngm nanogram
NGO nitroglycerin ointment
N. gonorrhoeae
Neisseria gonorrhoeae
(the causative agent
of gonorrhea)
NGPE neurogenic
pulmonary edema
NGR nasogastric replacement
NGSA nerve growth stimulating
activity
NGT nasogastric tube

normal glucose tolerance
NG tube nasogastric tube
NGU nongonococcal urethritis
NGVL National Gene Vector
Laboratories
NH natriuretic hormone
neonatal hepatitis
neurohormone
neurohypophysis
null hypothesis
(no association between
two variables)
nursing home
NH$_3$ ammonia
NHA National Health
Association
National Hearing
Association
NHAH National Hearing Aid
Helpline (800) 521-5247
NHBPEP National High Blood
Pressure Education
Program
NHC National Health Council
neonatal hypocalcemia
nursing home care
NHD Namaqualand hip dysplasia
normal hair distribution
NHF National Headache
Foundation
National Hemophilia
Foundation
NHG normal human globulin
NHH neurohypophyseal
hormone
NHIC National Health
Information Clearinghouse
(800) 336-4797
(assistance to
appropriate HOTLINES)
NHI national health insurance
NHIF National Head Injury
Foundation
NHL nodular histiocytic
lymphoma
non-Hodgkin lymphoma
normal hearing level
normal hormone level
NHLBI National Heart, Lung and

	Blood Institute (at NIH)
NHMC	National Hotline for Missing Children (800) 843-5678
NHML	non-Hodgkin's malignant lymphoma
NHP	nodular hyperplasia of prostate nonhemoglobin protein
NHPC	National Health Planning Council
NHR	net histocompatibility ratio
NHRA	Nursing Home Reform Act
NHS	normal human serum
NHSC	National Health Service Corps
NHSDA	National Household Survey on Drug Abuse
NHSS	National Health Screening Service
NHTR	nonhemolytic transfusion reaction
NI	neonatal isoerythrolysis neurologic improvement no improvement no information noise index not identified
Ni	nickel (metallic element)
NIA	National Institute on Aging (at NIH) noninflammatory acne no information available Nutritional Institute of America
nia	niacin (nicotinic acid)
NIAAA	National Institute on Alcohol Abuse and Alcoholism
NIAGRC	National Institute on Aging's Gerontology Research Center (at NIH)
NIAID	National Institute of Allergy and Infectious Diseases (at NIH)
NIAMSD	National Institute of Arthritis and Musculoskeletal and Skin

	Disorders (at NIH)
NIBP	non-invasive blood pressure
NIBSC	National Institute for Biological Standards and Control
NIC	neonatal inclusion conjunctivitis nursing interim care
NICC	neonatal intensive care center
NICD	National Information Center on Deafness (202) 651-5052
NICHHD	National Institute of Child Health and Human Development (at NIH)
NICODRD	National Information Center for Orphan Drugs and Rare Diseases
NICU	neonatal intensive care unit neurologic intensive care unit non-immunologic contact urticaria
NID	non-immunologic disease non-insulin dependent not in distress
NIDA	National Institute on Drug Abuse
NIDA Helpline	National Institute on Drug Abuse Helpline (800) 662-HELP
NIDA Screen	National Institute on Drug Abuse Screen (for cannabinoids, cocaine, metabolite, amphetamine, opiates and phencyclidine)
NIDCD	National Institute on Deafness and Other Communication Disorders (at NIH)
NIDD	non-insulin dependent diabetes

NIDDKD National Institute of Diabetes and Digestive and Kidney Diseases (at NIH)

NIDDM non-insulin dependent diabetes mellitus (type 2)

NIDDY non-insulin dependent diabetes in the young

NIDR National Institute of Dental Research (at NIH)

NIEHS National Institute of Environmental Health Sciences (at NIH)

NIF negative inspiratory force
neutrophil immobilizing factor

NIGMS National Institute of General Medical Sciences (at NIH)

NIH National Institutes of Health

NIHCC National Institutes of Health Clinical Center

NIHL noise-induced hearing loss

NIL noise interference level
nothing in light microscopy
not in labor

nil none

NIMBY not in my backyard (regarding medical waste disposal)

NIMH National Institute of Mental Health

NINDS National Institute of Neurological Disorders and Stroke (at NIH)

NINR National Institute for Nursing Research (at NIH)

NIOSH National Institute for Occupational Safety and Health (at CDC)

NIP negative inspiratory pressure
no infection present
no inflammation present
nonspecific interstitial pneumonitis

NIPS neuroleptic-induced

Parkinson syndrome

NIR nonionizing radiation

NIRD nonimmune renal disease

NIRMP National Intern and Resident Matching Program

NIS National Information System (for Health Related Services)
no inflammatory signs

NISS nosocomial infection surveillance system

NIST National Institute of Standards and Technology

NITD noninsulin-treated disease

NITR nonimmune transfusion reaction

Nitro nitroglycerin

NJD neuropathic joint disease (Charcot's joint)

NK natural killer (cells)
neurokinin
no ketones
not known

NK-1 neurokinin-1 (receptor)

NK-2 neurokinin-2 (receptor)

NKA no known allergies

NKB no known basis

NKC natural killer cells
nonketotic coma
null killer cells

NKCF natural killer chemotoxic factor

NKDA no known drug allergies

NKF National Kidney Foundation (212) 889-2210

NKFA no known food allergies

NKH nonketotic hyperglycemia

NKHA nonketotic hyperosmolar acidosis

NKMA no known medication allergies

NKRs neurokinin receptors

NKS needle-knife sphincterotomy

NL nasolacrimal
nephrolithiasis

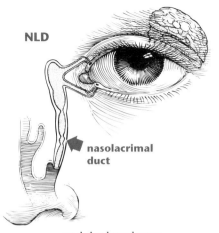

NLD

nasolacrimal
duct

nodular lymphoma
normal libido
normal limits

n.l.   *non licet* [Latin] it is
       not permitted

NLA   National Leukemia
       Association
       (516) 222-1944

NLB   needle liver biopsy

NLC   nocturnal leg cramps
       (recumbency
       night cramps)

NLC & C   normal libido, coitus,
       and climax

NLD   nasolabial distance
       nasolacrimal duct

NLDI   nasolacrimal duct
       impatency

NLDO   nasolacrimal duct
       obstruction

NLE   neonatal lupus
       erythematosus

NIe   norleucine (a nonessential
       amino acid)

NLEA   National Lupus
       Erythematosus
       Association

NLF   nasolabial fold
       neonatal lung fibroblast

NLK   neuroleukin

NLM   National Library of
       Medicine (at NIH)

NLMC   nocturnal leg muscle
       cramp

NLN   National League
       for Nursing
       no longer needed

NLP   no light perception
       normal light perception

NLS   normal lymphocyte
       supernatant

NLT   no later than
       normal lymphocyte
       transfer
       not less than

NLX   naloxone (a narcotic
       antagonist)

NM   neomycin (broad-spectrum
       antibiotic)
       neonatal meningitis
       neuromuscular
       nictitating membrane
       nitrogen mustard
       Nocardia madurae (causative
       agent of maduromycosis)
       nocturnal myoclonus
       nodular melanoma
       nonmalignant
       nuclear medicine
       nuclear membrane
       nurse midwife
       nursing mother

nM   nanomolar

nm   nanometer (one-billionth
       of a meter)

NMA   neurogenic muscular
       atrophy
       nonmedical attendent

NLD

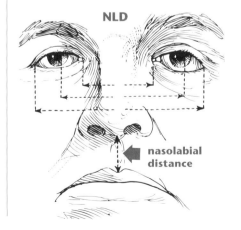

nasolabial
distance

NMD	neosynephrine/mydriacil dilation
	neuromuscular disease
	neuromyodysplasia
NMDA	*N*-methyl-*D*-aspartate
NMDP	National Marrow Donor Program (800) 654-1247
NME	neuromyeloencephalopathy
	nursemaid elbow
N. meningitidis	
	Neisseria meningitidis (leading cause of septicemia)
NMI	no meaningful improvement
	nonocclusive mesenteric infarction
	normal male infant
NMJ	neuromuscular junction
NMM	nodular malignant melanoma
NMN	nicotinamide mononucleotide
	Novy-MacNeal-Nicolle (culture medium)
nmol	nanomole
NMP	normal menstrual period
	nuclear matrix protein
	nucleoside monophosphate
NMR	neonatal mortality rate
	nuclear magnetic resonance (magnetic resonance imaging)
NMRI	nuclear magnetic resonance imaging
NMRS	nuclear magnetic resonance spectroscopy
NMS	neuroleptic malignant syndrome
	neuromuscular spindle
	neuromuscular system
NMSC	nonmelanoma skin cancer
NMSS	National Multiple Sclerosis Society (212) 986-3240
NMT	neuromuscular transmission
	no more than
	nuclear medicine

	technologist
NMTD	nonmetastatic trophoblastic disease
NN	neonatal
	nevocellular nevus
	normal nutrition
	nurse's notes
nn.	*nervi* [Latin] nerves
NNA	nonnarcotic analgesics
NNAC	neonatal narcotic abstinence syndrome
NNACS	neonatal neurologic and adaptive capacity score
NNBC	node-negative breast cancer
NNCC	neonatal chlamydial conjunctivitis
NND	neonatal death
	New and Nonofficial Drugs
NNE	neonatal necrotizing enterocolitis
NNF	National Neurofibromatosis Foundation (800) 323-7938
NNG	nonspecific, nonerosive gastritis
NNI	neonatal icterus
NNIS	National Nosocomial Infection Survey
NNIs	non-nucleoside inhibitors
NNL	no new laboratory (tests requested)
NNMC	National Naval Medical Center (Bethesda, MD)
NNO	no new orders
NNP	neonatal nurse practitioner
NNPBD	National Network to Prevent Birth Defects (202) 543-1070
NNS	neonatal screening
	nicotine nasal spray
NNT	neonatal tetanus
NO	nitric oxide
	nitroglycerin ointment
	nonobese
	number
NO₂	nitrogen dioxide
N₂O	nitrous oxide

N₂O₄ nitrogen peroxide

No nobelium (radioactive transuranic element)

number

NOA National Optometric Association

NOBT nonoperative biopsy technique

NOC night

noc nocturia

No-CPR no cardiopulmonary resuscitation

noct. *nocte* [Latin] at night

noct. maneq.

nocte maneque [Latin] at night and in the morning

NOD new-onset diabetes

non-obese diabetic

notified of death

NOE necrotizing otitis externa

NOF National Osteoporosis Foundation

(202) 223-2226

NOFAS National Organization on Fetal Alcohol Syndrome

NOG nuclear oncogenes

NOII nonocclusive intestinal ischemia

NOK next of kin

NOM nonsuppurative otitis media

normal extraocular movements

NOMI nonocclusive mesenteric infarction

NON nutritional optic neuropathy

non-REM

non-rapid eye movement

non rep. *non repetatur* [Latin] no refill; do not repeat

NOOB not out of bed

NOP not otherwise provided

NOR node of Ranvier

noradrenaline

normal

nortriptyline

nucleolar organizer region

NORD National Organization for Rare Disorders (ailments that affect less than 200,000 people)

(203) 746-6518

NorEpi norepinephrine

Norm normal

NOS nitric oxide synthase

nonobese subject

no organisms seen

NSAC nonsteroidal anti-inflammatory compound

NOS nonorgan-specific

NOSI nitric oxide synthase inhibitor

NOSIE nurse observation schedule for inpatient evaluation

NOT nocturnal oxygen therapy

NOTA National Organ Transplant Act

nova National Organization for Victim Assistance

(202) 393-6682

NOV 70/30

70 units/mL of isophane suspension human insulin + 30 units/mL of regular human insulin

NOV L Novolin L (zinc suspension human insulin)

NOV N Novolin N (isophane suspension human insulin)

NOV R Novolin R (regular human insulin)

NOVS National Office of Vital Statistics

NP nasal polyp

nasal polyp

nasopharyngeal
nasopharynx

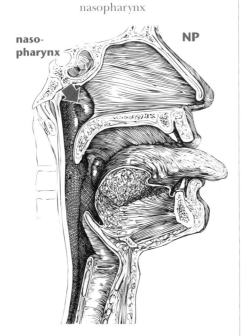

naso-
pharynx

NP

nerve palsy
neuropeptides
neurophysin
new patient
Niemann-Pick (disease)
noise pollution
nonpalpable
no pain
nonpathogenic
nonphagocytic
not pregnant
nucleus pulposus
nurse practitioner

Np neptunium (an unstable
radioactive element that
changes into plutonium)

n.p. *nomen proprium* [Latin]
proper name

NPA National Pharmaceutical
Association
no previous admission

NP-A Niemann-Pick disease, type
A (acute neuronopathy)

NPACs nonconducted premature
atrial contractions

NPB nodal premature beat

NP-B Niemann-Pick disease,
Type B (chronic non-
neuronopathy)

NPC nasal point of conversion
nasopancreatic catheter
nasopharyngeal carcinoma
nebulized prostacyclin
nodal premature
contractions
nonphysician clinician
nonproductive cough
no prenatal care
no previous complaint
nasopharyngeal carcinoma

NP-C Niemann-Pick disease,
type C (chronic
neuronopathy; common
cause of genetic liver
disease in infancy)

NPCa nasopharyngeal carcinoma

NPCC National Poison
Control Center

NPCP non-*Pneumocystis*
pneumonia

NP cult nasopharyngeal culture

NPD narcissistic personality
disorder
Niemann-Pick disease
(sphingomyelin lipidosis)
nocturnal paroxysmal
dystonia
nonprescription drug
no pathologic diagnosis

NPDL nodular poorly
differentiated
lymphocytic

NPDP National Practitioner Data
Bank (repository of
disciplinary actions and
malpractice payments
made by physicians)

NPDR nonproliferative diabetic
retinopathy

NPE neurogenic
pulmonary edema
nocturnal penile erection
normal pelvic examination

NPF nasopharyngeal fiberscope

National Parkinson
Foundation
National Psoriasis
Foundation
no predisposing factor
NPG nonpregnant
NPH National Pregnancy
Hotline (800) 852-5683
neutral protamine
Hagedorn (insulin)
noncirrhotic portal
hypertension
no previous history
normal-pressure
hydrocephalus
NPH insulin
neutral protamine
Hagedorn insulin
(neutral solution,
protamine zinc,
Hagedorn, MD, insulin)
NPhx nasopharynx
NPI nasopharyngeal intubation
no present illness
NPIC National Perinatal
Information Center
(401) 274-0650
neurogenic peripheral
intermittent claudication
NPK neuropeptide K
NPM neonatal-perinatal
medicine
nothing per mouth
NPN nasopalaine nerve
nonprotein nitrogen
n.p.o. *nulla per os* [Latin] nothing
by mouth
n.p.o.h.s. *nulla per os hora somni*
[Latin] nothing by
mouth at bedtime
NPP neuropathic pain
neuroperfusion pump
normal pool plasma
normal postpartum
NPPase nucleotide
pyrophosphatase
NP polio nonparalytic poliomyelitis
NPQ not physically qualified
NPR normal pulse rate

NPRI nasopharyngeal radium
irradiation
NPS nail-patella syndrome
(Osterreicher-Fong
syndrome)
nasopharyngeal secretions
nasopharyngeal stenosis
NPST nonparoxysmal
supraventricular
tachycardia
NPT neuroectodermal
pigmented tumor
nocturnal penile
tumescence (normal
periodic cycle of penile
erections during sleep)
normal pressure and
temperature
NPTN National Pesticide
Telecommunications
Network
NPTT nocturnal penile
tumescence test
NPV negative predictive value
(probability that the
person does not have the
disorder when the test
is negative)
negative pressure
ventilation
nothing per vagina
nuclear polyhidrosis virus
NPW nonpenetrating wound
NQA nursing quality assurance
NR negligible risk
nerve root
nodal rhythm
no radiation
nonreactive
no radiation
no recurrence
no refills
no respiration
no response
normal
normal range
normal reaction
not reacting
not readable

	not recorded
	not resolved
	nurse
nr	near
NRAF	nonrheumatic atrial fibrillation
NRB	nerve root block
	nonrejoining break
nRBC	nucleated red blood cell
NRC	National Rehabilitation Center
	National Research Council
	nerve root canal
	nerve root compression
	Nuclear Regulatory Commission
NRD	nerve root damage
NRDS	neonatal respiratory distress syndrome
NRE	negative regulatory element
	nonrandom error
NREH	normal renin essential hypertension
NREM	nonrapid eye movement (spindle sleep)
NREMS	nonrapid eye movement (spindle) sleep
NREM sleep	
	nonrapid eye movement (spindle) sleep
NRF	normal renal function
NRH	nodular regenerative hyperplasia
NRHA	National Rural Health Association
NRHSP	National Register of Health Service Providers
NRI	nerve root involvement
	nonrespiratory infection
	no recent illness
NRM	normal range of motion
NRMP	National Resident Matching Program
nRNA	nuclear ribonucleic acid
nRNP	nuclear ribonucleoprotein
NROM	normal range of motion
NRPC	nucleus reticularis pontis caudalis

NRPF	National Retinitis Pigmentosa Foundation
NRS	National Runaway Switchboard (800) 621-4000
	Newborn Rights Society (215) 323-6061
NRSF	National Reye's Syndrome Foundation
NRSL	nitroxide radical spin labels (measures translational and rotational diffusion in biological systems)
NRSP	nonrestorative sleep pattern
NRT	nicotine replacement therapy
NS	Naffziger syndrome (cervical rib syndrome; radiating shoulder pain due to compression of the nerves between a cervical rib and the anterior scalene muscle)
	neoplasm staging
	Neosporin
	nephrosclerosis
	nephrotic syndrome
	nervous system
	neurologic sign
	neurosecretion
	neurosurgery
	neurosyphilis
	Nikolsky's sign (separation of the epidermis)
	Nissl substance
	nodular sclerosis
	nonsmoker
	nonspecific
	nonsymtomatic
	Noonan syndrome (slant of the eyes and low set ears associated with valvular pulmonic stenosis)
	normal saline (0.9% sodium chloride solution)

no sample
no specimen
not seen
not significant
ns no specimen
not significant
NSA National Stroke
Association,
1-800-STROKES
Neurological Society
of America
normal serum albumin
no significant abnormality
nsa no salt added
NSAA nonsteroidal antiandrogen
NSAD no sign of acute disease
NSAIA nonsteroidal
antiinflammatory
analgesic
NSAID nonsteroidal
antiinflammatory drug
non-steroid anti-
inflammatory drug
NSAS nonsystemic antacid
suspension
NSC National Safety Council
nonspecific
suppressor cells
no significant change
nuclear sclerotic cataract
NSCIA National Spinal Cord
Injury Association
NSCLC non-small-cell lung cancer
NSCST nipple stimulation
contraction stress test
NSD nasal septal deviation
neonatal staphylococcal
disease
night sleep deprivation
no significant defect
no significant disease
nominal standard dose
normal standard dose
normal spontaneous
delivery
no significant deficiency
no significant difference
NSDA nonsteroid-dependent
asthmatic

NSE neuronal-specific enolase
(enzyme tumor marker)
neuron-specific enolase
(enzyme tumor marker)
normal saline enema
nsec nanosecond
NSF National Science
Foundation
National Sleep Foundation
nightstick fracture
NSFTD normal spontaneous
full-term delivery
NSG necrotizing sarcoidal
granulomatosis
NSGC National Society of Genetic
Counselors
(312) 791-4436
NSGI nonspecific genital
infection
NSHD nodular sclerosing
Hodgkin's disease
NSI negative self-image
nonspecific infection
nonstreptococcal infection
NSIDS near sudden infant death
syndrome
NSIDSF National Sudden Infant
Death Syndrome
Foundation
NSILA nonsuppressible insulin-
like activity
NSILP nonsuppressible insulin-
like protein
NS/LR normal saline/lactated
Ringer's solution
NSM nonantigenic specific
mediator
NSN nephrotoxic serum
nephritis
NSND nonsymptomatic and
nondisabling
NSO Neosporin ointment
Nursing Service Office
NSPB National Society to Prevent
Blindness (800) 221-3004
NSQ not sufficient quantity
NSR normal sinus rhythm
not seen regularly
NSS normal saline solution

(sodium chloride 0.9%)
normal size and shape
not statistically significant

1/2 NSS one-half normal saline
solution (sodium
chloride 0.45%)

NSSC normal size, shape and
consistency

NSSO National Second Surgical
Opinion Program
Hotline (800) 638-6833

NSSP normal size, shape and
position

NSSTT nonspecific ST and T (S-T
segment and T wave of
ECG cycle)

NST nonspecific therapy
nonstress test
not sooner than

NSTT nonseminomatous
testicular tumor

NSU nonspecific urethritis

NSV nonspecific vaginitis

NSVD normal spontaneous
vaginal delivery

NSVT nonsustained ventricular
tachycardia

NSX neurosurgical examination

NSY nursery

NT nasotracheal
nephrostomy tube
neurotensin
neurotransmitter
nicotine tartrate
nicotinc tcst
non-typable
normal temperature
normotensive
not tested
nucleotide

N & T nicotine and tobacco
nose and throat

nt nucleotide

NTA natural thymocytotoxic
autoantibody

NTBR not to be resuscitated

NTC neurotrauma center

NTCC National Type Culture
Collection

NTD negative to date
neural tube defect
nitroblue tetrazolium
dye (test)

NTDF National Transgenic
Development Facility

NTE neurotoxic esterase
neutral thermal
environment
not to exceed

NTF normal throat flora

NTG nitroglycerin
nontoxic goiter
nonthrombotic embolism
nontreatment group
normal tension glaucoma
normal triglyceridemia

NTGO nitroglycerin ointment

NTHi non-typable *H. influenzae*

NTI nasotracheal intubation
nerve trunk inflammation

NTIS National Technical
Information Services (at
CDC) (800) 232-1824

NTL nasotracheal lavage

NTM nontuberculous
mycobacteria

NTMI nontransmural myocardial
infarction

NTN nephrotoxic nephritis

NTOS neurogenic thoracic
outlet syndrome

NTP nitroprusside
normal temperature
and pressure

NTRC National Toxins
Research Center

NTS nasotracheal suction
nicotine transdermal
system
nontropical sprue
(celiac sprue)
nucleus of tractus solitarius
(solitary tract)

NTs nasal turbinates (conchae)
night terrors

NTSB National Transportation
Safety Board

NTT nasotracheal tube

nearly total thyroidectomy

nosocomial transmission of tuberculosis

NTV neurotransmitter vesicle

NTX naltrexone (a narcotic antagonist)

NU name unknown

nU nanounit

NUC nonspecific ulcerative colitis

nulliparous uterine cervix

nuc nucleoside

nucleus

Nuc Med nuclear medicine

NUD nonulcer dyspepsia

NUG necrotizing ulcerative gingivitis

nullip nullipara

NUT nonobstructive urinary tract

nutr nutrition

NV near vision

neurovascular

Newcastle virus

next visit

nonvaccinated

nonvenereal

normal value

Norwalk virus

not vaccinated

not verified

N & V nausea and vomiting

NVA near visual acuity

NVB neurovascular bundle

NVD nausea, vomiting and diarrhea

neck vein distention

neovascularization of the disk

neurovesicle dysfunction

new vessels that develop

nonvalvular disease (heart)

no venereal disease

N/V/D nausea/vomiting/diarrhea

NVE native valve endocarditis

neovascular edema

new vessels elsewhere

NVG neovascular glaucoma

NVI neurovascular injury

NVL no visible lesion

NVS neurologic vital signs

NVSS normal variant short stature

NVT nonvehicular trauma

NW nasal wash

NWB non-weight-bearing

NWCL new world cutaneous leishmaniasis

NWD normal well developed

NWDL nodular well-differentiated lymphocytic lymphoma

NWR normotensive Wistar rat

Nx nephrectomy

NYAM New York Academy of Medicine

NYAS New York Academy of Science

NYD neovascularization of optic disk

not yet diagnosed

not yet discharged

Nympho nymphomaniac

NYP not yet published

nyst nystagmus

NZB mice New Zealand black mice

NZO mice New Zealand obese mice

NZW mice New Zealand white mice

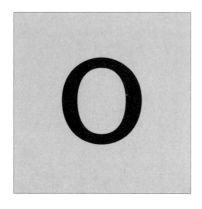

O   absence of a sex
        chromosome
        blood type
        none
        obesity
        objective
        occiput
        occlusal
        often
        ohm
        old
        Olestra (fat substitute)
        Oncovin (vincristine)
        oocyte
        open
        operon
        opium
        oral
        orbit
        osteoblast
        osteoclast
        osteocyte
        osteon
        other
        output
        ovary
        ovum
        oxygen
        zero
2O second opinion
O₂ (molecular) oxygen
O₃ ozone
o   opening
        oral

o.   *oculus* [Latin] eye
OA   obstructive apnea
         occipital artery
         occiput anterior
         ocular albinism
         old age
         oleic acid
         on admission
         ophthalmic assistants
         opioid analgesics
         optic atrophy
         oral administration
         osteoarthritis
         outcome assessment
         ovalbumin
         Overeaters Anonymous
         oxalic acid
         oxaloacetate
O & A observation and
         assessment
OAA old age assistance
         Older Americans Act
         Opticians Association of
         America
         oxaloacetic acid
OAD obstructive airway disease
         obstructive arterial disease
OAF osteoclast-activating factor
         osteoclastic activating
         factor
OAG open angle glaucoma
OAGV organoaxial gastric
         volvulus
OAH ovarian androgenic
         hyperfunction
OALL ossification of anterior
         longitudinal ligament
OAM oblique abdominal muscle
         Office of Alernative
         Medicine (to investigate
         and evaluate altenative
         medicine at NIH)
OAP old age pension
         old age pensioner
         ortho-amino-phenols
         Orthosorb absorbable pin
         (absorbable fracture
         fixation device)
         osteoarthropathy

oxidant air pollutant

OARs Ottawa ankle rules

OAS opiate abstinence
syndrome
oral allergy syndrome

OASDI old age, survivors and
disability insurance

OASI old age and survivors
insurance

OAT ornithine aminotransferase

OAV oculoauriculovertebral
(dysplasia)

OAW oral airways

OAWO opening abductory
wedge osteotomy

OB obese
obliterative bronchiolitis
obstetrics
occult bleeding
occult blood
olecranon bursa
olecranon bursitis
(student's elbow)
olfactory bulb

O & B opium and belladonna

ob obese

OBD organic brain disease

obese NIDDM
obese non-insulin-
dependent diabetes
mellitus

OBF open book fracture
organ blood flow

OBG obstetrics and gynecology

ob gene obese gene
obesity gene

OB/GYN obstetrician/gynecologist
obstetrics and gynecology

obl oblique

OBN occult blood negative

OBP occult blood positive
odorant-binding protein
osteoporosis and back pain

OBR osteoporosis from bed rest

OBRR obstetric recovery room

OBS obstetrical service
organic brain syndrome

Obs obstetrician

obs observation

obsolete

obsd observed

obst obstruction

OBT occult blood test

OC obstetrical conjugate
occipital condyle
Oedipus complex
office call
on call
onchocerciasis
(river blindness)
only child
open cholecystectomy
optic chiasma
oral cavity
oral contraceptive
ossification center
osteochondritis
osteochondroma
osteoclast
ovarian cancer
ovarian carcinoma
ovarian cyst
oxygen consumed

O & C onset and course

OCA oculocutaneous albinism
oral contraceptive agent

OCa ovarian carcinoma

OCAA ovarian
cystadenocarcinoma-
associated antigen

OCAD occlusive carotid
artery disease

OCaP occult cancer of prostate

O₂cap oxygen capacity

OCB obsessive-compulsive
behavior

OCC oat cell carcinoma
oral contraceptive

occ occasional
occipital

OCCC oocyte-cumulus-corona
complex
open chest cardiac
compression

occip occiput

occl occlusion

OCCM open chest cardiac
massage (resuscitation)

OccTh occupational therapy

Occup Hx
occupational history

OCD obsessive-compulsive
disorder
organ-confined disease
osteochondritis dissecans
osteochondrodysplasia
osteochondrodystrophy
outer canthal distance

OCD

outer canthal
distance

OCE osteocartilaginous
exostosis

OCETC S-(2-oxo-2-
carboxyethylthio)-
cysteine

OCG oral cholecystogram

OCIS Oncology Center
Information System

obl oblique

OCN obsessive-compulsive
neurosis
oculomotor nucleus

OCONUS
outside continental
United States

OCP oral contraceptive pill

OCPD obsessive-compulsive
personality disorder

OCR obsessive-compulsive
reaction
oculocardiac reflex
oculocephalic reflex
oculocerebrorenal
(syndrome)

OCRD oculocerebrorenal disease
(Lowe's syndrome)

OCRS oculocerebrorenal
syndrome

OCS occipital condyle syndrome
occult congenital syphilis

oral contraceptive steroid
orifice of coronary sinus

11-OCS 11-oxycorticosteroid

OCSE oral cancer screening
examination

OCT ornithine carbamyl
transferase
oxytocin challenge test

OCU observation care unit

OCV ordinary conversational
voice

OD Doctor of Optometry
obstructed defecation
occupational dermatitis
occupational disease
odontodysplasia
Ollier's disease
on duty
opioid dependence
optical density
optic disk
optimal dose
orphan drug
orthodiagraphy
osmotic diarrhea
osmotic diuretics
osteitis deformans
(Paget's disease of bone)
out-of-date
overdosage
overdose
oxygen deficiency
(hypoxia)

od outside diameter
overdose

o.d. *oculus dexter* [Latin]
right eye
omni die [Latin] every day

ODA on demand analgesia
Orphan Drug Amendment
overall disease assessment
occipito-dextra anterior
[Latin] right
occipitoanterior
(fetal position)

ODAT one day at a time

ODB opiate-directed behavior

ODC oligodendrocyte
ornithine decarboxylase

outpatient diagnostic
center
oxygen dissociation curve
oxyhemoglobin
dissociation curve
ODD oculodentodigital dysplasia
oxalate deposition disease
OD'd overdosed
ODDS oculodentodigital
syndrome
ODG oligodendroglial (cell)
ODH Organ Donor Hotline
(800) 24-DONOR
ODM ophthalmodynamometry
ODOD oculodentoosseous
dysplasia
ODP offspring of diabetic parent
occipito-dextra posterior
[Latin] right
occipitoposterior
(fetal position)
ODQ opponens digiti quinti
(opponens digiti minimi)
(muscle)
ODR oil droplet reflex
ODS Orton Dyslexia Society
ODSG ophthalmic Doppler
sonogram
ODT *occipito-dextra transversa*
[Latin] right
occipitotransverse
(fetal position)
OE on examination
orthopedic examination
otitis externa
O & E observation and evaluation
OEC oxygen equilibrium curve
OEE osmotic erythrocyte
enrichment
OEL occupational exposure
limit
OEP Office of Extramural
Programs
OER oxygen enhancement ratio
OES optical emission
spectroscopy
OET oral esophageal tube
organ extract therapy
OETT oral endotracheal tube

OF obturator foramen
occipitofrontal
occupational fatigue
Ogden fracture
olecranon fossa
olecranon fracture
open fracture

OF

**open
fracture**

optic foramen
optic fundus
ossifying fibroma
(fibrous osteoma)
osteitis fibrosa
ovalis fossa
ovarian follicle
OFA oncofetal antigen
OFC occipital frontal
circumference
osteitis fibrosa cystica (von
Recklinghausen disease
of bone)
OFD occipital frontal diameter
orofacial dyskinesia
oral-facial-digital (Mohr's
syndrome)
OFDS orofaciodigital syndrome
OFF orbital floor fracture
OFI overflow incontinence
OFM open face mask
orofacial malformation
OFR oxygen-free radical
OG oncogene
optic ganglion
oral gavage
orogastric (tube)

OGC	on-going care
OGDT	Ouchterlony gel diffusion test
OGF	ovarian growth factor
OGH	opera-glass hand
OGI	osteogenesis imperfecta (osteopenia)
OGP	oncogenic potential
OGS	osteogenic sarcoma
	osteogenic scoliosis
	oxygenic steroid
OGT	oculoglandular tularemia
OGTT	oral glucose tolerance test
OH	obstructive hypopnea
	ocular hypertension
	odontoid hypoplasia
	on hand
	open heart (surgery)
	oral hygiene
	outpatient hospital
17-OH	17-hydroxycorticosteroids
o.h.	*omni hora* [Latin] every hour
OHA	oral hyperglycemia agent
	oxyhemoglobin affinity
O₂Hb	oxyhemoglobin
OHC	outer hair cell (of inner ear)
OH-Cbl	hydroxocobalamin (hydroxo B_{12})
OHCC	hydroxycalciferol
OHCS	hydroxycorticosteroid
17-OHCS	17-hydroxycorticosteroid
OHD	hydroxyvitamin D
	Oast-house disease
	organic heart disease
25(OH)D	25-hydroxy vitamin D (major circulating metabolite)
25(OH)D₂	
	25-hydroxy vitamin D_2 (important metabolite of vitamin D)
1,25(OH)₂D₃	
	1,25-dihydroxy vitamin D_3
6-OHDA	6-hydroxydopamine
OHE	oxyhemoglobin equilibrium
OHFA	hydroxy fatty acid
OHG	oral hypoglycemic

OHH   orthopedic head halter

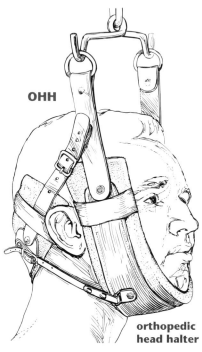

OHH

orthopedic head halter

OHIAA	hydroxyindolacetic acid
OHIVAT	oral HIV-1 antibody test (Orasure)
OHL	oral hairy leukoplakia
OHM	omohyoid muscle
OHN	occupational health nurse
OHP	hydroxyprogesterone
	oxygen under high pressure
	oxygen under hyperbaric pressure
OHS	obesity hypoventilation syndrome
	Occupational Health Services
	ocular hypoperfusion syndrome
	open heart surgery
OHSS	ovarian hyperstimulation syndrome
OHT	ocular hypertension
OHVS	obesity-hypoventilation syndrome

OI	obturator internus (muscle)
	occult injury
	opportunistic illness
	opportunistic infection
	orgasmic impairment
	osteogenesis imperfecta (osteopenia)
	otitis interna
	ovarian insufficiency
OIC	opioid-induced constipation
	osteogenesis imperfecta congenita
OIF	oil-immersion field
	Osteogenesis Imperfecta Foundation
OIH	orthoiodohippurate
	ovulation-inducing hormone
OILD	occupational immunologic lung disease
oint	ointment
OIT	oil immersion test
OIVABT	outpatient intravenous antibiotic therapy
OJ	obstructive jaundice
	orange juice
OK	okay; all right; all correct (derived from Old Kinderhook, a town in New York State)
OKN	optokinetic nystagmus
OKS	oral Kaposi's sarcoma
O & L	osteoporosis and leukemia
o.l.	*oculus laevus* [Latin] left eye
ol.	*oleum* [Latin] oil
OLA	*occipito-laeva anterior* [Latin] left occipito-anterior (fetal position)
	oligonucleotide ligation assay
OLACLI	open-loop anterior chamber lens implantation
OLB	open liver biopsy
	open lung biopsy
OLCA	orifice of left

	coronary artery
OLD	obstructive lung disease
	occupational lung disease
oleo	oleomargarine
olf	olfactory
OLIDS	open loop insulin delivery system
OLM	ocular larva migrans (syndrome)
	ophthalmologic laser microendoscope
OLP	*occipito-laeva posterior* [Latin] left occipitoposterior (fetal position)
OLT	*occipito-laeva transversa* [Latin] left occipitotransverse (fetal position)
	orthotopic liver transplant
	orthotopic liver transplantation
OLV	one-lung ventilation
OM	occupational medicne
	onychomycosis
	oral mucositis
	osteomalacia
	osteomyelitis
	otitis media
	ovulation method (birth control technique)
o.m.	*omni mane* [Latin] every morning
OMAC	otitis media, acute catarrhal
OMAR	Office of Medical Applications of Research (at NIH)
OMB	Office of Management and Budget
OMD	ocular muscular dystrophy
	organic mental disorder
	oromandibular dystonia
OME	Office of Medical Examiner
	orbicular muscle of eye
	otitis media with effusion
OMH	omohyoid (muscle)
OMI	old myocardial infarct

oocyte-maturation
  inhibitor
oocyte-meiotic inhibitor
OMM orbicular muscle of mouth
OMN oculomotor (3rd
  cranial) nerve
oculomotor nucleus
omn. bih. *omni bihors* [Latin]
  every two hours
omn. hor. *omni hora* [Latin]
  every hour
omn. man.
  omni mane [Latin]
  every morning
omn. noct.
  omni nocte [Latin]
  every night
omn. quar. hor.
  omni quadrante hora [Latin]
  every quarter of an hour
OMO oral malodor
OMP obstetrical measuring plate
oculomotor (3rd cranial
  nerve) palsy
orotidine-5'-
  monophosphate
outer membrane protein
OMPA octamethyl
  pyrophosphoramide
otitis media, purulent, acute
OMPC otitis media, purulent,
  chronic
om. quar. hor.
  omni quadrante hora [Latin]
  every quarter of an hour
OMR operative mortality rate
OMS opsocionus-myoclonus
  syndrome (dancing eyes,
  dancing feet)
oral morphine sulfate
organic mental syndrome
osteomalacia senile
osteomeatal stent
osteomyelosclerosis
otomandibular syndrome
OMSA otitis media,
  suppurative, acute
OMSC otitis media,
  suppurative, chronic

OMT Oriental movement
  therapy (qigong)
osteopathic manipulative
  therapy
OMwE otitis media with effusion
ON obstructive nephropathy
oculomotor nerve
  (3rd cranial nerve)
office nurse
olfactory nerve
  (1st cranial nerve)
optic nerve
  (2rd cranial nerve)
optic neuritis
Osler node (small, tender,
  and discolored node
  usually appearing on the
  pads of fingers and toes
  in individuals with
  subacute endocarditis)
osteonecrosis
overnight
o.n. *omni nocte* [Latin]
  every night
ONB obturator nerve block
ONC oncology
oncology nurse, certified
Oncovin (vincristine)
over-the-needle catheter
ONCO oncology
OND organic nervous disease
other neurologic disorders
ONDCP Office of National Drug
  Control Policy
ONM oronasal membranes
ONP oxalate nephropathy
ONTG oral nitroglycerin
ONTR order not to resuscitate
OO oophorectomy
oral order
osteoid osteoma
OOB out of bed
OOC onset of contractions
organ of Corti
out of control
OOD overdose of drugs
OOHCA out-of-hospital cardiac
  arrest
OOL onset of labor

OOR	out of room
OORA	oligoarticular onset rheumatoid arthritis
OORR	orbicularis oculoreflex response
OOS	occupational overuse syndrome
OOT	out of town
OOW	out of wedlock
OP	obstructive pancreatitis
	occiput posterior
	odontoid process
	open
	operation
	operative procedure
	opiate poisoning
	opponens pollicis (muscle)
	optical pachometer
	organophophorus
	oropharynx
	osmotic pressure
	osteopetrosis
	osteoporosis
	outpatient
	oxidative phosphorylation
op	operation
OPC	oculopalatocerebral (syndrome)
	outpatient catheterization
	outpatient clinic
OPCA	olivopontocerebellar atrophy
op. cit.	*opus citatum* [Latin] in the work cited
OPD	otopalatodigital (syndrome)
	outpatient department
	outpatient dispensary
OPEN	Oncovin (vincristine) + prednisone + etoposide + Novantrone (mitoxantrone) (combination chemotherapy)
OPG	ocular plethysmography
	oculoplethysmography
opg	opening
OPGA	outpatient general anesthesia

OPH	obliterative pulmonary hypertension
	ophthalmology
Oph	ophthalmoscope
Ophth	ophthalmology
OPL	outer plexiform layer (of retina)
OPLL	ossification of the posterior longitudinal ligament
OPM	occult primary malignancy
	oculopharyngeal myopathy
	ophthalmoplegic migraine
OPO	organ procurement organization
	oropharyngeal candidiasis
OPP	opposite
	organophosphorous poisoning
	oxygen partial pressure
OPRDU	outpatient renal dialysis unit
OPRR	Office for Protection from Research Risk (at NIH)
OPRT	orotate phosphoribosyltransferase
OPS	organic personality disorder
	outpatient service
	outpatient surgery
OPSA	ovarian papillary serous adenocarcinoma
OPSI	overwhelming postsplenectomy infection
OPSR	Office of Professional Standards Review
OPT	open pneumothorax
	outpatient
	outpatient treatment
OPt	outpatient
opt	optimum
OPTHD	optimal hemodialysis
OPTN	Organ Procurement and Transplantation Network
OPV	oral polio vaccine
	oral poliovirus vaccine
OPWL	opiate withdrawal
OR	odds ratio
	open reduction (of a fracture)

	operating room
	optic radiation
	oral rehydration
	orienting reflex
	own recognizance
O-R	oxidation-reduction
ORA	opiate receptor agonist
ORBC	Orthoset radiopaque bone cement
ORCA	orifice of right coronary artery
ORCH	orchiectomy
orch	orchitis
ORD	oral radiation death
OR & F	open reduction and fixation
ORFs	open reading frames
org	organic
ORIF	open reduction and internal fixation
ORL	otorhinolaryngology
ORM	other regulated material
ORN	operating room nurse osteoradionecrosis
Orn	ornithine (an amino acid)
ORP	opioid-resistant pain oxidation-reduction potential
ORS	oral rehydration solution oral surgery orthopedic surgery ovarian remnant syndrome
ORT	operating room technician oral rehydration therapy
Ortho	orthodontics orthopedics
ORWH	Office of Research on Women's Health (at NIH)
OS	occupational safety office surgery Ogilvie's syndrome opening snap (diastolic heart sound) oral surgery OraSure (oral HIV test) orthopedic surgery Osgood-Schlatter (disease)

	osteogenic sarcoma
	osteosarcoma
	osteosclerosis
	oxidant stress (damage to cells caused by free radicals, i.e., unstable oxygen molecules)
	oxygen saturation
Os	osmium (hard metallic element)
o.s.	*oculus sinister* [Latin] left eye
OSA	obstructive sleep apnea Optical Society of America
OSAP	Office of Substance Abuse Prevention
OSAS	obstructive sleep apnea syndrome
OSD	optical scanning device Osgood-Schlatter disease
OSF	organ system failure
OSH	outside the hospital
OSHA	Occupational Safety and Health Act Occupational Safety and Health Administration
OSHT	orthostatic hypotension
OSI	Office of Scientific Integrity (at NIH) open systems interconnections
OSIR	Office of Scientific Integrity Review
OSL	Osgood-Schlatter lesion
OSM	osteosclerotic myeloma
Osm	osmolarity osmole (mole is preferred)
Osmol	osmole (mole is preferred)
Osm S	osmolarity serum
Osm U	osmolarity urine
OSO	Osgood-Schlatter osteochondritis
OSRD	Office of Scientific Research and Development
oss	osseous
OSSP	open-set speech perception
OST	occlusal splint therapy

Office of Science
and Technology

Osteo osteoarthritis
osteomyelitis
osteopath

OT objective test
occupational therapist
occupational therapy
ocular tension
old tuberculin
optic tract
oral temperature
orotracheal
ortolani's test (maneuver)
oxygen therapy

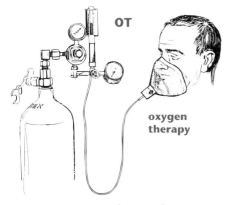

OT

**oxygen
therapy**

oxygen transport
oxytocin

OTA Office of Technology
Assessment
ornithine transaminase
ovarian tumor-associated
antigen

OTABN ortho-tolueno-azo-
beta-naphthol
(poisonous dye)

OTC Online Training Center
ornithine
transcarbamoylase
over-the-counter (drugs)
oxytetracycline

OTC DA over-the-counter drug abuse

OTC drugs
over-the-counter drugs
(nonprescription drugs)

OTD organ tolerance dose

out the door
Registered Occupational
Therapist

oth other

OTI Office for Treatment
Improvement
orotracheal intubation
ovomucoid trypsin
inhibitor

OTO otology

Otol otology

OTR organ transplant rejection
ovarian tumor registry
registered occupational
therapist

OTS orotracheal suction

OTSC Office of the
Surgeon General

OTT one-tail test (to determine
a statistical difference in
only one direction)
orotracheal tube

OTW over-the-wire

OU obstructive uropathy

o.u. *oculus uterque* [Latin]
both eyes

O₂UC O_2UC oxygen utilization
coefficient

OUI operating (a vehicle)
under influence

OURQ outer upper right quadrant

OUS overuse syndrome

OV office visit
Onchocerca volvulus
(causative agent of
onchocerciasis)
ovary
ovulation
ovum

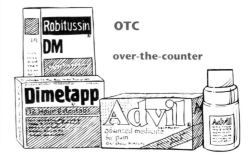

OTC

over-the-counter

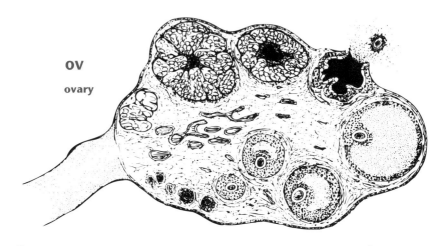

OV

ovary

Ov	ovary
	ovum
Ova	ovalbumin
OVC	ovarian cancer
OVD	obliterative vascular disease
	occlusal vertical dimension
OVLA	oblique vein of left atrium
OVLT	organum vasculosum laminae terminalis
O. volvulus	
	Onchocerca volvulus (causative agent of onchocerciasis)
OVR	Office of Vocational Rehabilitation
OVX	ovariectomy
OW	open wedge (osteotomy)
	open wound
	out-of-wedlock
	oval window (between middle ear chamber and vestibule of inner ear)
OWB	oscillating waterbed (to stimulate the newborn in an extrauterine environment)
OWCL	old world cutaneous leishmaniasis
OWCP	Office of Worker's Compensation Program
OWR	Osler-Weber-Rendu (syndrome; hereditary hemorrhagic telangiectasia)
OX	optic chiasma
	oxacillin (a semi-synthetic penicillinase-resistant penicillin)
	oxytocin (hormone formed by the neuronal cells of the hypothalamic nuclei)
oxi	oximeter
OXP	oxypressin
OXT	oxytocin
OXY	oxygen (O_2)
OXZ	oxazepam
oz	ounce (30 ml)

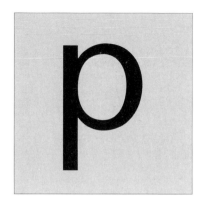

P   pain
pancreas
para
part
passive
Pasteurella (genus of
ellipsoidal or rod-shaped
gram-negative bacteria
that usually occur singly;
some species cause
tularemia)
patella

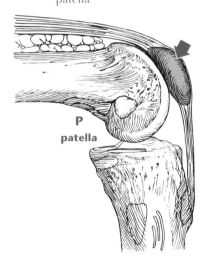

P
patella

paternal
pellagra (dietary niacin
deficiency)
percussion
perforation

peripheral
peritoneum
permeability
pharynx
phenotype
phosphate
phosphorus
physostigmine
pint
placebo
plasma
Plasmodium (a genus of the
class Sporozoa; some
species cause malaria)
platelet

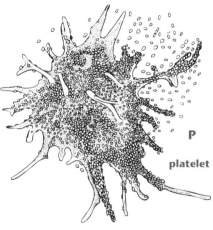

P
platelet

Pneumocystis (a genus of
microorganisms thought
to be either protozoa or
yeastlike fungi)
pollicis (thumb)
polymyxin
position
positive
posterior
precursor
prednisone
premolar
presbyopia
pressure
primipara
prions (slow viruses)
probability
progesterone

	prolactin		peritoneal adhesions
	proline		pernicious anemia
	proprionate		phakic-aphakic
	prostate		phenol alcohol
	protein		phenylalkylamine
	Proteus (a genus of gram-negative bacteria commonly associated with urinary tract and wound infections)		Phobics Anonymous
			photoallergenic
			Physician Assistant
			pituitary adenoma
			placenta accreta
	psychiatry		plasma aldosterone
	pubis		plasminogen activator
	pulmonary		platelet adhesiveness
	pulse		platelet aggregation
	pupil		pleomorphic adenoma
p	partial pressure		polyarteritis
P1	first parental generation		popliteal artery
P₁	first pulmonic heart sound		posteroanterior (x-ray)
P₂	second pulmonic heart sound		prealbumin
			pregnancy-associated
P₅₀	partial pressure of oxygen with hemoglobin half-saturated with oxygen		primary aldosteronism
			primary amenorrhea
			primary anemia
P/3	proximal third		prior to admission
³²P	radioactive phosphorus		prolonged action
p	after		prostate antigen
	page		protective antigen
	papilla		proteolytic action
	pico (prefix denoting decimal factor 10⁻¹²)		prothrombin activity
			protrusio acetabuli
	pint		*Pseudomonas aeruginosa* (major cause of nosocomial infection)
	pressure		
	proton		
	pulse		psoriatic arthritis
	pupil		psychoanalysis
	short arm of chromosome		psychoanalyst
PA	pancreatic ascites		pulmonary artery
	panic attack		pulmonary atelectasis
	panniculus adiposus		psychogenic aspermia
	pantothenic acid		pyogenic arthritis
	paralysis agitans		pyruvic acid
	paranoia	**P-A**	posteroanterior (x-ray)
	paranoid	**P & A**	percussion and auscultation
	parenteral alimentation		
	passive-aggressive	**Pa**	Pascal (SI unit of pressure)
	pendulous abdomen		protactinium (radioactive metallic element)
	perennial allergy		
	periarteritis	**pA**	picoampere
	periodontal abscess	**pa**	pascal

p.a. *per anum* [Latin] by way of the anus

PAA peri-appendicular abscess
phenylacetic acid
plasma angiotensinase activity
polyammino acid

PAB para-aminobenzoic (acid)
pes anserinus bursa
premature atrial beat

PABA para-aminobenzoic acid

PABD predeposited autologous blood donation

PABP pulmonary artery balloon pump

PAC papillary adenocarcinoma
papular acrodermatitis of childhood
periapical cyst
phenacetin, aspirin, and caffeine
Platinol (cisplatin)
+ Adriamycin (doxorubicin)
+ cyclophosphamide (combination chemotherapy)
premature atrial contraction

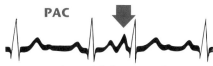

PAC

premature atrial contraction

prostatic adenocarcinoma
pulmonary adenocystic carcinoma
pulmonary artery catheter
pulmonary artery catheterization

PACATH pulmonary artery catheter

PACC pediatric acute care clinic

PACE pulmonary angiotensin I converting enzyme

PaCO$_2$ arterial partial pressure of carbon dioxide (in blood gases)

PACU post-anesthesia care unit (recovery room)

PACP pulmonary alveolar-capillary permeability

PACT papillary carcinoma of thyroid

PAD pelvic adhesive disease
percutaneous abscess drainage
peripheral arterial disease
phlegmasia alba dolens
photon absorption densitometry
physician-assisted death
preoperative autologous donation
primary affective disorder
probable Alzheimer's disease

PADI Professional Association of Diving Instructors

PADP pulmonary artery diastolic pressure

PADS pectoral aplasia dysdactyly syndrome (Poland's syndrome)

PAE passive assistive exercise
positive affect enhancement
postantibiotic effect
progressive assistive exercise

p.ae. *partes aequales* [Latin] in equal parts

PAEDP pulmonary arterial end diastolic pressure

P. aeruginosa *Pseudomonas aeruginosa* (a major agent of nosocomial infections, especially in elderly debilitated individuals)

PAES popliteal artery entrapment syndrome

PAF paroxysmal atrial fibrillation
platelet-activating factor
platelet-aggregating factor
pollen adherence factor

prostatic antibacterial
fraction

pseudoamniotic fluid

pulmonary arteriovenous
fistula

PAF-AH platelet activating factor
acetylhydrolase

PAFI platelet-aggregation factor
inhibitor

PAFIB paroxysmal atrial
fibrillation

PAFs platelet activating factors

PAG pneumatic antishock
garment

pregnancy-associated
globulin

PAGE polyacrylamide gel
electrophoresis

PAH para-aminohippurate

para-aminohippuric acid

Parents Anonymous
Hotline (800) 421-0353

phenylalanine hydroxylase

primary alveolar
hypoventilation

pulmonary artery
hypertension

pulmonary artery
hypotension

PAHA para-aminohippuric acid

PAHO Pan American Health
Organization

PAHVC pulmonary alveolar
hypoxic vasoconstrictor

PAHS primary alveolar
hypoventilation syndrome

PAI plasminogen activator
inhibitor

platelet accumulation
index

Pseudomonas aeruginosa
infection

PAI-1 plasminogen activator
inhibitor- type 1 (crucial
enzyme to the balance
between clotting and
bleeding)

PAIDS pediatric AIDS

PAIRS pain and impairment

relationship scale

PAIT passive adoptive
immunotherapy

PAJ paralysis agitans juvenilis

PAL plasma ammonia level

posterior axillary line

pregnancy-associated
listeriosis

pyogenic abscess of liver

PALNs para-aortic lymph nodes

Palp palpable

palpate

palpated

palpation

PALS periarteriolar lymphatic
sheath

posterior axillary line

Palv alveolar pressure

PAM phenylalanine mustard

preanesthetic medication

pregnancy-associated
macroglobulin

primary amebic
meningoencephalitis

pulmonary alveolar
macrophage

pulmonary alveolar
microlithiasis

pulmonary artery mean
pressure

PAMD prelingually acquired
meningitic deafness

primary adrenocortical
micronodular dysplasia

PAME primary amebic
meningoencephalitis

PAMP pulmonary artery mean
pressure

PAMS periodic acid-
methenamine silver stain

PAN periarteritis nodosa
(necrotizing arteritis)

periodic alternating
nystagmus

polyarteritis nodosa

positional alcohol
nystagmus

pan pancreas

PAND primary adrenocortical

nodular dysplasia

PANESS physical and neurologic
examination for soft signs

PANS peripheral autonomic
nervous system
puromycin
aminonucleoside

PANs periaortic nodes
positive axillary nodes
primary afferent
nociceptors
(pain receptors)

PAO peak acid output
peripheral airway
obstruction
plasma amine oxidase
power already on
pustulotic arthro-osteitis

Pao pressure at airway opening

PaO₂ arterial partial pressure
of oxygen

PAOD peripheral arterial
occlusive disease

PAOJA pauciarticular onset
juvenile arthritis

PAOP pulmonary artery
occlusion pressure

PAP Papanicolaou (test)
passive-aggressive
personality
periarticular arthritic pain
peroxidase-antiperoxidase
(complex)
phosphoadenosine
phosphate
placental acid phosphatase
placental alkaline
phosphatase
positive airway pressure
primary atypical
pneumonia
prostatic acid phosphatase
pseudoachondroplasia
pulmonary alveolar
proteinosis
pulmonary artery pressure
pyelonephritis-
associated pili

pap papilla

PAPD passive-aggressive
personality disorder
postaxial polydactyly
preaxial polydactyly

PAPF platelet adhesiveness
plasma factor

PAPP pregnancy-associated
plasma protein

PAPS papillomas
3'-phosphoadenosine-5'-
phosphosulfate

PA/PS pulmonary atresia/
pulmonary stenosis

Pap sm Papanicolaou smear

Pap smear
Papanicolaou smear

Pap test Papanicolaou test
(stain test)

PAPVR partial anomalous
pulmonary venous return

PAR arteriolar resistance
paraffin
passive avoidance reaction
People Against Rape
perennial allergic rhinitis
photoallergic reaction
platelet aggregate ratio
population attributable
risk
postanesthesia recovery
(room)
post-anesthesia room
probable allergic rhinitis
program for alcoholic
recovery
pulmonary arteriolar
resistance

PAR% population attributable
risk percentage

PARA number of pregnancies

PARA I having borne one child
(unipara)

PARA II having borne two children
(bipara)

PARA III having borne three
children (tripara)

PARA IV having borne four children
(quadripara)

para paraplegic

paracent paracentesis

par. aff. *pars affecta* [Latin] the part affected

parasym parasympathetic

parent parenteral

PARF parenchymatous acute renal failure

parox paroxysmal

PARR postanesthesia recovery room

part. aeq.
partes aequales [Latin] in equal parts

part. dolent.
partes dolentes [Latin] painful parts

part. vic. *partitis vicibus* [Latin] in divided doses

PARU postanesthetic recovery unit

PAS pain amplification syndrome
painful arc syndrome
para-aminosalicylic acid (Pamisyl)
periodic acid-Schiff (stain)
personality assessment schedule
phosphatase acid serum
physician-assisted suicide
postadrenalectomy syndrome
postanesthesia shivering
premature atrial stimulus
progressive accumulated stress
pulmonary artery stenosis
pulmonary aspiration syndrome
pulsatile antiembolic system

PASA para-aminosalicylic acid (Pamisyl)
primary acquired sideroblastic anemia

PASD phytanic acid storage disease

PASG pneumatic antishock garment

pass passive

PAT pancreatic aberrant tissue
paroxysmal atrial tachycardia
patella
platelet aggregation test
polyamine acetyltransferase
potassium antimony tartrate
preadmission testing
pregnancy at term
prophylactic antibiotic therapy
psychoacoustic test

pat patella
patent

PATC pain-anxiety-tension cycle

PATE pulmonary artery thromboembolism

PATH pituitary adrenotropic hormone

Path pathogenic
pathologic
pathology

PATI penetraing abdominal trauma index

PATS Parsonage-Aldren-Turner syndrome

PAVF pulmonary arteriovenous fistula

PA view posteroanterior view (patient position for x-ray)

PAW peripheral airways

PAWP pulmonary artery wedge pressure

PB paraffin bath
peripheral blood
peroneus brevis (muscle)
phenobarbital
pigeon breast (pectus carinatum; congenital chondrocostal prominence)
placental barrier
placentation bleeding
polymyxin B
premature beat

premature birth
protein-bound
pudendal block
punch biopsy

P & B pain and burning
phenobarbital and
belladonna

Pb *plumbum* [Latin] lead
phenobarbital

PBA partial-birth abortion
percutaneous bladder
aspiration
pressure breathing assister
prolactin-binding assay
pudendal block anesthesia

PBAL protected brancho-
alveolar lavage

PBAR post-balloon angioplasty
restenosis

PBBs polybrominated biphenyls
(causes chronic health
effects in humans)

PBC peripheral blood cells
primary biliary cirrhosis
progestin-binding
complement

PBCC pigmented basal
cell carcinoma

PBD percutaneous biliary
drainage
pigeon breeder's disease
postburn day
primary blistering disorder
proliferative breast disease
prostatic balloon dilation

PBE partial breech extraction

PBF peripheral blood flow
pharyngobasilar fascia
placental blood flow
pulmonary blood flow
punch biopsy forceps

PBFe protein-bound iron

PBG porphobilinogen (organic
compound present in
large quantities in the
urine of patients with
acute or congenital
porphyria)

PBI penile brachial index

protein-bound iodine; also
called protein-bound
radioactive iodine
Pseudoallesceria boydii
infection

PbI lead intoxication

PBK phosphorylase B kinase

PBL palmar beak ligament
peripheral blood leukocyte
peripheral blood
lymphocyte
pigeon breeder's lung

PBLC peripheral blood
lymphocyte count
premature-birth
living child

PBM placental basement
membrane

PBMCs peripheral blood
mononuclear cells

PBMV percutaneous balloon
mitral valvoplasty

PBN peripheral benign
neoplasm
polymyxin B sulfate,
bacitracin and neomycin
postburn neuralgia
polymyxin, bacitracin
and neomycin

PBND pollybeak nasal deformity

PBO placebo

PBP penicillin-binding protein
postural back pain
progressive bulbar palsy
prostate-binding protein

PBPC peripheral blood
progenitor cells

PBPS penicillin-binding protein
periodic blood pressure
surveillance

PBR Patient's Bill of Rights

Pb-RBC lead red blood cell count

PBS phenobarbital sodium
phosphate-buffered saline
phosphate buffer system
polymyxin B sulfate
(Aerosporin)
powder burn spots
prune-belly syndrome

	pulmonary branch stenosis
Pbs	pressure at body surface (of chest)
PBSC	peripheral blood stem cells
PBT$_4$	protein-bound thyroxine
PBV	percutaneous balloon valvuloplasty
	pulmonary blood volume
PBx	prostate biopsy
	punch biopsy
PBY	postgraduate year
PBZ	phenylbutazone
	pyribenzamine
PC	paccinian corpuscle
	pain control
	pancreatic carcinoma
	pancreatic cholera
	paper chromatography
	pectus carinatum
	pedigree chart
	penicillin
	pentose cycle
	percent
	periosteal chondroma
	phosphate cycle
	phosphatidylcholine
	phosphocreatine choline
	phosphorylcholine
	phytochemicals
	pilonidal cyst (hair-containing cyst in the dermis or subcutaneous tissue, usually connected to the surface of the skin by a sinus tract)
	plasma cell
	plasma cortisol
	plasma creatinine
	platelet count
	Platinol (cisplatin) + cyclophosphamide (combination chemotherapy)
	pneumotaxic center
	polyposis coli (familial intestinal polyposis; many potentially malignant adenomatous polyps lining the mucous

	membrane of the intestine, especially the colon)
	popliteal cyst
	portal cirrhosis
	postcoital
	posterior capsule
	posterior chamber (of eye)
	postcoital
	precordium
	premature contraction
	prenatal care
	present complaint
	primary care
	procollagen
	productive cough
	prostate cancer
	protein C
	pubococcygeus (muscle)
	Purkinje cell
	pyloric canal
P/C	posterior chamber of eye
P & C	precautions and contraindications
	pevention and control
pc	picocurie
p.c.	*post cibum* [Latin] after meals
PCA	papillary cystadenoma
	para-chloroamphetamine
	parent-controlled analgesia
	passive cutaneous anaphylaxis
	patient care aide
	patient-controlled analgesia
	patient-controlled anesthesia
	perchloric acid
	percutaneous carotid angiography
	physician's comparability allowance
	posterior cerebral artery
	posterior communicating artery
	President's Council on Aging

procoagulation activity

prostatic carcinoma

PCAD premature coronary artery disease

PCAG primary closed-angle glaucoma

PCAN potential child abuse and neglect

PCAPI postcentral anterior parietal infarction

P. carinii *Pneumocystis carinii* (the causative agent of a contagious, interstitial plasma cell pneumonia)

PCB paracervical block

paracolon bacilli

placebo

polychlorinated biphenyl (widespread environmental contaminant)

portacaval bypass

postcoital bleeding

PCBs polychlorinated biphenyls (widespread environmental contaminants)

PCBZ polychlorobenzene

PCC pericardial constriction

pericardiocentesis

pheochromocytoma

plasma catecholamine concentration

Pneumocystis carinii (the causative agent of a contagious, interstitial plasma cell pneumonia)

Poison Control Center

postcoital contraception

Pregnancy Crisis Center (800) 368-3336

primary care center

PCCS postcholecystectomy syndrome

PCCU postcoronary care unit

PCD pacer-cardioverter defibrillator

percutaneous diskectomy

pericardial disease

phlegmasia cerulea dolens

plasma cell dyscrasia

polycystic disease

posterior corneal deposits

primary ciliary dyskinesia

pseudocholinesterase deficiency

PCDDs polychlorinated dibenzodioxins (environmental contaminant formed when polychlorobenzene (PCBZ) is heated)

PCDFs polychlorinated dibenzofurans (environmental contaminant formed when polychlorinated biphenyl (PCB) is heated)

PCDT Pacific Coast dog tick (*Dermacentor occidentalis*)

PCE perchloroethylene

physical capacities evaluation

pericardial effusion

posterior chamber of eye

PCEA patient-controlled epidural analgesia

PCEC pneumococcal endocarditis

P cells principal cells (in renal tubules)

PCES pain control by electrical stimulation

p.c. et h.s.

post cibos et hora somni [Latin] after meals and at bedtime

PCF peripheral circulatory failure

pharyngoconjunctival fever

posterior cervical fusion

posterior cranial fossa

procoagulant factor

prothrombin conversion factor

PCG paracervical ganglion

pericardial graft

phonocardiogram
piezocardiogram
postcentral gyrus

PCG
postcentral gyrus

primary congenital
  glaucoma
primate chorionic
  gonadotropin
pubococcygeus (muscle)
PCH   paroxysmal cold
  hemoglobinuria
PChe   pseudocholinesterase
PCheD   pseudocholinesterase
  dficiency
PCHRG   Public Citizen Health
  Research Group
PCI   pneumococcal
  immunization
  positive chemical
  ionization
  prophylactic cranial
  irradiation
pCi   picocurie
PCIA   pneumococcal infectious
  arthritis
PCIC   Poison Control
  Information Center
PCIOL   posterior chamber
  intraocular lens
PCIS   post-cardiac injury
  syndrome
PCK   polycystic kidney
PCKD   polycystic kidney disease
PCL   papillary cystadenoma
  lymphomatosum
  (Warthin's tumor)

persistent corpus luteum
plasma cell leukemia
plasma cholesterol level
posterior chamber lens
posterior cruciate ligament
  (of knee joint)
precancerous lesion
precordial leads
PCLD   polycystic liver disease
PCM   patellar chondromalacia
  phase contrast microscope
  plasma cell myeloma
  (plasmacytoma)
  pneumococcal meningitis
  primary cutaneous
  melanoma
  protein-calorie
  malnutrition
PCN   papillary-cystic neoplasm
  penicillin
  percutaneous nephrostomy
  primary care nursing
PCNB   pentachloronitrobenzene
PCNL   percutaneous
  nephrostolithotomy
  plantar calcaneonavicular
  ligament
PCNV   postchemotherapy nausea
  and vomiting
PCO   patient complains of
  polycystic ovary
pCO$_2$ partial pressure of carbon
  dioxide (in blood gases)
PCOD   polycystic ovarian disease
PCOS   polycystic ovary syndrome
PCP   partial cleft palate
  pentachlorophenol
  percutaneous pinning
  pericardial pressure
  persistent cough and
  phlegm
  phencyclidine pill
  (phencyclidine
  hydrochloride)
  plasma cell pneumonia
  pneumococcal peritonitis
  pneumococcal pneumonia
  Pneumocystis carinii
  pneumonia
  postoperative

constrictive pericarditis
primary care physician
principal care provider
prochlorperazine
pulmonary capillary
   pressure

PCPA para-chlorophenylalanine
pericardiacophrenic artery

PCPF percutaneous pin fixation

PCPGV postchallenge plasma
   glucose value

PCPS percutaneous
   cardiopulmonary support

PCQs polychlororinated
   quaterphenyls

PCR plasma clearance rate
polymerase chain reaction
porphyria cutanea tarda
posterior cruciate rupture
postinfarction cardiac
   rehabilitation
protein catabolic rate

PCr phosphocreatine (along
   with ATP, it provides the
   energy that makes the
   heart contract and pump
   blood into the arteries)
plasma creatinine

PCr/ATP phosphocreatine-
   adenosine triphosphate
   ratio (an indicator of the
   heart's ability to cope
   with low oxygen
   concentrations in the
   blood)

PCS pelvic congestion
   syndrome
pericordial catch syndrome
pharmacogenic
   confusional syndrome
portacaval shunt
postcardiotomy syndrome
postcentral sulcus
postcholecystectomy
   syndrome
post-coital syndrome
post-concussion syndrome
posterior crus of stapes
preconscious

primary cancer site
prolonged crush syndrome
prostatic cryosurgery
Purkinje conducting
   system

Pcs preconscious

PCT painful cervical trauma
patient care technician
pericardial tamponade
peripheral carcinoid tumor
photochemotherapy
plasma clotting time
polychlorinated triphenyl
porphyria cutanea tarda
postcoital test
photochemotherapy
   (treatment with drugs
   that react to sunlight)
precentral sulcus
prepared childbirth
   training
progestin challenge test
prothrombin
   consumption time
proximal convoluted
   tubule (of kidney)

pct percent

PCTA percutaneous transluminal
   angioplasty

PCU pain control unit
palliative care unit
primary care unit
protective care unit

PCV packed cell volume
   (hematocrit)
polychlorinated vinyl
polycythemia vera
postcapillary venule
pressure-control
   ventilation

PCVP procarbazine +
   cyclophosphamide +
   vinblastine + prednisone
   (combination
   chemotherapy)

PCW pulmonary capillary
   wedge (pressure)

PCWP pulmonary capillary
   wedge pressure

PCZ procarbazine (an
antineoplastic agent)
PD interpupillary distance
Paget's disease
(osteitis deformans)
pancreatic duct
panic disorder
Panner disease
papillary duct (of kidney)
parkinsonism dementia
Parkinson's disease
partial denture
patent ductus
pelvic diaphragm
Penrose drain
(cigarette drain)
periodontal disease
peritoneal dialysis
personality disorder
Perthes' disease
Peyronie's disease
phosphate dehydrogenase
phosphodiesterase
photoderm
photosensitivity dermatitis
physical dependence
Pick's disease
pituitary dwarfism
Plummer's disease
Pompe's disease
poorly differentiated
postnasal drainage
postnasal drip
postural drainage
potassium depletion
potential difference
Pott's disease
preexisting disease
pregnanediol
premature delivery
problem drinker
progesterone deficiency
protein diet
psychotic depression
pulmonary disease
pupillary distance
pyloric dilator
pyoderma (any pus-
producing skin disorder)

P/D packs per day (cigarettes)
Pd palladium (an inert
metallic element)
pd papilla diameter
potential difference
prism diopter
pupillary distance
PDA Parenteral Drug
Association
patent ductus arteriosus

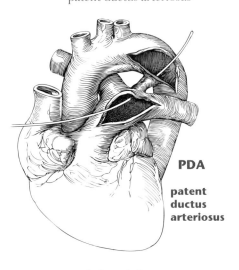

PDA

**patent
ductus
arteriosus**

periodontal abscess
polydrug abuse
posterior descending
(coronary) artery
prescription drug abuse
PDAB paradimethylamino-
benzaldehyde
PD-ALS Parkinson-dementia-
amyotrophic lateral
sclerosis
PDAS pulmonary disease-
anemia syndrome
PDB Paget's disease of bone
papillary duct of Bellini
(of kidney)
periodic drinking bout
protein data bank
PDBRCA
posterior descending
branch of right
coronary artery

PDC parkinsonism dementia
complex
patient denies condition
postductal coarctation
private diagnostic clinic

PD & C postural drainage
and clapping

PDCA posterior descending
coronary artery
primary degenerative
cerebral disease

PD CSE pulsed Doppler
crosssectional
echocardiography

PDD percent depth dose
peridontal disease
pervasive developmental
disorder
polydystrophic dwarfism
(Marateaux-Lamy
disease)
primary degenerative
dementia
progressive
diaphyseal dysplasia
(Engelmann's disease)
pyridoxine-deficient diet

PDE paroxysmal dyspnea
on exertion
personality disorder
examination
phosphodiesterase
progressive dialysis
encephalopathy
pulsed Doppler
echocardiography

PD Echo pulsed Doppler
echocardiography

PDEGF platelet-derived epidermal
growth factor

PDF Parkinson's Disease
Foundation
peritoneal dialysis fluid
pigmented
dermatofibroma

PDGF platelet-derived growth
factor

PDH phosphate dehydrogenase
progressive disseminated
histoplasmosis

pyruvate dehydrogenase

PDHC pyruvate dehydrogenase
complex

PDI periodontal disease index
psychomotor develop-
ment index

Pdi transdiaphragmatic
pressure

PDIGC patient discharged in
good condition

P-diol pregnanediol

PDK polycystic kidney disease

PDK1 gene
gene of polycystic
kidney disease

PDL periodontal ligament
poorly differentiated
lymphocyte
progressively diffused
leukoencephalopathy

PDLC poorly differentiated
lung cancer

PDLL poorly differentiated
lymphocytic lymphoma

PDLN poorly differentiated
lymphocytic-nodular

PDN prednisone
private-duty nurse
private-duty nursing

PDP peptidyl dipeptidase
periodontal pain
periodontal pocket

perio-dontal pocket   **PDP**

platelet-derived plasma
Product Development
Protocol

PD & P   postural drainage
     and percussion
PDPD   prolonged-dwell
     peritoneal dialysis
PDPH   post-dural puncture
     headache
PDQ   personality diagnostic
     questionnaire
     physician data query
     pretty darn quick
     (immediately)
PDR   peripheral diabetic
     retinopathy
     Physicians' Desk Reference
     postdelivery room
     proliferative diabetic
     retinopathy
pdr   powder
PDS   pain dysfunction syndrome
     paroxysmal
     depolarizing shift
     patient data system
     peritoneal dialysis system
     pigment dispersion
     syndrome
     plasma derived serum
PDs   personality disorders
PDT   percutaneous dilational
     tracheostomy
     photodynamic therapy
     (cancer treatment
     modality)
     posterior drawer test
     preimplantation
     diagnostic test
PDU   pulsed Doppler
     ultrasonography
PDV   peak diastolic velocity
PE   painful engorgement
     paper electrophoresis
     partial epilepsy
     passive exercise
     pectus excavatum
     (funnel chest)
     pelvic examination
     pericardial effusion
     peritoneal exudate
     phakoemulsification
     pharyngoesophageal

     phenylephrine
     phosphatidyl ethanolamine
     phycoerythrin
     physical education
     physical examination
     phytoestrogens
     pigmented epithelium
     pitcher's elbow
     plasma expander
     Platinol (cisplatin) +
     etoposide (combination
     chemotherapy)
     pleural effusion
     polyethylene
     pre-eclampsia
     premature ejaculation
     present evaluation
     probable error
     protein electrophoresis
     psychiatric evaluation
     psychological evaluation
     pulled elbow (nursemaid's
     elbow; transient
     subluxation of head of
     radius of young children)
     pulmonary edema
     pulmonary embolectomy
     pulmonary embolism
     pulmonary emphysema
     pyramidal eminence
     pyrogenic exotoxin
P & E   pneumonia and empyema
PEA   pelvic examination while
     anesthetized
     phosphoethanolamine
     phosphorylethanolamine
PEAP   positive end-airway
     pressure
PEARL   pupils equal and react
     to light
PEARLA   pupils equal and react to
     light and accommodation
PEB   Platinol (cisplatin) +
     etoposide + bleomycin
     (combination
     chemotherapy)
PEC   pelvic cramps
     pre-existing condition

premature epiphyseal
  closure
pulmonary endothelial cell

PECHO prostatic echogram

PECO₂R partial extracorporeal
  carbon dioxide removal

PECT progestin-estrogen
  cyclic therapy

PED pediatrics
  pre-existing disease

Peds pediatrics

PEE punctate epithelial erosion

PEEP positive end-expiratory
  pressure (breathing)

PEF peak expiratory flow
  pharyngo-epiglottic fold
  pulmonary edema fluid

Peff effective filtration pressure

PEFR peak expiratory flow rate

PEFV partial expiratory
  flow volume

PEG percutaneous endoscopic
  gastrostomy (implanted

feeding tube)
pneumoencephalogram
polyethylene glycol
pneumoencephalogram

PEG tube
  percutaneous endoscopic
  gastrostomy tube

PEH papillary endothelial
  hyperplasia

PEI pancreatic exocrine
  insufficiency
  percutaneous ethanol
  injection
  phosphate excretion index
  polyethyleneimine

PEJ percutaneous endoscopic
  jejunostomy
  pharyngo-esophageal
  junction

PEL peritoneal exudate
  lymphocyte
  permissible exposure limit
  phreno-esophageal
  ligament

PELs peak exposure levels
  permissible exposure limits

PEM peritoneal exudate
  macrophage
  probable error of
  measurement
  protein-energy
  malnutrition
  pulmonary embolism

PEMA phenyl ethylmalonamide

PEMF pulsating electromagnetic
  field (treatment)

PEMS postencephalic myalgia
  syndrome

PEN parenteral and enteral
  nutrition

Pen penicillin

PENS percutaneous epidural
  nerve stimulator

Pent Pentothal (thiopental)

PEO progressive external
  ophthalmoplegia

PEP painful erection of penis
  pancreatogenic enzymatic
  peritonitis

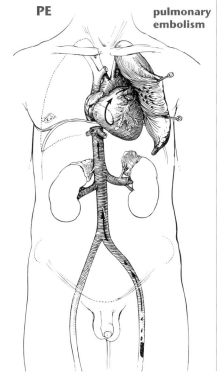

PE   **pulmonary embolism**

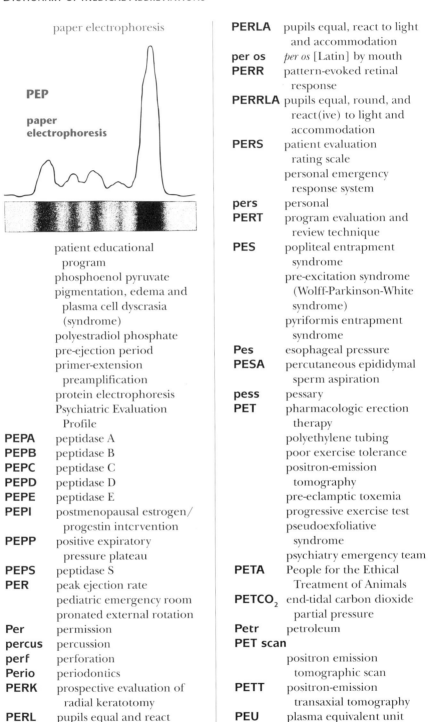

paper electrophoresis

PEP

paper electrophoresis

patient educational
program
phosphoenol pyruvate
pigmentation, edema and
plasma cell dyscrasia
(syndrome)
polyestradiol phosphate
pre-ejection period
primer-extension
preamplification
protein electrophoresis
Psychiatric Evaluation
Profile
PEPA   peptidase A
PEPB   peptidase B
PEPC   peptidase C
PEPD   peptidase D
PEPE   peptidase E
PEPI   postmenopausal estrogen/
progestin intervention
PEPP   positive expiratory
pressure plateau
PEPS   peptidase S
PER   peak ejection rate
pediatric emergency room
pronated external rotation
Per   permission
percus   percussion
perf   perforation
Perio   periodontics
PERK   prospective evaluation of
radial keratotomy
PERL   pupils equal and react
to light

PERLA   pupils equal, react to light
and accommodation
per os   *per os* [Latin] by mouth
PERR   pattern-evoked retinal
response
PERRLA   pupils equal, round, and
react(ive) to light and
accommodation
PERS   patient evaluation
rating scale
personal emergency
response system
pers   personal
PERT   program evaluation and
review technique
PES   popliteal entrapment
syndrome
pre-excitation syndrome
(Wolff-Parkinson-White
syndrome)
pyriformis entrapment
syndrome
Pes   esophageal pressure
PESA   percutaneous epididymal
sperm aspiration
pess   pessary
PET   pharmacologic erection
therapy
polyethylene tubing
poor exercise tolerance
positron-emission
tomography
pre-eclamptic toxemia
progressive exercise test
pseudoexfoliative
syndrome
psychiatry emergency team
PETA   People for the Ethical
Treatment of Animals
PETCO₂   end-tidal carbon dioxide
partial pressure
Petr   petroleum
PET scan
positron emission
tomographic scan
PETT   positron-emission
transaxial tomography
PEU   plasma equivalent unit
PEV   peak expiratory velocity

PEW	pulmonary extravascular water
PEx	physical examination
PF	pacemaker failure
	palmar fibromatosis
	paratrooper fracture
	peak factor
	peak flow
	pelvis fracture
	peritoneal fluid
	permeability factor
	personality factor
	Piedmont fracture
	Pipkin fracture
	plantar fascia
	plantar fasciitis
	plantar flexion
	platelet factor
	pleural fluid
	posterior fontanel
	Pott's fracture

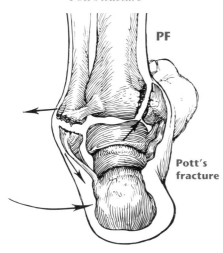

PF

Pott's fracture

	power failure
	prostatic fluid
	pseudofracture
	pulmonary fibrosis
	pump failure
	Purkinje fibers
	purpura fulminans
	push fluids
PF1	platelet factor one
PF2	platelet factor two
PF3	platelet factor three

PF4	platelet factor four
	repligen
PFA	patellofemoral arthrosis
	phosphonoformate
P. falciparum	*Plasmodium falciparum* (causative agent of malaria)
PFB	pseudofolliculitis barbae
PFC	patellofemoral chondrosis
	pelvic flexion contracture
	persistent fetal circulation
	plaque-forming cell
	press-fit component
PFD	perfluorodecalin
	polyostotic fibrous dysplasia
PFE	proximal femoral epiphysis
PFES	pelvic floor electrical stimulation
PFFD	proximal femoral focal deficiency
PFG	peak flow gauge
PFGE	pulsed-field gel electrophoresis
PFIB	perfluoroisobutylene
PFJ	patellofemoral joint
PFK	phosphofructokinase
PFKD	phosphofructokinase deficiency (type VII glycogenosis)
PFL	Platinol (cisplatin) + fluorouracil + leucovorin (combination chemotherapy)
	profibrinolysin
PFM	peak flow meter
	pelvic floor myalgia
PFO	patent foramen ovale
PFOV	posterior fornix of vagina
PFP	peripheral facial paralysis
	platelet-free plasma
	pore-forming protein
PFPS	patellofemoral pain syndrome
PFR	peak flow rate
	pericardial friction rub
PFS	prefilled syringe
	primary fibromyalgia syndrome

protein-free supernatant
P-FSH plasma follicle-stimulating
hormone
PFT pancreatic function test
platelet-fibrin-thrombi
posterior (cranial)
fossa tumor
pulmonary function test
PFTBE progressive form of tick-
borne encephalitis
PFU plaque-forming unit
PFUO prologed fever of
unknown origin
PG paregoric (anhydrous
morphine)
parotid gland
pigmentary glaucoma
pelvic girdle
peptidoglycan
phosphate glutamate
phosphatidylglycerol (fetal
lung maturity test)
pituitary gland
(hypophysis)
pituitary gonadotropin
placentogram
plasma glucose
polyposis gastrica
postgraduate
pregnant
progesterone
prostaglandin
pyoderma gangrenosum
Pg pregnant
pg page
picogram
pregnant
PGA phosphoglyceric acid
polyglandular autoimmune
(syndrome)
prostaglandin A
pteroylglutamic acid
(folic acid)
PGA$_1$ prostaglandin A$_1$
PGA$_2$ prostaglandin A$_2$
PGA$_3$ prostaglandin A$_3$
PGAM phosphoglycerate mutase
PGAS persisting galactorrhea–
amenorrhea syndrome

PGB paravertebral
ganglion block
prostaglandin B
PGB$_1$ prostaglandin B$_1$
PGB$_2$ prostaglandin B$_2$
PGBG postgastrectomy bile
gastritis
PGC periglomerular cell
postganglionic cell
primordial germ cell
prostaglandin C
PGC$_1$ prostaglandin C$_1$
PGC$_2$ prostaglandin C$_2$
PGC$_3$ prostaglandin C$_3$
PGD phosphogluconate
dehydrogenase
pluriglandular dosing
polygenic disorder
primary glomerular disease
prostaglandin D
pure gonadal dysgenesis
PGD$_1$ prostaglandin D$_1$
6PGD 6-phosphogluconate
dehydrogenase
PGD$_2$ prostaglandin D$_2$
PGDH prostaglandin
dehydrogenase
PGDS postgastrectomy dumping
syndrome
PGDU$_{2u}$ prostaglandin DU$_{2u}$
PGE platelet granule extract
posterior
gastroenterostomy
prostaglandin E
PGE$_1$ prostaglandin E$_1$
(alprostadil)
PGE$_2$ prostaglandin E$_2$
(dinoprostone)
PGEU$_{1u}$ prostaglandin EU$_{1u}$
PGEU$_{2u}$ prostaglandin EU$_{2u}$
PGF palatoglossal fold
PGF prostaglandin F
PGF$_1$ prostaglandin F$_1$
PGF$_{1\alpha}$ prostaglandin F$_1$alpha
PGF$_2$ prostaglandin F$_2$
PGF$_{2\alpha}$ prostaglandin F$_2$ alpha
PGF$_3$ prostaglandin F$_3$
PGFs postganglionic fibers
preganglionic fibers

PGFU$_{2u}$ prostaglandin FU$_{2u}$
PGG prostaglandin G
   polyclonal gamma globulin
PGG$_2$ prostaglandin G$_2$
PGH pituitary growth hormone
   prostaglandin H
PGH$_2$ prostaglandin H$_2$
   (endoperoxide)
P. gingivalis
   Porphyromonas gingivalis
PGI potassium, glucose,
   and insulin
   prostaglandin I
PGI$_2$ prostacyclin (prosta-
   glandin I$_2$)
PGIU$_{2u}$ prostaglandin IU$_{2u}$
PGK phosphoglycerate kinase
PGKD phosphoglycerate kinase
   deficiency (type IV
   glycogenosis)
PGL persistent generalized
   lymphadenopathy
   phosphoglycolipid
PGlyM phosphoglyceromutase
PGM phosphoglucomutase
pgm picogram
PGMD phosphoglycerate mutase
   deficiency (type X
   glycogenosis)
PGME propylene glycol
   monomethyl ether
P-G mutase
   phosphoglucomutase
PGN proliferative
   glomerulonephritis
   Punctur-Guard needle
PGO ponto-geniculo-occipital
   (EEG waves)
PGO spikes
   ponto-geniculo-occipital
   spikes (in REM sleep)
PGP prepaid group practice
   progressive general
   paralysis
PGR psychogalvanic response
PgR progesterone receptor
PGS postsurgical gastroparesis
   syndrome
   prostaglandin synthetase

PGSI prostaglandin synthetase
   inhibitor
PGTR plasma glucose
   tolerance rate
PGTT prednisolone glucose
   tolerance test
PGU peripheral glucose uptake
   postgonococcal urethritis
PGV proximal gastric vagotomy
   psychogenic vomiting
PGWV Persian Gulf war veteran
PSY-1 postgraduate year one
PGY-2 postgraduate year two
PGY-3 postgraduate year three
PGY-4 postgraduate year four
PGY-5 postgraduate year five
PH partial hysterectomy
   passive hemagglutination
   past history
   Pavlik harness
   persistent hepatitis
   personal history
   poor health
   porphyria hepatica
   posterior hypothalamus
   postural hypotension
   prostatic hypertrophy
   psychotic hallucinations
   public health
   pulmonary hemorrhage
   pulmonary hypertension
Ph phalanx
Ph[1] Philadelphia chromosome
   (long arm of chromo-
   some 22 is translocated
   onto the long arm of
   chromosome 9)
pH hydrogen-ion
   concentration
   (measurement of acidity
   or alkalinity; pH7 is
   neutral; above 7,
   alkalinity increases;
   below 7, acidity increases)
PHA arterial pH
   parental hyperalimentation
   passive hemagglutination
   Pelger-Huet anomaly
   peripheral

hyperalimentation
phenylalanine (an essential
   amino acid)
phytohemagglutinin
   antigen
postsurgery holding area
primary
   hyperaldosteronism
pseudohypoaldosteronism

PHACO phacoemulsification
PHAL phytohemagglutinin-
   stimulated lymphocyte
phal phalanges
   phalanx
PHAP phytohemagglutinin
   protein
PHAR pharynx
phar pharmaceutical
pharm pharmacy
Pharm B Bachelor of Pharmacy
Pharm D Doctor of Pharmacy
PHASE Pre-Hospital Arrest
   Survival Evaluation
PHBB propylhydroxybenzyl
   benzimidazole
PHC posthospital care
   prehospital care
   primary health care
   primary hepatocellular
      carcinoma
   proliferative helper cell
Ph¹C Philadelphia chromosome
   (long arm of chromo-
   some 22 is translocated
   onto the long arm of
   chromosome 9)
PHCC primary hepatocellular
   carcinoma
PHCG parahippocampal gyrus
PHD pathological habit disorder
   potentially harmful drug
   pulmonary heart disease
PhD Doctor of Philosophy
Phe phenylalanine (an essential
   amino acid)
Phen phenotype
Pheno phenobarbital (a long-
   acting barbiturate)

Phenob phenobarbital (a long-
   acting barbiturate)
Pheo pheochromocytoma
phg phagosome
PHI past history of illness
   phosphohexose isomerase
   physiologic hyaluronidase
      inhibitor
   protein hydrolysate
      injection
PHIA profoundly hearing-
   impaired adult
PHK postmortem human kidney
PHLP primary
   hyperlipoproteinemia
PHM pulmonary hyaline
   membrane
PHN postherpetic neuralgia
   public health nurse
phono phonocardiogram
phos phosphate
PHP Pillet hand prosthesis
   pooled human plasma
   postheparin plasma
   prepaid health plan
   primary
      hyperparathyroidism
   pseudohypoparathyroidism
PHPA *p*-hydroxyphenylacetate
PHPPA *p*-hydroxyphenylpyruvic
   acid
PHPT primary
   hypoparathyroidism
   pseudohypoparathyroidism
PHR Physicians for Human
   Rights
   peak heart rate
PHS phenylalanine hydroxylase
   stimulator
   pineal hypertrophy
      syndrome
   posthypnotic suggestion
   US Public Health Service
PHSC pleuripotent hemopoietic
   stem cell
   posterior horn of
      spinal cord
PHT portal hypertension
   primary hyperthyroidism

provocative histamine test
pulmonary hypertension

P. humanus

Pediculus humanus
(human lice)

PHV prosthetic heart valve
PHX pilmonary histiocytosis X
Phx pharynx
Phys physical
physician
PhysEd physical education
Phys Med
physical medicine
physio physiotherapy
PhysTh physical therapy
PhysTher physical therapy
PI package insert
pancreatic insufficiency
parainfluenza
paranoid ideation
pars intermedia
(of hypophysis)
passive immunity
patient's interests
perinatal injury
periodontal index
peripheral iridectomy
persistent illness
personal injury
physically impaired
physician intervention
pneumatosis intestinalis
poison ivy
postinfection
pregnancy induced
premature infant
present illness
primary infarction
primary infection
principal investigator
product information
proinsulin
prolactin inhibitor
protamine insulin
protease inhibitor
puerperal infarction
pulmonary infarction
pulmonary insufficiency
P & I pneumonia and influenza

probe and irrigation
Pi inorganic orthophosphate
inorganic phosphate
PIA photoelectric intravenous
angiography
plasma insulin activity
preinfarction angina
Psychiatric Institute of
America
PIB percutaneous intra-aortic
balloon
PIBC plasma iron-binding
capacity
PIC peripherally inserted
catheter
potassium ion channels
potentially ineffective care
PICA percutaneous transluminal
coronary angioplasty
posterior inferior
cerebellar artery
posterior inferior
communicating artery
PICD primary irritant contact
dermatitis
PICFS postinfective chronic
fatigue syndrome
PICSO pressure-controlled
intermittent coronary
sinus occlusion
PICT pancreatic islet cell tumor
PICU pediatric intensive
care unit
PID pelvic inflammatory
disease
primary irritant dermatitis
prolapsed intervertebral
disk
protruded intervertebral
disk
PIDS primary immunodeficiency
syndrome
PIE preimplantation embryo
prosthetic infectious
endocarditis
pulmonary infiltration with
eosinophilia
pulmonary interstitial
edema

pulmonary interstitial
emphysema

PIF Pacific Islander female
peak inspiratory flow
proinsulin-free
prolactin-inhibiting factor
(inhibits release of the
milk hormone prolactin
from the anterior
pituitary)
proliferation inhibitory
factor
prostatic interstitial fluid

PIFA pain-inhibition fear
avoidance

PIFG poor intrauterine fetal
growth

PIFR peak inspiratory flow rate

PIFT platelet
immunofluorescence test

PIGI pregnancy-induced glucose
intolerance

PIGN postinfectious
glomerulonephritis

PIH post-inflammatory
hyperpigmentation
pregnancy-induced
hypertension
prolactin-inhibiting
hormone

PII plasma inorganic iodine

PIIID peripheral indwelling
intermediate infusion
device

PIIP portable insulin infusion
pump

PIIS posterior inferior
iliac spine

PIL patient information leaflet

PILC Pregnancy and Infant
Loss Center

PILOT programmed inquiry,
learning or teaching

PILOTS published international
literature on traumatic
stress (bibliographic
database)

PIM Pacific Islander male

PIN product

identification number
prostatic intraepithelial
neoplasia

PINS patient in need of
supervision
posterior interosseous
nerve syndrome

PINT posterior internodal tract
(between S-A node and
A-V node)

PIO pemoline (central nervous
system stimulant)

PIO$_2$ partial pressure of inspired
oxygen

PIP peak inspiratory pressure
positive inspiratory
pressure
postinfusion phlebitis
preinfarction pain
proximal interphalangeal
(joint)

PIP$_2$ phosphatidylinositol
diphosphate

PIPE persistent interstitial
pulmonary emphysema

PIPJ proximal interphalangeal
joint

PIRG Public Interest Research
Group

PIRI plasma immunoreactive
insulin

P. irritans
Pulex irritans (human flea)

PIQ performance IQ
posterior inferior quadrant

PIS preinfarction syndrome
primary immunodeficiency
syndrome

PISI palmar intercalated
segemtal instability

PIT pancreatic islet tumor
Pitocin (oxytocin)
pituitary
plasma iron turnover
polyoma-induced tumor

PITP pseudo-idiopathic
thrombocytopenic
purpura

PIU polymerase-inducing unit

PITR	plasma iron turnover rate
PIV	parainfluenza viruses
	primate immuno-deficiency virus
PIVD	protruded intervertebral disk
PIVH	peripheral intravenous hyperalimentation
PIVI	parainfluenza virus infection
PIVOT	prostate cancer intervention versus observation trial
PIWT	partially impacted wisdom tooth (3rd molar)
PIXE	proton-induced x-ray emission
PIXEA	proton-induced x-ray emission analysis
Pixel	picture element
PJ	pancreatic juice
	Peutz-Jeghers (syndrome)
	porcelain jacket (tooth crown reconstruction)
PJB	premature junctional beat
PJC	premature junctional contractions
PJO	pancreatico-jejunostomy
PJS	Peutz-Jeghers syndrome
PJT	paroxysmal junctional tachycardia
	peritoneojugular shunt
PK	pain-killer
	penetrating keratoplasty
	plasma potassium
	protein kinase
	psychokinesis
	pyruvate kinase
PKA	prekallikrein activator
PKase	protein kinase
PKB	prone knee bend
PKC	protein kinase C
PKD	polycystic kidney disease
	proliferative kidney disease
	pyruvate kinase deficiency
PKDL	post-kala azar dermal leishmaniasis
PKF	permanent kidney failure
PKN	phenylketonuria

PKP	penetrating keratoplasty
PKR	Polycystic Kidney Research (Foundation)
	Prausnitz-Kustner reaction
PKS	pseudo-Kaposi's sarcoma (acroangiodermatitis)
PKU	phenylketonuria
PKU-P	Phenylketonuria Parents
PKV	killed poliomyelitis vaccine
PL	palmaris longus (muscle)
	patellar ligament
	perception of light
	peritoneal lavage
	peroneus longus (muscle)
	phospholipid
	place
	placebo
	placental lactogen
	plantar
	plasma level
	preleukemia
PLA	pelvic lymphadenectomy
	peripheral laser angioplasty
	phospholipid antibody
	plasminogen activator
	platelet antigen
PLAP	placental alkaline phosphatase
Plat P	platelet pheresis
PLB	phospholipase B
	pursed-lip breathing
PLC	phospholipase C
	primary liver cancer
	protein-lipid complex
PLCC	primary liver cell cancer
PLD	parenchymal lung disease
	patellar ligament disruption
	percutancous laser diskectomy
	platelet defect
	polycystic liver disease
	potentially lethal damage
	prelingually deaf
PLDH	plasma lactic dehydrogenase
PLE	protein-losing enteropathy
	pseudolupus erythematosus

PLEDs periodic lateralized
epileptiform discharges
PLEVA *pityriasis lichenoides et
varioliformis acuta*
PI fl pleural fluid
PLG plasminogen (the inactive
precursor of plasmin)
P-LGV psittacosis-
lymphogranuloma
venereum
PLH paroxysmal
localized hyperhidrosis
placental lactogenic
hormone
posterior lobe of
hypophysis (pituitary)
PLI pancreatic lymphocytic
infiltration
professional liability
insurance
PLIF posterolateral
interbody fusion
postlumbar
interbody fusion
PLISSIT permission, limited
information, structured
suggestions, intensive
therapy
PLL posterior longitudinal
ligament (connects the
posterior body of the 2nd
vertebra to the posteror
bodies of the sacrum on
the inside of the
vertebral canal)
prolymphocytic leukemia
PLM percent-labeled mitosis
periodic leg movement
plasma level monitoring
polarized light microscopy
PLMS periodic limb movement
when sleeping
PLN pancreatic lymph nodes
pelvic lymph nodes
peripheral lymph node
popliteal lymph node
pudendal lymph nodes
PLND pelvic lymph node
dissection

PLO polycystic lipomembranous
osteodysplasia
PLP parathyroidlike protein
phantom limb pain
phospholipid
plasma leukapheresis
proteolipid protein
(myelin)
PLR patellar lateral retinaculum
product liability risk
pronation/lateral rotation
pupillary light reflex
PLRI posterolateral rotary
instability
PLS perfusion lung scan
phantom limb sensation
phantom limb syndrome
plastic surgery
polydactyly-luxation
syndrome
preschool language scale
primary lateral sclerosis
prostaglandinlike
substance
PLT platelet

PLT

platelet

primed lymphocyte test
Plts platelets
plumb *plumbum* [Latin] lead
PLV poliomyelitis live vaccine
panleukopenia virus
partial liquid ventilation

	phenylalanine, lysine,		Pharmaceutical
	vasopressin		Manufacturers
	posterior left ventricle		Association
plx	plexus		phorbol myristate acetate
PM	afternoon		pre-market approval
	evening		premenstrual asthma
	mean pressure		Prinzmetal's angina
	pacemaker		progressive muscular
	pansystolic murmur		atrophy
	papillary muscle		pyridylmercuric acetate
	partial mastectomy	**PMB**	papillomacular bundle
	partial meniscectomy		polymorphonuclear
	perinatal morbidity		basophil (white
	petit mal (epilepsy)		blood cell)
	Phalen's maneuver		polymyxin B (antibiotic
	(full flexion of wrist for		substance derived from
	1 minute)		strains of the soil
	physical medicine		bacterium *Bacillus*
	pia mater		*polymyxa*)
	pituitary myxedema		postmenopause bleeding
	plasma membrane	**PMBV**	percutaneous mitral
	Plasmodium malariae		balloon valvotomy
	(causative agent	**PMC**	pilomatrix carcinoma
	of malaria)		premature mitral (left
	platysma muscle		atrioventricular valve)
	pneumomediastinum		closure
	poliomyelitis		pseudo-membranous colitis
	polymorph		pseudomeningocele
	polymyositis		pseudomucinous
	postmenopause		cystadenoma
	postmenstrual	**PMCI**	postmyocardial infarct
	postmortem	**PMCIS**	post-myocardial
	premenstrual		infarction syndrome
	premolar (bicuspid)		(Dressler's syndrome)
	presystolic murmur	**PMCs**	Patient Management
	preventive medicine		Categories
	prostatic massage	**PMD**	Pelizaeus-Merzbacher
	pseudomonas		disease
	pterygoid muscle		permanent
	pulmonic murmur		maxillary dentition
Pm	promethium (radioactive		premenstrual depression
	metallic element)		primary myocardial disease
pm	picometer		private medical doctor
p.m.	*post meridiem* [Latin]		progressive muscular
	afternoon		dystrophy
	post mortem [Latin]	**PMDS**	persistent müllerian duct
	after death		syndrome
PMA	paramethoxyamphetamine	**PME**	pelvic muscle exercise
	peroneal muscular atrophy		(Kegel technique)

polymorphonuclear eosinophil (white blood cell)
postmenopausal estrogen
premature ejaculation
progressive myoclonus epilepsy
pseudomembranous enterocolitis

PMF platelet membrane fluidity
Platinol (cisplatin) + mitomycin C + fluorouracil (combination chemotherapy)
primary myelofibrosis
progressive massive fibrosis
pterygomaxillary fossa

PMF LE progressive multifocal leukoencephalopathy

PMGA pteroylmonoglutamic acid (folic acid)

PMGV postmeal glucose value

PMH previous medical history
pseudomyocardial hypertrophy

PMHx past medical history

PMI past medical illness
patient medication information
patient medication instruction
perioperative myocardial infarction
place of maximal impulse
posterior myocardial infarction
premature infant
previous medical illnesses

PMIS postmyocardial infarction syndrome

PML polymorphonuclear leukocyte
posterior mitral (left atrioventricular valve) leaflet
premature labor
progressive multifocal leukoencephalopathy
prolapsed mitral (left

atrioventricular valve) leaflet
promyelocyte leukemia
pulmonary microlithiasis

PMLE polymorphous light eruption

PMM pentamethylmelamine
post-menopausal mother
psoas major muscle

PMMA polymethylmethacrylate (self-curing acrylic)

PMN polymorphonuclear (leukocyte)

PMN

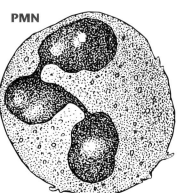

polymorphonuclear (leukocyte)

polymorphonuclear neutrophil
polymorphonuclear neutrophilic leukocyte
polymorphonucleotide

PMO postmenopausal osteoporosis

PMOC pseudomembranous oral candidiasis

PMP pain management program
patient medication profile
plantar metatarsal padding
premenstrual pain
previous menstrual period
plasma membrane protein
postmastectomy pain
prior menstrual period
pseudomyxoma peritonei
pulse methylprednisolone

PMR	pacemaker rhythm
	patellar medial retinaculum
	perinatal mortality rate
	physical medicine and rehabilitation
	polymyalgia rheumatica
	progressive muscle relaxation
	pterygomandibular raphe
PM & R	physical medicine and rehabilitation
PMRI	posteromedial rotary instability
PM RS	physical medicine and rehabilitation services
PMS	patient management system
	passive maternal smoking
	patella malalignment syndrome
	periodic movement of sleep
	petit mal seizure
	phenazine methosulfate
	postmenopausal syndrome
	postmenstrual stress
	pregnant mare serum
	premenstrual syndrome
	psychotic motor syndrome
PMS A	Premenstrual Syndrome Access (800) 222-4767
PMSC	pluripotent myeloid stem cell
PMSU	peripheral motor-sensory unit
PMT	phenol O-methylltransferase
	place of maximum tenderness
	premenstrual tension
	psychogenic muscle tension
PMTS	prementrual tension syndrome
PMTs	photomultiplier tubes
PMV	paramyxovirus
	prolapse of mitral (left atrioventricular) valve

PMVL	posterior mitral (left atrioventricular) valve leaflet
PMW	post-menopausal women
	premenopausal women
PN	parenteral nutrition
	penicillin
	perenteral nutrition
	periarteritis nodosa
	peripheral nerve
	peripheral neuropathy
	phrenic nerve
	pneumonia
	polyarteritis nodosa
	polyneuritis
	poorly nourished
	positional nystagmus
	posterior nares
	postnasal
	postnatal
	practical nurse
	progress notes
	prostatic neoplasm
	psychoneurosis
	pulmonary nodule
	pyelonephritis
PN$_2$	partial pressure of nitrogen
Pn	pain
	pneumonia
PNA	pentosenucleic acid
PNa	plasma sodium
PNAB	percutaneous needle aspiration biopsy
PNB	penile nerve block
	percutaneous needle biopsy
	perineal needle biopsy
	prematue newborn
	premature nodal beat
	prophylactic nerve block
	prostatic needle biopsy
	pudendal nerve block
PNBI	premature newborn infant
PNC	penicillin
	percutaneous nephrostomy catheter
	peripheral nerve conduction
	postnecrotic cirrhosis

premature nodal
contraction
prenatal care
prenatal clinic

pNCS p-nitrocatechol sulfate

PND paroxysmal nocturnal
dyspnea (acute dyspnea
occurring suddenly at
night, caused by
pulmonary congestion
and edema)
postnasal drainage
postnasal drip
postnatal depression
prenatal diagnosis
purulent nasal discharge

PNE peripheral
neuroepithelioma
plasma norepinephrine
pseudomembranous
necrotizing enterocolitis

PNET primitive neuroectodermal
tumor

pneu pneumonia

PNF proprioceptive
neuromuscular
facilitation (reaction)

PNG penicillin G

PNH paroxysmal nocturnal
hemoglobinuria
(acquired clonal disease)
polynuclear hydrocarbons

PN HIV I perinatal HIV infection

PNI peripheral nerve injury
postnatal infection
psychoneuroimmunology

PNK polynucleotide kinase

PNL percutaneous
nephrolithotomy
peripheral nerve lesion

PNLA percutaneous needle lung
aspiration

PNM perinatal mortality
peripheral nerve myelin

PNMG persistent neonatal
myasthenia gravis

PNMR postneonatal mortality rate

PNMT phenylethanolamine- N-
methyltransferase

PNP para-nitrophenol
pediatric nurse
practitioner
peripheral neuropathy
psychogenic nocturnal
polydipsia
purine nucleoside
phosphorylase

PNPB positive-negative
pressure breathing
postnatal pain behavior

pNPS *p*-nitrophenyl sulfate

PNS paraneoplastic syndrome
parasympathetic nervous
system
partial nonprogressing
stroke
peripheral nerve
stimulator
peripheral nervous system
posterior nasal spine

PNSL papulonodular skin lesion

PNT partial nodular
transformation
percutaneous
nephrostomy tube

PNTX pneumothorax

PNU protein nitrogen unit

PNV prenatal vitamins

PNVX pneumococcus vaccine

Pnx pneumothorax

PNZ posterior necrotic zone

PO period of onset
postoperative
project officer
prophylactic
oophorectomy
pulse oximetry

P/O phone order

PO₂ partial pressue of oxygen
(in blood gases)

P & O prosthetics and orthotics

Po polonium (a rare metallic
element)

p.o. *per os* [Latin] by mouth

POA pancreatic oncofetal
antigen
phalangeal osteoarthritis
point of application

posterior osseous ampulla
power of attorney
preoptic area
primary optic atrophy
POAG primary open angle
    glaucoma
POB phenoxybenzamine
place of birth
prevention of blindness
POBP preoperative bowel
    preparation
POBs postolympic blues
POBT postoperative
    bleeding time
POC para-ovarian cyst
point of care
postoperative care
postoperative complication
probability of chance
products of conception
POD period of disability
peroxidase
place of death
podiatry
polycystic ovary disease
postobstructive diuresis
postoperative day
POD1 postoperative day 1
POD 2 postoperative day 2
POD 3 postoperative day 3
PODx preoperative diagnosis
    (before surgery)
POE pediatric orthopedic
    examination
postoperative exercise
proof of eligibility
POEMS polyneuropathy,
    organomegaly,
    endocrinopathy,
    monoclonal gammopathy
    and skin changes (plasma
    cell dyscrasia syndrome)
POF physician's order form
premature ovarian failure
pyruvate oxidation factor
POFTTB postoperative flexor
    tendon traction brace
POG polyethylene oxide gel
proto-oncogenes (help

embyonic cells grow and
divide; they shut down
soon after birth, and if
accidently reactivated can
result in cancer)
pog pogonion (craniometric
    landmark)
POH personal oral hygiene
POHA preoperative holding area
POHS presumed ocular
    histoplasmosis syndrome
POI postoperative instructions
proof of illness
P of ILL proof of illness
POIK poikilocytosis
POL politics online
premature onset of labor
polio poliomyelitis
poly-A polyadenylic acid
poly-C polycytidylic acid
poly-G polyguanylic acid
poly-I polyinosinic acid
polys polymorphonuclear
    leukocytes
polymorphonuclear
    neutrophils
poly-T polythymidylic acid
poly-U polyuridylic acid
POM pain on motion
prescription-only
    medication
POMC pro-opiomelanocortin
POMD patent omphalomesenteric
    duct
POMP prednisone + Oncovin
    (vincristine) +
    methotrexate +
    mercaptopurine
    (combination
    chemotherapy)
POMR problem-oriented
    medical record
PONA progressive optic nerve
    atrophy
pond. *pondere* [Latin] by weight
PONV postoperative nausea and
    vomiting
POP pain on palpation
plaster of Paris (anhydrous

calcium sulfate)
point-of-purchase
postoperative pain
POp postoperative
POR physician of record
polymyositis ossificans
progressiva
problem-oriented record
PORP partial ossicular
replacement prosthesis
PORT postoperative respiratory
therapy
POS parieto-occipital sulcus
parosteal osteosarcoma
(juxtcortical osteogenic
sarcoma)
patella overload syndrome
periosteal osteosarcoma
physician's order sheet
point-of-service
(health care plan)
polycystic ovary syndrome
preovulatory swelling
pos positive
poss possible
POST peritoneal oocyte and
sperm transfer
post posterior
postmortem
postgangl
postganglionic
post-op postoperative; after surgery
post-stim
post-stimulation
POT postoperative treatment
pulmonary oxygen transfer
pot potential
potion
pot. *potus* [Latin] a drink
powd powder
POX point of exit
PP pancreatic polypeptide
paradoxical pulse
paralytic polio
paraplegia
paraquat poisoning
partial pressure
pedal pulse
penile prosthesis

periodic peritonitis
permanent pacemaker
Peyer's patches
pharyngeal paralysis
pink puffer (refers to some
emphysema patients)
pinprick
placental protein
placenta previa
plasmapheresis
plasma protein
plaster of Paris
pleural pressure
posterior pituitary
postpartum
postprandial
post-test probability
precocious puberty
preferred provider
presenting part
pretest probability
primapara
primary payer
private patient
private practice
probe patency
prothrombin-proconvertin
protoporphyria
proximal phalanx
pterygoid process
pulse point
pulse pressure
pulsus paradoxus
pyrophosphate
P & P policy and procedure
P-5'-P pyridoxal-5'-phosphate
P & P pyelitis and pyelonephritis
P-p P-pulmonale (in
electrocardiography, the
P-wave pattern
characteristic of cor
pulmonale; a tall peaked
P wave, usually seen in
leads II, III, and aVF)
pp postprandial
postpartum
p.p. *punctum proximum* [Latin]
near point of
accommodation
PPA pediatric pain assessment

phenylpropanolamine

phenylpyruvic acid

polyphosphoric acid

postpartum amenorrhea

postpill amenorrhea

PP & A palpation, percussion and auscultation

p.p.a. *phiala prius agitate* [Latin] shake bottle first

PPAR peroxisome proliferator-activated receptor

PPAS peripheral pulmonary artery stenosis

postpolio atrophy syndrome

PPB parts per billion

platelet-poor blood

positive pressure breathing

prepatella bursa

prepatellar bursitis (housemaid's knee)

PPB

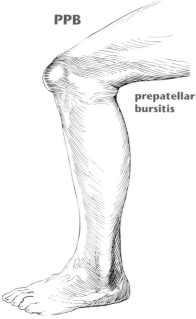

prepatellar bursitis

ppb parts per billion

PPBE postpartum breast engorgement

PPBS postprandial blood sugar

PPBTL postpartum bilateral tubal ligation

PPC plasma prothrombin conversion

pluripotential cell

polypeptide chain

proximal palmar crease

pyogenic pericarditis

PPCD polymorphous posterior corneal dystrophy

PPCF plasma prothrombin conversion factor

PPCM postpartum cardiomyopathy

PPCS postpericardiotomy syndrome

PPD packs (of cigarettes) per day

paranoid personality disorder

percussion and postural drainage

permanent partial disability

posterior polymorphous dystrophy

postpartum day

postpartum depression

progressive perceptive deafness

purified protein derivative (TB skin test)

P & PD percussion and postural drainage

PPDR preproliferative diabetic retinopathy

PPE palmoplantar erythrodysesthesia

personal protective equipment

postictal pulmonary edema

postpartum eclampsia

PPES palmoplantar erythrodysesthesia syndrome

pedal pulses equal and strong

PPF palatopharyngeal fold

pellagra preventive factor

phagocytosis promoting

factor

ping-pong fracture (pond fracture)

plasma protein fraction

posterior pillar of fauces

pterygopalatine fossa

PPG photoplethysmographic

photoplethysmography

postprandial glucose

pterygopalatine ganglion

PPGA postpill galactorrhea-amenorrhea

PPGD pelvic plane of greatest dimension

PPGF polypeptide growth factor

PPGM photoplethysmographic monitoring

PPGP prepaid group practice

PPGS postpartum glomerulosclerosis

PPH persistent pulmonary hypertension

postlumbar puncture headache (postpuncture headache)

postpartum hemorrhage

primary pulmonary hypertension

PPHN persistent pulmonary hypertension of the neonate

persistent pulmonary hypertension of the

newborn

PPHPT pseudo-pseudohypo-parathyroidism

PPI partial permanent impairment

patient-package insert

pelvic plane of inlet

permanent pacemaker implantation

pleuropulmonary infection

proton pump inhibitor

purified porcine insulin

PPi inorganic pyrophosphate

PPICC plasma proinflammatory cytokine concentration

PPIDs pulse polio immunization days

PPIE prolonged postictal encephalopathy

PPK palmoplantar keratosis

PPL pars planus lensectomy

posterior palpebral ligament

postpartum lactation

puboprostatic ligament

PPLO pleuropneumonia-like organisms

PPLOV painless progressive loss of vision

PPLV pars plana lensectomy-vitrectomy

PPM parts per million

permanent pacemaker

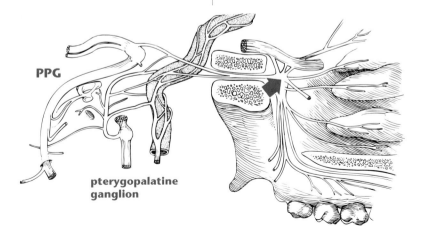

PPG

pterygopalatine ganglion

posterior papillary muscle
pulse per minute
ppm parts per million
pulses per minute
PPMA postpoliomyelitis
muscular atrophy
PPMS postpoliomyelitis syndrome
PPN partial parenteral nutrition
peripheral parenteral
nutrition
peripheral polyneuropathy
PPO pelvic plane of outlet
preferred-provider
organization
PPP palatopharyngoplasty
pentose phosphate
pathway
peripheral pulses palpable
platelet-poor plasma
polyphoretic phosphate
positionable penile
prosthesis
postpartum psychosis
purified placental protein
PPPA Poison Prevention
Packaging Act
PPPBL peripheral pulses palpable
on both legs
PPPD pylorus-preserving
pancreatoduodenectomy
PPPG postprandial plasma
glucose
PPPPPP pain, pallor, paresthesia,
pulselessness, paralysis,
prostration (mnemonic
of 6 symptoms of acute
arterial occlusion)
PPR physician-patient relation
PPRC Physician Payment Review
Commission
PPRF postpartum renal failure
PPROM prolonged premature
rupture of membranes
PPRP pontine paramedian
reticular formation
PPS pap plus speculoscopy
pepsin (an enzyme present
in gastric juice; it converts
proteins into peptones

and proteoses)
peripheral pulmonary
stenosis
plasminogen-plasmin
system
popliteal pterygium
syndrome
postpartal state
postpartum sterilization
postpartum syndrome
postperfusion syndrome
postphlebitic syndrome
post-polio syndrome
protein plasma substitute
pulses per second
PPs Peyer's patches
PPSC prostaglandin-producing
suppressor cell
PPT palmitoyl-protein
thioesterase
partial thromboplastin
time
pleuropulmonary
tuberculosis
postpartum thyroiditis
primary pure teratoma
pyopneumothorax
ppt parts per thousand
precipitate
PPTL postpartum tubal ligation
PPU perforated peptic ulcer
postpartum uterus
PPV pars plana vitrectomy
pneumococcal
polysaccharide vaccine
positive predictive value
(probability that the
person has the disorder)
positive pressure
ventilation
pulmonary vein venting
Ppv portal venous pressure
PPVR pruritic papulovesicular
rash
PPWI pregnant and postpartum
women and their infants
PPY packs (of cigarettes)
per year
pancreatic polypeptide

PQ	paraquat
	permeability quotient
	plastoquinone
	pronator quadratus
	(muscle)
PR	palindromic rheumatism
	partial remission
	partial response
	Passavant's ridge
	(on pharyngeal wall)
	pathology report
	peer review
	peripheral resistance
	per rectum
	pesticide residue
	physical rehabilitation
	pityriasis rosea
	pleural reflection
	polyribosome (polysome)
	posterior root
	postmyalgia rheumatica
	postural reflex
	pregnancy rate
	premature
	pressor receptor
	prevalence rate
	proctologist
	progesterone receptor
	proliferative retinopathy
	prolonged remission
	prosthion
	pulse rate
P & R	pulse and respiration
Pr	praseodymium (rare earth
	element)
	prednisolone
	presbyopia
	pressure
	prolactin
pr	pair
	prism
p.r.	*per rectum* [Latin] through
	the rectum
PRA	phosphoribosylamine
	plasma renin activity
	postrenal azotemia
	progesterone
	receptor assay
PrA HPA	protein A hemolytic

	plaque assay
PRAT	platelet radioactive
	antiglobulin test
p.rat.aetat.	
	pro ratione aetatis [Latin]
	in proportion to age
PRBC	packed red blood cells
PRBV	placental residual
	blood volume
PRC	packed red cells
	photo receptor cell
	plasma renin
	concentration
	proximal row carpectomy
	(of wrist)
PRCA	pure red cell aplasia
PRCP	percutaneous renal
	cyst puncture
PRD	polycystic renal disease
	postradiation dysplasia
	pressure relieving device
PRDPC	pooled random donor
	platelet concentrates
PRE	passive resistance exercise
	peptic regurgitant
	esophagitis
	pigmented retinal
	epithelium
	progressive resistive
	exercise
pre	preliminary
precip	precipitation
PRED	prednisone
Pred	prednisone
preemy	premature newborn
	(infant)
prefd	preferred
Preg	pregnant
	Pregestimil
prelim	preliminary
PREMI	premature newborn
	(infant)
pre-op	preoperative; before surgery
prep	preparation (usually
	for surgery)
PRERLA	pupils round, equal,
	react to light and
	accommodation
PRF	placental

respiratory function

prolactin releasing factor
(stimulates release of the
milk hormone
prolactin from the
anterior pituitary)

pubic rami fracture

PREs progressive resistive
exercises

prev prevention
previous

prev AGT previous abnormality of
glucose tolerance

PRF progressive renal failure
prolactin-releasing factor

pRF polyclonal rheumatoid
factor

PRFM prolonged rupture of
fetal membranes

PRG peer review group
purge

PRH preretinal hemorrhage
prolactin-releasing
hormone

PRI pain rating index
phosphoribose isomerase

PRIDE Parents' Resource
Institute for Drug
Education
(800) 677-7433

PRIH prolactin release-inhibiting
hormone

prim primary

primip primiparous
(first pregnancy)

prim. m. *primo mane* [Latin] first
thing in the morning

prin principal

PRIND prolonged reversible
ischemic neurologc
deficit

P-R interval
the P wave and P-R
segment of the ECG
cycle; it is a measure of
the time interval from the
beginning of atrial
depolarization to the
beginning of

ventricular depolarization

PRIST paper radioimmunosorbent test

priv private

PRJs peer-reviewed journals

PRK photorefractive
keratectomy
photorefractive keratotomy

PRL prolactin (mammotrophic
hormone)
prolonged response
latency

PRM phosphoribomutase
premature rupture of
membranes

PrM preventive medicine

PRMF preretinal macular fibrosis

PRM-SDX
pyrimethamine-
sulfadoxine

PRMSS pregnancy-related
mortality surveillance
system (of CDC)

PRN polyradiculoneuritis

p.r.n. *pro re nata* [Latin] as
needed, according to
circumstances; whenever
necessary

PRND prophylactic regional node
dissection

PRO Peer Review Organization
Professional Review
Organization
pronation
protein

Pro prolactin (a hormone
produced by the anterior
lobe of the pituitary that
stimulates and sustains
milk secretion in
postpartum women)
proline (an amino acid
present in collagen)
pronation
pronator
protein
prothrombin

prob probable

Proc procarbazine

proceedings
Procto proctology
proctoscopic
PROG progesterone
prognosis
program
prog prognosis
PROLAC prolactin (a hormone
produced by the anterior
lobe of the pituitary that
stimulates and sustains
milk secretion in
postpartum women)
PROM passive range of motion
premature rupture of
membranes
prolonged rupture of
membranes
PROMIS Problem-Oriented Medical
Information System
PROMM passive range of motion
machine
proximal myotonic
myopathy
pron pronation
pronator
Prop propranolol
proph prophylactic
PROS prostate
prosth prosthesis
prot protein
pro time prothrombin time
(blood clotting test)
proto oxidase
protoporphyrinogen
oxidase
pro-UK pro-urokinase
pro us. ext.
pro usu externo [Latin]
for external use
prov provisional
prox proximal
prox/3 proximal third
prox RTA
proximal renal
tubular acidosis
PRP panretinal
photocoagulation
penicillinase-resistent

penicillin
pityriasis rubra pilaris
platelet-rich plasma
polyribose ribitol
phosphate
postural rest position
primary Raynaud's
phenomenon
procedure-related pain
progressive rubella
panencephalitis
proliferative retinopathy
photocoagulation
psychotic reaction profile
PRPE progressive rubella
panencephalitis
5-PRPP 5-phosphoribosyl
pyrophosphate
PRPT polyribosylribitol
phosphate-tetanus
PrR progesterone receptor
PRRE pupils round, regular,
and equal
PRS personality rating scale
Pierre Robin syndrome
prolonged respiratory
support
P-R segment
the part of the ECG cycle
that measures from the
end of atrial
depolarization (A wave)
to the beginning of
ventricular depolarization
PRSs polyribosomes
positive rolandic spikes
(in EEG)
PRT phosphoribosyl transferase
postoperative respiratory
therapy
PRTA proximal renal
tubular acidosis
PRTH prothrombin time
PRTH-C prothrombin time control
PRU peripheral resistance unit
PRV polycythemia rubra vera
pseudorabies virus
PRW polymerized ragweed
PRZF pyrazofurin

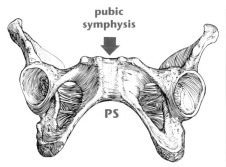

pubic symphysis

PS

pubic symphysis
puerperal sepsis
pulmonary sequestration
pulmonary stenosis

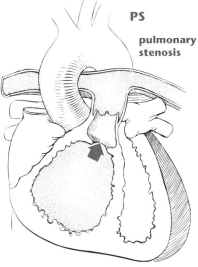

PS

pulmonary stenosis

(antineoplastic agent)

PRZs pressoreceptor zones

PS pacemaker syndrome
Pancoast's syndrome
Papanicolaou stain
paradoxical sleep
paranoid schizophrenia
paranoid state
parasympathetic
Parents of Suicides
Parinaud's syndrome
parotid sialography
partial seizure
passive smoke
passive smoking
patient survival
phosphoserine
phrenic stimulation
physical status
physiologic saline
pickwickian syndrome
pineal syndrome
plastic surgery
plica syndrome
Poland's syndrome
(pectoral aplasia
dysdactyly syndrome)
polysaccharide
population sample
presenting symptom
pressure sore
(decubitus ulcer)
prevalence study
(cross-sectional study)
primary syphilis (chancre)
primitive streak
prostatic secretion
protein S

pulmonary surfactant
pyloric stenosis

PS-I physical status I; healthy
patient with minor
localized pathology
(ASA scale)

PS-II physical status II; patient
with moderate systemic
disorder (ASA scale)

PS-III physical status III; patient
with nonincapacitating
severe systemic disorder
(ASA scale)

PS-IV physical status IV; patient
with incapacitating severe
systemic disorder
(ASA sale)

PS-V physical status V;
moribund patient with
short life expectancy
(ASA scale)

P/S ratio of polyunsaturated to
saturated fatty acids

P & S pain and suffering
paracentesis and suction

Ps *Pseudomonas* (some species

are pathogenic)

PSA poly-substance abuse
prepseudoarthrosis
*Progetto Sistematica
Actinomiceti* (Milan)
progressive spinal ataxia
prolonged sleep apnea
prostate-specific
antigen (test)
public service
announcement

PsA psoriatic arthritis

PSA-ACT
prostate specific antigen
bound to alpha-1-
antichymotrypsin (test)

PSAC President's Science
Advisory Committee

PSACO papillary serous
adenocarcinoma of ovary

PSAD prostate-specific antigen
density

PSAGN poststreptococcal acute
glomerulonephritis

PSAP pulmonary surfactant
apoprotein

PSAT prostate-specific
antigen test

PSbetaG
pregnancy-specific beta-1-
glycoprotein

PSBO partial small bowel
obstruction

PSC papillary serous cyst
peptostreptococcus
percutaneous suprapubic
cystostomy
pluripotential stem cell
posterior subcapsular
cataract
poststreptococcal
postsynaptic cell
Pott spinal curvature
primary sclerosing
cholangitis
primary spermatocyte
pulse synchronized
contractions

PSCC posterior

semicircular canal
posterior subcapsular
cataract

PsChE pseudocholinesterase

PSCT peripheral stem cell
transplant

PSD partial sleep deprivation
Patient Self-Determination
Act
Pelligrini-Stieda disease
photosensitivity dermatitis
poststenotic dilatation
postsurgical distress
protein S deficiency
psychoactive substance
dependence

PSDA Patient Self-Determination
Act
psychoactive substance
dependence and abuse

PSE passive smoke exposure
portal-systemic
encephalopathy

PSF posterior spinal fusion
pseudosarcomatous
fasciitis

PSFs parasympathetic fibers

PSG parasympathetic ganglion
peak systolic gradient
polysomnogram
presystolic gallop

PSGN poststreptococcal
glomerulonephritis

PSH postspinal headache

PSI Parona space infection
Pollutant Standards Index
pounds per square inch
problem solving
information
prostaglandin synthase
inhibitor

psi pounds per square inch

PSIFT platelet suspension
immunofluorescence test

PSIN presynaptic interneuron

PSIS posterior sacroiliac spine
posterior superior
iliac spine

PSL parasternal line

	prednisolone
PSLD	parasympatholytic drug
PSM	portal-systemic myelopathy
	presystolic murmur
	purse-string mouth
PSMA	progressive spinal
	muscular atrophy
	progressive streptococcal
	muscular atrophy
	prostate specific
	membrane antigen
PSMed	psychosomatic medicine
PSN	postsynaptic neuron
	presynaptic neuron

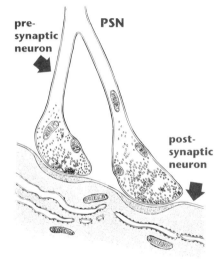

	phosphoserine
	phosphatase
	positive spike pattern
	(on EEG)
	postsynaptic potential
	progressive supranuclear
	palsy
	prone sleeping position
	pseudopregnancy
	pseudosexual precocity
PSPS	postsurgical pain syndrome
PSQ	patient satisfaction
	questionnaire
PSR	pain sensitivity range
	Physicians for Social
	Responsiblity
	portal systemic resistance
	pulmonary stretch
	receptor

PSR BOW

	premature spontaneous
	rupture of bag of waters
PSRO	Professional Standards
	Review Organization
PSS	painful shoulder syndrome
	perisinusoidal space
	physiologic saline solution
	polysplenia syndrome
	Ponceau-S stain
	posterior sag sign
	primary Sjogren syndrome
	progressive systemic
	scleroderma
	progressive systemic
	sclerosis
	pulmonary sling syndrome
	purse-string sutures
PST	pancreatic suppression test
	paroxysmal
	supraventricular
	tachycardia
	phenolsulfotransferase
	pivot shift test
	platelet survival time
	protein-sparing therapy
	proximal straight tubule
	(thick descending limb of
	kidney's nephron)
PSTI	pancreatic secretory

PSNS	parasympathetic nervous
	system (craniosacral)
PSNs	parasympathetic nerves
	peripheral spinal nerves
PSO	pelvic stabilization orthosis
	pilonidal sinus opening
	proximal subungual
	onychomycosis
pSO$_2$	arterial oxygen saturation
PSP	painful sterile prostate
	parathyroid secretory
	protein
	phenolsulfonphthalein
	(excretion test dye for
	determining kidney
	impairment)

trypsin inhibitor

PSTM paraspinal soft tissue mass

PSTT placental-site trophoblastic
tumor

PSU primary site undetermined

PSUDs psychoactive substance
use disorders

PSV pressure-supported
ventilation
pressure-support
ventilation

PSVT paroxysmal
supraventricular
tachycardia

psych psychology

psy-path psychopathic

PT paclitaxel (Taxol); alkaloid
derived from the
Pacific Yew
pain threshold
parathormone
parathyroid
paroxysmal tachycardia
part-time
patch test

PT

patch test

patient
pericardial tamponade
peroneal tendonitis
pertussis toxin
phlebothrombosis
physical therapist

physical therapy
pigeon-toed
pneumothorax
post-transfusion
post-transplantation
post-traumatic
pronator teres (muscle)
prothrombin time
psychotherapy
pulmonary thrombus
pulmonary trunk
pulmonary tuberculosis
pulmonary tularemia

P & T permanent and total
(disability)
pharmacy and therapeutics

Pt platinum
(metallic element)

pt patient
pint (a unit of measure
equal to 16 fluid ounces)

PTA pantothenic acid
parathyroid adenoma
percutaneous transluminal
angioplasty
peritonsillar abscess
persistent truncus
arteriosus
phosphotungstic acid
plasma thromboplastin
antecedent (clotting
factor XI)
post-traumatic amnesia
pretreatment anxiety
prior to admission
prior to arrival
pure tone audiometry
pure-tone threshold
average

PTAH phosphotungstic acid
hematoxylin

PTB partial-thickness burn
patellar tendon (weight)-
bearing (cast or
prosthesis)
pretibial bearing
prior to birth

PTb pulmonary tuberculosis

PTBA percutaneous transluminal

	balloon angioplasty
PTBD	percutaneous transhepatic biliary drainage
	percutaneous transluminal balloon dilatation
PTBDEF	percutaneous transhepatic biliary drainage – enteric feeding
PTBE	pyretic tick-borne encephalitis
PTBPD	post-traumatic borderline personality disorder
PTBS	post-traumatic brain syndrome
PTC	patient to call
	percutaneous transhepatic cholangiography
	phenothiocarbazine
	phenylthiocarbamide (clotting factor IX)
	pheochromocytoma-thyroid carcinoma
	pigtail catheter
	plasma thromboplastin component (clotting factor IX)
	plugged telescoping catheter
	post-traumatic confusion
	premature tricuspid closure
	prior to conception
	prothrombin time control
	proximal transverse crease (of the palm)
	pseudotumor cerebri
PTCA	percutaneous transluminal coronary angioplasty
PTCR	percutaneous transluminal coronary recanalization
PTD	permanent and total disability
	personality trait disorder
	prior to delivery
	prior to discharge
Ptd	phosphatidyl
PTE	parathyroid extract
	post-traumatic epilepsy
	proximal tibial epiphysis

	pulmonary thromboembolism
PTED	pulmonary thromboembolic disease
PTF	patient treatment file
	plasma thromboplastin factor
PTFE	polytetrafluoroethylene
PTFE graft	polytetrafluoroethylene graft
PTFS	post-traumatic fibromyalgia syndrome
PTG	papaverine topical gel
	teniposide (chemotherapy)
PTGs	parathyroid glands
PTH	parathormone (parathyroid hormone)
	parathyroid (gland)
	parathyroid hormone (maintains extracellular fluid and calcium concentration; increases resorption of bone)
	plasma thromboplastin component
	post-transfusion hepatitis
	post-traumatic headache
	post-traumatic hypersomnia
	prior to hospitalization
PTHC	parathyroid carcinoma
	percutaneous transhepatic cholangiography
PTHrP	parathyroid hormone-related peptide
	parathyroid hormone-related protein
PTHS	parathyroid hormone secretion
	profile total hip system
PTI	pancreatic trypsin inhibitor
	persistent tolerant infection
	preterm infant
PTK	phototherapeutic keratectomy

	protein tyrosine kinase
PTL	pain tolerance level
	posterior tricuspid leaflet
	preterm labor
PTLC	precipitation thin-layer chromatography
PTLD	post-transplant lymphoproliferative disorder
	prescribed tumor lethal dose (radiation therapy)
PTM	patient monitored
	post-transfusion mononucleosis
	post-traumatic meningitis
PTMA	phenyltrimethyl-ammonium
PTMDF	pupil, tension media, disk and fundus
PtmF	pterygomaxillary fissure
PTN	phenytoin (diphenylhydantoin)
	posterior tibial nerve
PTNB	preterm newborn
PTNS	pain transmission neurons
PTO	personal time off
PTOA	post-traumatic osteoarthritis
PTP	posterior tibial pulse
	post-transfusion purpura
	proximal tubular pressure
PTPD	post-traumatic personality defect
PTPI	post-traumatic pulmonary insufficiency
PTPM	post-traumatic progressive myelopathy
PTPN	peripheral (vein) total parenteral nutrition
PTPS	post-thrombophlebitis syndrome
PTR	patella tendon reflex
	patient to return
	peripheral total resistance
	prothrombin time ratio
P-triol	pregnanetriol
PTS	Parson-Turner syndrome
	passive tobacco smoke
	Pediatric Trauma Score

	permanent threshold shift
	placental transfusion syndrome (intrauterine parabiotic syndrome)
	post-thrombotic syndrome
	post-tonsillitis septicemia
	post-traumatic syndrome
	prior to surgery
	pronator teres syndrome
	pseudothalidomide syndrome
Pts	patients
PTSD	post-traumatic stress disorder
PTSS	post-traumatic stress syndrome
PTT	partial thromboplastin time
	patellar tendon transfer
	platelet transfusion therapy
	pulmonary transit time
ptt	partial thromboplastin time
PTU	pain treatment unit
	propylthiouracil
PTW	pork tapeworm (*Taenia solium*)
PTX	pneumothorax
PTx	parathyroidectomy
	pelvic traction
	pneumothorax
PTZ	pentylenetetrazol
	phenothiazine
PU	passed urine
	patent urachus
	peptic ulcer
	per urethra
	pregnancy urine
	pressure ulcer
	pressure urticaria
	prostatic urethra
Pu	plutonium (a transuranic radioactive element)
	purine
PUB	pubic
PUBS	percutaneous umbilical (cord) blood sampling
PUC	pediatric urine collector
PUD	para-urethral duct

peptic ulcer disease
PuD pulmonary disorder
PUE pyrexia of unknown
etiology
PUFA polyunsaturated fatty acids
PUH pregnancy urine hormone
PUI platelet uptake index
PUL percutaneous ultrasonic
lithotripsy
pulm pulmonary
pulv. *pulvis* [Latin] powder
PUN plasma urea nitrogen
PUNL percutaneous ultrasonic
nephrolithotripsy
PUO pyrexia of undetermined
origin
pyrexia of unknown origin
PUP percutaneous ultrasonic
pyelolithotomy
PUPPP pruritic urticarial papules
and plaques of pregnancy
PUR polyurethane
Pur purine
purulent (containing or
secreting pus)
PUREX plutonium-uranium
extraction facility
purg purgative
PUS post-ulcer surgery
PUVA psoralen (plus)
ultraviolet A
PV papillomavirus
paravertebral

pemphigus vulgaris
peripheral vein
peripheral vessels
pityriasis versicolor
plasma volume
polio vaccine (attenuated
or killed poliomyelitis
viruses)
poliovirus
polycythemia vera
(myeloproliferative
disorder)
polyoma virus
polyvinyl
portal vein
postvoiding
predictive value
pulmonary valve
pulmonary vein
P & V pyloroplasty and vagotomy
p. v. *per vaginam* [Latin]
through the vagina
PVA polyvinyl acetate
polyvinyl alcohol
Prinzmetal's variant angina
provitamin A
PVB Platinol (cisplatin) +
vinblastine + bleomycin
(combination
chemotherapy)
premature ventricular beat
PVC polyvinyl chloride
postvoiding cystogram
predicted vital capacity
premature ventricular
contraction

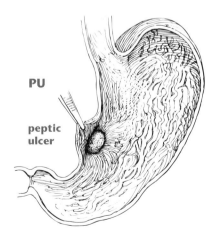

PU

peptic ulcer

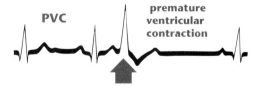

PVC premature ventricular contraction

primary visual cortex
pulmonary-valve cusps
pulmonary
venous congestion
PVD patient very disturbed
peripheral vascular disease

posterior vitreous
    detachment
postvagotomy diarrhea
pulmonary vascular disease
pulmonary vascular
    disorder

PVE passive vascular exercise
plasma volume expander
    (artificial plasma
    extender)
prosthetic valve
    endocarditis
premature ventricular
    extrasystole
prosthetic valve
    endocarditis

PVEM postvaccinal
    encephalomyelitis

PVF peripheral visual field
portal venous flow

PVFS postviral fatigue syndrome

PVG pulmonary valve gradient

PVH periventricular
    hemorrhage
pulmonary vascular
    hypertension

PVI peripheral vascular
    insufficiency
placental villus
    inflammation
post-vaccination immunity

PVK penicillin V potassium

PVL periventricular
    leukomalacia
pubovesical ligament

PVLV posterior vein of
    left ventricle

PVM preventive medicine

PVN paraventricular nucleus

PVNS pigmented villonodular
    synovitis

PVO peripheral vascular
    obstruction
pulmonary venous
    occlusion
pyogenic vertebral
    osteomyelitis

PVOD pulmonary vascular
    obstructive disease

pulmonary venous
    occlusive disease

PVP penicillin V potassium
peripheral venous pressure
polyvinylpyrrolidone
    (povidone)
portal venous pressure
pulmonary venous
    pressure

PVR peripheral vascular
    resistance
portal venous pressure
postvoiding residual
proliferative
    vitreoretinopathy
pulmonary vascular
    resistance

PVRI pulmonary vascular
    resistance index

PVRs pressure-volume
    relationships

PVS percussion, vibration
    and suction
peripheral vascular surgery
persistent vegetative state
pigmented villonodular
    synovitis
Plummer-Vinson syndrome
poliovirus susceptibility
premature ventricular
    systole
pulmonic valve stenosis

PVSS post-Vietnam stress
    syndrome

PVT paroxysmal ventricular
    tachycardia
pelvic vein
    thrombophlebitis
persistent vegetative state
portal vein thrombosis
previous trouble
private (patient)

pvt private (patient)

P. vulgaris
Proteus vulgaris (species
    found in putrefying
    tissues and abscesses;
    certain strains are

	agglutinated by typhus serum and therefore are used in diagnosing the disease)
PVW	posterior vaginal wall
PW	penetrating wound
	pinworm (*Enterobius vermicularis*)
	plantar wart (verruca plantaris)
	psychological warfare
	pulmonary wedge (pressure)
	puncture wound
Pw	progesterone withdrawal
PWA	person with AIDS
P wave	an upward deflection of the ECG cycle caused by atrial depolarization
PWB	partial weight-bearing
PWBC	peripheral white blood cell
PWC	peak work capacity
pwdr	powder
PWDS	postweaning diarrhea syndrome
PWFT	Phalen's wrist flexion test
PWI	posterior wall infarct
PWLV	posterior wall of left ventricle
PWM	pokeweed mitogen
PWMI	posteror wall myocardial infarction
PWP	Parents Without Partners
	pulmonary wedge pressure
PWS	port-wine stain
	Prader-Willi syndrome
Px	physical examination
	pneumothorax
	prognosis
PXAT	paroxysmal atrial

	tachycardia
PXE	pseudoxanthoma elasticum
PXE-AS	pseudoxanthoma elasticum and angioid streak
PxI	pyridoxal (a form of vitamin B$_6$)
Pxm	pyridoxamine (one of the active forms of vitamin B$_6$)
PXS	pseudoexfoliation syndrome
PYA	psychoanalysis
PYLL	potential years of life lost
PYP	pyrophosphate (a salt of pyrophosphoric acid)
PYR	pyruvic acid (an intermediate product in the metabolism of carbohydrate)
Pyr	pyruvate (used interchangeably with pyruvic acid)
PYY	peptide YY
PZ	pancreozymin (a hormone, secreted by the mucosa of the small intestine, that stimulates the secretion of pancreatic enzymes)
	peripheral zone
	proliferative zone
PZA	pyrazinamide (an antibacterial agent)
	pyrazinoic acid
PZ CCK	pancreozymin-cholecystokinin
PZE	piezoelectric
PZI	protamine zinc insulin
PZQ	praziquantel (an anthelmintic agent)
PZI	protamine zinc insulin

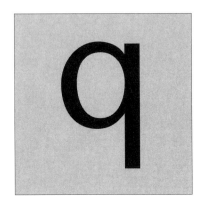

Q   cardiac output
coenzyme Q
coulomb
electric quantity
flow/cardiac output
glutamine
quadrant
quality
quantity
quart
quarter
question
quickening
quinidine
quotient
reactive power
ubiquinone
volume of blood

Q_{10}   temperature coefficient

q   each
every
long arm of chromosome
quart

q.   *quaque* [Latin] each, every

QA   quality assurance

QALE   quality-adjusted life expectancy

QALYs   quality-adjusted life years

QAM   quality assurance monitoring

q^{AM}   *quaque ante meridiem* [Latin] every morning

q.a.m.   *quaque ante meridiem* [Latin] every morning

QAP   quality assurance program

QAUR   quality assurance and utilization review

QAS   quality assurance standards

QB   whole blood

QBV   whole blood volume

QC   quality control
quick catheter
quinine colchicine

Qc   pulmonary capillary blood flow

QCA   quantitative coronary angiography

QCIM   *Quarterly Cumulative Index Medicus*

QCT   quantitative computed tomography

QD   *Questionable Doctors* (published by the Public Citizen Health Research Group)

q.d.   *quaque die* [Latin] every day

q.d.s.   *quater die sumendum* [Latin] to be taken four times daily

QEA   quick electrolyte analyzer

QEE   quadriceps extension exercise

QEEG   quantitative electroencephalography

QENF   quantitative examination of neurologic function

QEW   quick early warning

QF   quality factor
Q (query) fever
quick freeze

Q fever   query (Q) fever

q.h.   *quaque hora* [Latin] every hour

q.2h.   *quaque secunda ora* [Latin] every two hours

q.3h.   *quaque tertia hora* [latin] every three hours

q.4h.   *quaque quarta hora* [Latin] every four hours

q.h.s.   *quaque hora somni* [Latin] every night at bedtime

q.i.d.   *quater in die* [Latin] four

times a day

QIG quantitative immunoglobulin

QJ quadriceps jerk

QL quality of life

q.l. *quantum libet* [Latin] as much as desired

QLI quality of life index

QLM quadratus lumborum muscle

qlty quality

q.m. *quaque mane* [Latin] every morning

QMI Q-wave myocardial infarction

QMT quantitative muscle test

QMWS quasi-morphine withdrawal syndrome

q.n. *quaque nocte* [Latin] every night

q.n.s *quantum non sufficiat* [Latin] quantity not sufficient

QO₂ oxygen consumption

q.o.d *quaque other die* [Latin] every other day

q.o.h. *quaque other hora* [Latin] every other hour

QOL quality of life

q.o.n. *quuaque other nocte* [Latin] every other night

Qp pulmonary blood flow

q.p. *quantum placeat* [Latin] as much as desired

QPC quality of patient care

q.p.m. *quaque post meridiem* [Latin] every evening

Q & Q quinidine and quinine

qq. *quaque* [Latin] every

qq.d. *quaque die* [Latin] every day

q.q.h. *quaque quarta hora* [Latin] every four hours

qq.hor. *quaque hora* [Latin] every hour

QR quality review
quick recovery
quiet room

QRS ventricular electrical

segment of the ECG cycle including the Q wave, R wave, and S wave; it normally does not exceed 0.1 second

Q.R.Z. *qaddel reaktion zeit* [German] wheal reaction time

QS quiet sleep
quinine sulfate
quota sampling

QS₂ electromechanical systole

q.s. *quantum satis* [Latin] sufficient quantity
quantum sufficit [Latin] as much as will suffice

QSAR quantitative structure – activity relationships

Q-SHP qualified student health plan

Qsma superior mesenteric artery blood flow

QSS quantitative sacroiliac scintigraphy

QST quantitative sensory test

q. suff. *quantum sufficit* [Latin] as much as will suffice

QT Q-Tip
Quick's test
quiet

qt quantity
quart (32 oz)
quiet

QTB quadriceps tendon bearing

Q-T interval
the segment of the ECG cycle measured from the beginning of the QRS complex to the end of the T wave

QTPS QT prolongation syndrome

Q-TWST time without symptoms or toxicity

quad quadrant
quadriceps
quadriplegic

quad atrophy
quadriceps atrophy

quads quadriceps

qual   quality
qual anal
        quality analysis
quant   quantity
quant suff
        quantity sufficient
quar   quarantine
QUART   quadrantectomy, axillary
        dissection and
        radiotherapy (breast
        cancer treatment)
quat.   *quater* [Latin] four times
quint   quintuplet

quot   quotient
quotid.   *quotidie* [Latin] daily
quot. o. s.
        quoties opus sit [Latin] as
        often as needed
q.v.   *quantum volueris* [Latin] as
        much as wanted
        quod vide [Latin] which see
Q wave   the first downward
        deflection of the QRS
        complex of the ECG
        cycle, due to septal
        depolarization

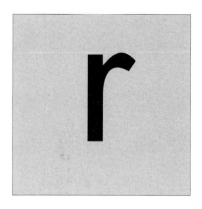

R arginine (amino acid)
electrical resistance
gas constant
organic radical
race
radial
radiation absorbed dose
radical
radioactive
radiology
radius
rate
ratio
reaction
recapitulation
receptor
rectum
refraction
regular insulin
regulator
relapse
remission
replication
resident
residue
resistance
respiratory rate/minute
response
rest
retching
retinol (vitamin A)
reverse
review
rhythm
ribosome

Rickettsia (a genus of gram-
negative, pathogenic,
intracellular parasitic
bacteria that are
transmitted to humans
through the bites of
infected fleas, ticks, mites,
and lice)
right
roentgen (unit of
radiation quantity)
rough
rub
rubella (German measles)

R1 1st year resident
R2 2nd year resident
R3 3rd year resident
R4 4th year resident
r correlation coefficient
oxidation-reduction
potential
radius
recombinant
respiration
ribose
ring chromosome

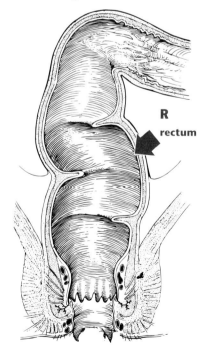

RA
roentgen
radioactive
radiographic
    absorptiometry
ragweed antigen
refractory anemia
refractory ascites
regression analysis
renal artery
repeat action
residual air
respiratory acidosis
respiratory alkalosis
retinoic acid (tretinoin)
rheumatoid arthritis

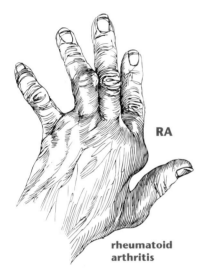

RA

**rheumatoid
arthritis**

right atrium
right auricle
risk assessment
ruptured appendix

R_A   airway resistance

Ra   radium (a radioactive
    metallic element that
    emits alpha, beta, and
    gamma radiation and a
    radioactive gas called
    radon; it is used in the
    treatment of some
    malignancies)

rA   riboadenylate
RAA   renin-angiotensin-
    aldosterone (system)
    restenosis after angioplasty
    right atrial appendage
    (auricle)

RAAA   ruptured abdominal aortic
    aneurysm

RAAG   rheumatoid arthritis
    agglutination

RAAM   renin-angiotensin-
    aldosterone mechanism

RAAS   renin-angiotensin-
    aldosterone syndrome

RA & AS   rheumatoid arthritis and
    ankylosing spondylitis

RAB   risk assessed by

RAC   Recombinant DNA
    Advisory Committee
    right atrial catheter

RAD   radiation
    radiation absorbed dose
    (of ionizing radiation)
    radiology
    reactive airway disease
    reactive attachment
    disorder
    right axis deviation
    roentgen administered
    dose

rad   radial
    radiation absorbed dose

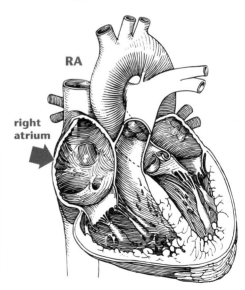

RA

**right
atrium**

	(of ionizing radiation)
	radical
	right axis deviation
rad.	*radix* [Latin] root
RADAR	Regional Alcohol and Drug Awareness Resources
RADCA	right anterodescending coronary artery
Radiol	radiology
RADISH	rheumatoid arthritis diffuse idiopathic skeletal hyperostosis
RadLV	radiation leukemia virus
RADP	right acromiodorso-posterior (fetal position)
RADS	rapid assay delivery system reactive airways dysfunction syndrome
rad/s	rad per second
Rad Ther	radiation therapy
RAE	right atrial enlargement right atrium enlargement
RAEB	refractory anemia with excess of blasts
RAEB-T	refractory anemia with excess of blasts in transformation
RAEM	refractory anemia with excess myeloblasts
RAF	rapid atrial fibrillation rheumatoid arthritis factor
RAFS	recurrent afebrile flulike symptoms
RAH	right atrial hypertrophy
RA & H	rheumatoid arthritis and hypersplenism (Felty's syndrome)
RAI	radioactive iodine
RAID	radioimmunodetection
RAIR	rectoanal inhibitory reflex
RAIS	reflection-absorption infrared spectroscopy
RAIU	radioactive iodine uptake (test)
RALN	retro-auricular lymph node
RALT	routine admission lab tests
RAM	radioactive material random access memory

	random alternating movements
	rapid alternating movements
	rectus abdominis muscle
ram	relative atomic mass (new term for atomic weight)
RAMP	right atrial mean pressure
RAN	resident's admission notes
RANA	rheumatoid agglutinin nuclear antigen
rand	random
RAO	renal artery obstruction right anterior-oblique (view)
RaONC	radiation oncology
RAP	recurrent abdominal pain rheumatoid arthritis precipitin right atrial pressure
RAPD	relative afferent pupillary defect (sign of ipsilateral optic neuropathy)
RAPS	Resource Analysis and Planning System
RAQ	right anterior quadrant
RARA	retinoid acid receptor alpha
RARS	refractory anemia with ringed sideroblasts
RAS	recurrent aphthous stomatitis renal artery stenosis renin-angiotensin system reticular activating system rheumatoid arthritis serum rheumatoid arthritis synovectomy
RA slide	rheumatoid arthritis slide (test)
RAST	radioallergosorbent test
RAT	rheumatoid arthritis test
RATx	radiation therapy
RAU	radioactive uptake recurrent aphthous ulceration recurrent aphthous ulcers
RAV	recurrent aural vertigo Rous-associated virus

RAVC retrograde atrioventricular conduction

RAVV right atrioventricular (tricuspid) valve

Raw airway resistance (resistance of tracheobronchial tree to flow of air into lungs)

RB radiation burn
rectal bleeding
recurrent bacteriuria
relieved by
respiratory bronchiole
retinoblastoma
Rickettsial burnetii (*Coxiella burnetii*; the etiologic agent of Q fever)
right bronchus
right bundle
right buttock
runner's bump

R & B risks and benefits

Rb rubidium (rare metallic element)

RBA relative binding affinity
rescue breathing apparatus
right brachial artery

RBB right breast biopsy
right bundle branch

RBBB right bundle branch block

RBBx right breast biopsy

RBC red blood cell (erythrocyte)
red blood count

rbc red blood cell (erythrocyte)

RBCM red blod cell mass

RBCV red blood cell volume

RBD recurrent brief depression
relative biologic dose
REM sleep behavior disorder
round-back deformity

RBE relative biological effectiveness

RBF rat bite fever
renal blood flow

RBG random blood glucose

RBg retinoblastoma gene

(recessive mutation of a tumor-suppressor gene that leads to tumor formation)

RBN retrobulbar neuritis

RBOW ruptured bag of waters

RBP resting blood pressure
retinoid-binding protein
retinol-binding protein
riboflavin-binding protein

RBRVS resource-based relative value scale (Medicare)

RBS random blood sugar
rigid bronchoscopy

rBST recombinant bovine somatotropin

RBT Rochester bone trephine

RBV right brachial vein

RBW relative body weight

RC radial-carpal
radiation cystitis
rectocele
red cell
Red Cross
referred case
retention catheter
reticulocyte count (red blood cell count)
retrograde cystogram
rheumatic carditis
rib cage
right coronary

rbc

red blood cell

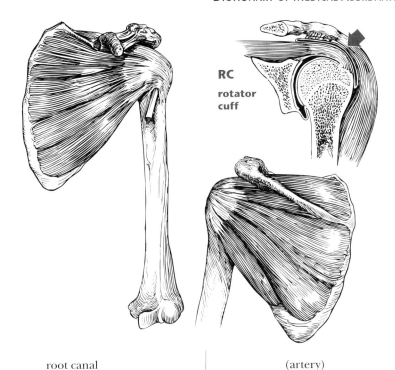

RC
rotator
cuff

root canal
rotator cuff (supraspinatus
  tendon)
routine cholecystography
R & C   referral and consultation
        risks and complications
RCA   radiographic
        contrast agent
        red cell agglutination
        relative chemotactic
          activity
        right carotid artery
        right coronary artery
        rotational coronary
          atherectomy
        rotator cuff arthropathy
          (cuff-tear arthropathy)
RCBV regional cerebral blood
        volume
RCC   rape crisis center
        receptor-cyclase-coupling
        red cell casts
        red cell count
        renal cell carcinoma
        rickets and chronic cough
        right common carotid

(artery)
RCCT randomized controlled
        clinical trial
RCD   relative cardiac dullness
        renal cystic disease
        right crus of diaphragm
        rotator cuff disease

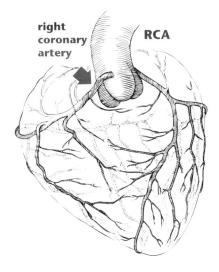

**right
coronary
artery**   **RCA**

	ruptured cevical disk
rCD4	recombinant CD4
RCDA	recurrent chronic dissecting aneurysm
RCE	right carotid endarterectomy
RCF	relative centrifugal force
	reverse Colles' fracture
	root canal filling
RCG	radiocardiography
RCH	rectocolic hemorrhage
RCHF	right-sided congestive heart failure
RCHSA	Radiation Control for Health and Safety Act
RCI	red cell index
	rotator cuff injury
RCIA	red cell immune adherence
RCJ	radiocarpal joint
RCL	radial collateral ligament
	renal clearance
RCM	radiographic contrast medium
	retinal capillary microaneurysm
	right costal margin
RCP	red cell protoporphyrin
	respiratory care plan
	riboflavin carrier protein
rcp	reciprocal translocation
RCPD	relative cephalopelvic disproportion
RCPT	registered cardiopulmonary technician
RCR	rod cell of retina
	rotator cuff repair
RCS	reticulum-cell sarcoma
	right coronary sinus
R/CS	repeated cesarean section
RCT	randomized clinical trial
	randomized controlled trial
	registered care technician
	root canal therapy
	rotator cuff tear
	rotator cuff tendinitis
RCV	red cell volume

RD	radiation damage
	rate difference
	Raynaud's disease (Raynaud's gangrene, a vascular disorder)
	reaction of degeneration
	rectal dysfunction
	recurrent depression
	Refsum's disease (phytanic acid storage disease, an inborn error of metabolism)
	registered dietician
	Reiter's disease (Reiter's syndrome, a triad of symptoms comprising arthritis, urethritis and conjunctivitis)
	related donor
	renal dialysis
	resistance determinant
	respiratory distress
	retinal detachment
	Reye's disease (Reye's syndrome, an acute and frequently fatal childhood syndrome marked by encephalopathy, hepatitis and fatty accumulations in the viscera)
	rheumatoid disease
	ruptured disk
R & D	research and development
	risk and death
rd	rutherford (unit of radioactive disintegration)
RDA	recommended daily allowance
	recommended dietary allowance
	right dorsoanterior (fetal position)
RD-BS	randomized double-blind study
RDDA	recommended daily dietary allowance
RDE	receptor-destroying

enzyme

RDFC recurring digital fibroma of childhood

RDFS ratio of decayed and filled surfaces

RDFT ratio of decayed and filled teeth

RDH registered dental hygienist

RDI recommended daily intake
relative dose intensity
respiratory disturbance index
rupture–delivery interval

RDIH right direct inguinal hernia

RDM readmission

RDMS registered diagnostic medical sonographer

rDNA ribosomal deoxyribonucleic acid

RDOD retinal detachment, right eye (*oculus dexter*)

RDOS retinal detachment, left eye (*oculus sinister*)

RDP right dorsoposterior (fetal position)

RDPE reticular degeneration of the pigment epithelium

RDS respiratory distress syndrome
Riley-Day syndrome (familial dysautonomia)

RDSN respiratory distress syndrome of newborn

RDT *Rational Drug Therapy*
regular dialysis treatment (hemodialysis)
routine dialysis therapy

RDVT recurrent deep vein thrombosis

RDW red cell distribution width

RE radiation enteritis
random error
rectal examination
reflux esophagitis
regional enteritis
resistive exercise
restriction enzyme
reticuloendothelial
retinol equivalent

retrograde ejaculation
rheumatic endocarditis
right eye

R & E rest and exercise

Re rhenium (chemical element, atomic number 75)

REA radioenzymatic assay
restriction endonuclease analysis

ReA reactive arthritis

readm readmission

REAS reasonably expected as safe

REAT radiologic emergency assistance team

REB roentgen-equivalent biologic

REC radioelectrocardiogram
receptor
record
recovery

Rec recent
recommendation

rec recombinant
recurrence

rec. *recens* [Latin] fresh

RECAL rheumatic endocarditis of aortic leaflets

RECCE right extracapsular cataract extraction

rec'd received

RECG radioelectrocardiogram

recip recipient

rect rectum
rectus (muscle)

recumb recumbent

recur recurrence

RED rapid erythrocyte degeneration
rolled edge deformity (of aortic valve cusps caused by syphilis)

red. in pulv.
reductus in pulverem [Latin] reduced to powder

redox reduction-oxidation

REE rare earth element
resting energy expenditure

REEG radioelectroencephalogram

REEGT registered electro-encephalography technician

ReEND reproductive endocrinology

re-ev re-evaluate

REF referred
renal erythropoietic factor (erythrogenin)

ref reference

Ref Doc referring doctor

refl reflex

REG radiation exposure guide
radioencephalogram

Reg registered

reg region
regular

reg diet regular diet

regurg regurgitation

rehab rehabilitation

REL rate of energy loss
recommended exposure limit
relative
religion

RELE resistive exercise of lower extremity

REM rapid eye movement (sleep)
recent-event memory
remission
reticular erythematous mucinosis
roentgen-equivalent-man (the absorbed ionizing radiation equivalent to one roentgen of x-rays) now obsolete, having been superceded by the sievert = 100 rem

rem roentgen-equivalent-man (the absorbed ionizing radiation equivalent to one roentgen of x-rays) now obsolete, having been superceded by the sievert = 100 rem

REMAB radiation-equivalent-manikin absorption

REMCAL radiation-equivalent-manikin calibration

remP roentgen-equivalent-man period

REMS rapid eye movement sleep

REM sleep rapid eye movement sleep

REN renal

ren renal

ren.sem. *renovetum semel* [Latin] renew only once

REO respiratory enteric orphan (virus)

reovirus respiratory enteric orphan virus

REP repair
report
rest exercise program
roentgen equivalent physical

rep repetition
report

rep. *repetatur* [Latin] let it be renewed

repol repolarization

REPR rough (granular) endoplasmic reticulum

req requisition

requ requirement

RER renal excretion rate
respiratory exchange ratio
rough (granular) endoplasmic reticulum

RERF Radiation Effects Research Foundation

RES research
resident
reticulo-endothelial system

res residue

resp respiration

REST regressive electroshock therapy

Resus resuscitation

RET retention
reticulocyte
reticulo-endothelial tumor
retina
return
right esotropia

ret	rad equivalent therapeutics
	retired
retard	retardation
ret cath	retention catheter
Ret Detach	
	retinal detachment
retic	reticulocyte
	reticulum
retro	retrograde
REU	rectal endoscopic ultrasonography
REV	reticuloendotheliosis viruses
	reverse
	review
REVL	reviewed by laboratory (pathologist)
re-x	re-examination
RF	radiofrequency (portion of electromagnetic spectrum between 10^6 and 10^8 hertz)
	rat flea (*Xenopsylla cheopis*)
	regurgitant factor
	relapsing fever
	relative flow
	releasing factor
	renal failure
	resistance factor
	respiratory failure
	reticular formation
	rheumatic fever (febrile disease associated with previous hemolytic streptococcal infection)
	rheumatoid factor
	riboflavin (vitamin B_{12})
	risk factor
	Rolando fracture
	Rubens flap
R & F	radiographic and fluoroscopic
Rf	rutherfordium (transuranic element, atomic number 104)
rf	radiofrequency
RFA	radio-frequency ablation
	request for application
	right femoral artery

	right frontoanterior (fetal position)
RFB	retained foreign body (in surgery)
RFC	radiofrequency coagulation
	right flexure of colon
RFCA	radiofrequency catheter ablation
RFD	radiofrequency destruction
RFE	relative fluorescence efficiency
	residual fibroemphysema
	return flow enema
RFFIT	rapid fluorescent focus inhibition test
RFI	renal failure index
rFIX	recombinant factor IX (bloodclotting protein)
RFL	right frontolateral (fetal position)
RFLA	rheumatoid factor-like activity
RFLP	restriction fragment length polymorphism
RFM	radio-frequency modulator
RFOL	results to follow
RFOU	retroflexion of uterus
RFP	recurrent facial paralysis
	request for payment
	request for proposal
	right frontoposterior (fetal position)
RFR	refraction
RF radiation	
	radiofrequency radiation
RFS	rapid frozen section
RFT	renal function test
	respiratory function test
	right frontotransverse (fetal position)
	routine fever therapy
RFUO	recurrent fever of unknown origin
RG	recessive gene
	renal glycosuria
	retrograde
rG	regulator gene
RGBM	renal glomerular basement membrane

RGC	radio-gas chromatography
RGM	right gluteus maximus (muscle)
	right gluteus medius (muscle)
	right gluteus minimus (muscle)
rGM CSF	recombinant granulocyte-macrophage colony-stimulating factor
RGO	reciprocating gait orthosis
RGP	retrograde pyelogram
RGR	relative growth rate
RH	radiation hazard
	reactive hyperemia
	recurrent herpes
	regulatory hormone
	relative humidity
	releasing hormone
	renal hypercalciuria
	respiratory hypoxia
	rest home
	retinal hemorrhage
	rheumatism
	right hand
	room humidifier
	Runaway Hotline (800) 231-6946
Rh	Rhesus factor in blood
	rhodium (a rare metallic element)
rh	relative humidity
	rheumatic
RHA	right hepatic artery
RhA	rheumatoid arthritis
RHB	raise head of bed
	right heart bypass
rhBMP-2	recombinant human bone morphogenetic protein-two
RHC	respiration has ceased
	right heart catheterization
RHD	radiological health data
	relative hepatic dullness
	renal hypertensive disease
	rheumatic heart disease
rheo	rheology
rhEPO	recombinant human erythropoietin

rheum	rheumatoid
RHF	refractory heart failure
	right heart failure
RHf	Rhesus factor
rhG-CSF	recombinant granulocyte-colony stimulating factor
RHH	right homonymous hemianopsia
Rhig	Rh immunoglobulin
rhIL-11	recombinant human interleukin-eleven
rhIL-12	recombinant human interleukin-twelve
RHL	recurrent herpes labialis
	right hepatic lobe
RhMk	rhesus monkey
Rh Neg	Rhesus factor negative
RH & PND	
	radical hysterectomy and pelvic-node dissection
Rh Pos	Rhesus factor positive
RHR	resting heart rate
RHS	Ramsay Hunt syndrome (geniculate neuralgia)
RHT	radiant heat therapy
	renal homotransplantation
	retinohypothalamic tract
	right hypertropia
rhTNF	recombinant human tumor-necrotic factor
RHU	Registered Heath Underwriter
	rheumatology
rHuEPO	recombinant human erythropoictin (humoral

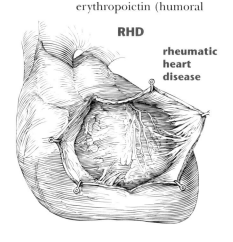

RHD

rheumatic heart disease

regulator of
erythropoiesis)
RHx   radical hysterectomy
RI   radiation injury
          radiation intensity
          radioactive isotope
          radioisotope
          rape injury
          rectal incontinence
          refractive index
          regional ileitis
          regular insulin
          remission induction
          renal insufficiency
          respiratory illness
          respiratory infection
          ribosome
RIA   radioimmune assay
          radioimmunoassay
RIAT   radioimmune anti-
          globulin test
Rib   riboflavin (vitamin B$_2$)
          ribose (a five-carbon
          sugar present in
          ribonucleic acid)
RIBA   recombinant immunoblot
          assay
RIC   radiation-induced
          carcinogenesis
          right iliac crest
          right internal carotid
          (artery)
RICCE   right intracapsular cataract
          extraction
RICE   rest, ice, compression and
          elevation (initial
          treatment regimen for
          sprains and strains)
RICM   right intercostal margin
RICS   right intercostal space
RICU   respiratory intensive
          care unit
RID   radial immunodiffusion
          Remove Intoxicated
          Drivers (518) 372-0034
          ruptured intervertebral
          disk
RIF   release inhibiting factor
          rifampin (rifampicin)

right iliac fossa
RIFA   radioiodinated fatty acid
rIFN   recombinant interferon
RIG   rabies immune globulin
RIH   right inguinal hernia
RIHS   recurrent intraoral
          herpes simplex
RIHSA   radioactive iodinated
          human serum albumin
RIIH   right indirect
          inguinal hernia
RIJ   right internal
          jugular (vein)
rIL   recombinant interleukin
RIM   radioisotope medicine
RIMA   reversible inhibitors of
          MAO type A
RIMR   Rockefeller Institute for
          Medical Research
RIND   reversible ischemic
          neurologic deficit
RINI   radiation-induced nerve
          injury
RIOJ   recurrent intrahepatic
          obstructive jaundice
RIP   radioimmunoprecipitin
          (test)
          rapid infusion pump
          reflex inhibiting pattern
RIPA   radioimmunoprecipitation
          assay
RIPP   resistive intermittent
          positive pressure
RIR   radioisotope renography
          right inferior rectus
          (eye muscle)
RIS   radioactive isotope scan
          (scintigraphy)
          radioisotope scan
          (scintigraphy)
RISA   radioiodinated serum
          albumin
RIST   radioimmunosorbent test
RIT   radioiodine treatment
          Rorschach inkblot test
RIU   radioactive iodine uptake
RIVD   ruptured intervertebral
          disk
RIX   radiation-induced

xerostomia

RK radial keratoplasty
radial keratotomy
right kidney
runner's knee

RKW renal potassium wasting

RKY roentgenkymography

RL Radiation Laboratory
right lung
right leg
Ringer's lactate (solution)
Roeder loop (slipknot used
in surgery)

RLBP recurrent low back pain

RLC radial longitudinal crease
(of the palm)
residual lung capacity

RLD related living donor
ruptured lumbar disk

RLE right lower extremity

RLF retained lung fluid
retrolental fibroplasia

RLL right lower limb
right lower lobe (of lung)

RLM restless legs movement
(sleep disorder)

RLN recurrent laryngeal nerve
regional lymph nodes
Rotter's lymph nodes
(occasionally seen
between the pectoral
muscles, often containing
metastases from
mammary cancer)

RLQ right lower quadrant

RLR right lateral rectus
(eye muscle)

RLQ right lower quadrant
(of abdomen)

RLS radial ligament sprain
restless legs syndrome
(irresistible urge to move
the legs due to an
annoying discomfort
inside the calves when
sitting or lying down)
Ringer's lactate solution

RLSB right lower scapular border

RLT right lateral thigh

RLX relaxin (a polypeptide
ovarian hormone
secreted by the corpus
luteum of pregnancy;
it facilitates delivery of
the fetus)

RM radical mastectomy
range of motion
red marrow (bone)
relative mobility
repetition maximum
resistive movement
respiratory movement
risk management
room

R & M routine and microscopic

Rm remission

RMA radiculomedullary artery
retinal microaneurysm
right mentoanterior
(fetal position)

RMB right main bronchus

RMC reticularis magnocellularis

RMCA right middle
cerebral artery

RMCL right midclavicular line

RMD rapid movement disorder

RME right mediolateral
episiotomy

RMEE right middle ear
exploration

RMI repetitive motion injury

r/min revolutions per minute

RML radiation myeloid
leukemia
Regional Medical Library
right middle lobe (of lung)

RMLB right middle
lobe bronchus

RMLE right medial lateral
episiotomy

RMLS right middle lobe
syndrome

RMP Regional Medical Program
resting membrane
potential
rifampin (rifampicin, a
semisynthetic derivative
of the broad-spectrum
antibiotic rifamycin)

	right mentoposterior (fetal position)
RMR	resting metabolic rate
RMRI	remote magnetic resonance imaging
RMS	rectal morphine sulfate (analgesic suppository)
	renal medullary syndrome
	repetitive motion syndrome
	rhabdomyosarcoma
	rheumatic mitral stenosis
	root mean square
RMSF	Rocky Mountain spotted fever (tick-borne disease)
RMT	registered music therapist
	right mentotransverse (fetal position)
RMV	respiratory minute volume
RMW	renal magnesium wasting
RMWT	Rocky Mountain wood tick (*Dermacentor andersoni*)
RMx	radical mastectomy
RN	radiation nephritis
	radionuclide
	random noise
	Ranvier's node (an interruption occurring at regular intervals in the myelin sheath of a nerve fiber)
	red nucleus
	reflux nephropathy
	registered nurse
	rheumatoid nodules (Schmorl's nodules)
R/N	renew
Rn	radon (radioactive element produced by the decay of radium)
RNA	radionuclide angiography
	registered nurse anesthetist
	ribonucleic acid
RNAase	ribonuclease
RNA dDNA	
	ribonucleic acid-dependent DNA
RNA-TVs	ribonucleic acid tumor viruses
RNBS	radionuclide bleeding scan
RNC	radionuclide cineangiography
	registered nurse, certified
	rubella nuclear cataract
RND	radical neck dissection
RNEF	radionuclide ejection fraction
RNES	radial nerve entrapment syndrome
RNMD	respiratory neuromuscular disorder
RNMT	registered nuclear medicine technologist
RNP	registered nurse practitioner
	ribonucleoprotein
RNR	radionuclide renogram
	residual nuclear radiation (fallout)
	ribonucleotide reductase
RNS	radionuclide scanning
	radionuclide scintigraphy
rNTP	ribonuclease-5'-triphosphate
RNV	radionuclide venography
	radionuclide ventriculography
	retinal neovascularization
RO	radiation oncology
	radiation output
	reality orientation
	relative odds
	right occipital
	routine order
	rule out
R/O	rule out
ROA	right occipitoanterior (fetal position)
ROAD	reversible obstructive airway disease
ROC	receiver operator characteristic (plot of true positive versus false positive results)
	resident on call
ROD	renal osteodystrophy
roent	roentgenology
ROH	rubbing alcohol

ROI   reactive oxygen
intermediates
region of interest
ROL   right occipitolateral
(fetal position)
ROM   range of motion (joint
movements quantified
in degrees)
range of movement
read only memory
right otitis media
rupture of membranes
ROM/CPF
range of motion, complete
and pain free
ROMI   rule out myocardial
infarction
RON   rule of nine
ROO   register of operations
ROP   retinopathy of prematurity
(retrolental fibroplasia)
right occipitoposterior
(fetal position)
right occiput posterior
(fetal position)
RorschT Rorschach test
ROS   review of (organ) systems
ROSC   return of spontaneous
circulation
ROSS   review of subjective
symptoms
ROT   registered occupational
therapist
right occipitotransverse
(fetal position)
ROU   recurrent oral ulcers
ROW   Rendu-Osler-Weber
(syndrome)
RP   rachitic potbelly
radial pulse
radiation proctitis
radical prostectomy
Rathke's pouch
(outpouching of
embryonic oral cavity)
Raynaud's phenomenon
reactive protein
rectal pain (dyschezia)
rectal prolapse

referred pain
referring physician
registered pharmacist
relapse prevention
relapsing polychondritis
renin profiling
retinitis pigmentosa
retinitis proliferans
retrograde pyelogram
retroperitoneal
rheumatic pain
rheumatoid polyarthritis
ring pessary
R-5-P   ribose-5-phosphate
RPA   registered physician's
assistant
reverse passive anaphylaxis
right pulmonary artery
rPA   recombinant plasminogen
activator (clot buster)
RPase   ribonucleic acid
polymerase
RPC   relapsing polychondritis
RPCF   Reiter protein complement
fixation (test)
RPD   recurrent psychotic
depression
removable partial denture
rPDGF   recombinant platelet-
derived growth factor
RPE   rating of perceived
exertion
recurrent pulmonary
embolism
retinal pigment epithelium
rubella panencephalitis
RPED   retinal pigment epithelial
detachment
RPEE   rectal probe
electroejaculation
RPF   radium placement film
relaxed pelvic floor
renal plasma flow (rate)
retroperitoneal fibrosis
RPG   retrograde pyelogram
RPGN   rapidly progressive
glomerulonephritis
RPH   retroperitoneal
hemorrhage

RPh	registered pharmacist		rate ratio
RPHA	reverse passive hemagglutination		recovery room
			referred pain
RPI	reticulocyte production index		regular respirations
			regular rhythm
RPL	renal phosphate leak		relative risk
RPLAD	retroperitoneal lymphadenectomy		renin release
			respiratory rate
RPLC	reverse phase liquid chromatography		retinal reflex
			Rickettsia rickettsii (the
RPLN	retropancreatic lymph node		causative agent of Rocky Mountain spotted fever;
	retroperitoneal lymph node		transmitted through the bites of infected ticks)
	retropharyngeal lymph node		risk of recurrence
			road rage
RPLND	retroperitoneal lymph node dissection	**R & R**	rate and rhythm (pulse)
			rest and recuperation
rpm	revolutions per minute	**RR-1**	first recovery room
RPN	renal papillary necrosis	**RR-2**	second recovery room
RPP	radical perineal prostatectomy	**RRA**	radioreceptor assay
			registered record administrator
RPR	rapid plasma reagin (test)		renal renin activity
	Reiter protein reagin		right renal artery
RPr	retinitis proliferans	**RRAM**	rapid and repetitive alternating movements
RPRTs	rapid plasma reagin tests		
RPS	refractory partial seizure	**RRC**	Residency Review Committee
	renal perfusion scan		
	renal pressor substance		routine respiratory care
	retroperitoneal sarcoma	**RRCA**	Road Runners Club of America
	routine preventive screening	**RR&E**	round, regular and equal (pupils)
rps	revolutions per second		
RPT	registered physical therapist	**RREF**	resting radionucleic ejecton fraction
	ring precipitin test	**RRI**	recurrent respiratory infection
	Rorschach psychodiagnostic test		
RPTA	renal percutaneous transluminal angioplasty	**RRIS**	recurrent respiratory infection syndrome
RPTC	regional poisoning treatment centers	**RRMS**	relapsing-remitting multiple sclerosis
Rptd	ruptured	**rRNA**	ribosomal ribonucleic acid
RPU	retropubic urethropexy	**rRNP**	ribosomal ribonucleoprotein
RPV	retropubic vein		
	right pulmonary vein	**RROM**	resistance in range of motion
RPVs	right pulmonary veins		
RQ	respiratory quotient	**RRP**	radical retropubic prostatectomy
RR	radiation reaction		

	recurrent respiratory papillomatosis
	relative refractory period
RRpm	respiratory rate per minute
RRR	recovery room routine
	regular rate and rhythm
	renin-release rate
RR & R	regular rhythm and rate
RRRN	round, regular, and react normally (pupils during eye examination)
RRS	retrorectal space
	Richards-Rundle syndrome
RRT	registered respiratory therapist
RRV	rhesus rotavirus
RS	radiation safety
	radiomimetic substance
	random sample
	Raynaud's syndrome
	rectal sinus
	rectal suppository
	rectosigmoid
	Reed-Sternberg (cell)
	refractive surgery (corneal surgery for vision correction)
	Reifenstein syndrome (incomplete male pseudohermaphroditism)
	Reiter's syndrome
	respiratory sounds
	retinal stroke
	review of systems
	Reye's syndrome (an acute and frequently fatal childhood syndrome marked by encephalopathy, hepatitis and fatty accumulations in the viscera)
	rheumatoid spondylitis
	right sacral
	right side
	Ringer's solution
	Rotor's syndrome
	Rous sarcoma
	rubella syndrome
R/S	resuscitation status (scaled from one to three)
R & S	rest and sleep
RSA	Rehabilitation Services Administration
	relative standard accuracy
	reticulum cell sarcoma
	right sacroanterior (fetal position)
	right subclavian artery
	roentgen stereophotogrammetric analysis
RSB	right sternal border
	right subclavian artery
RSC	Reed-Sternberg cell
	rested-state contraction
	reversible sickle-cell
	right subclavian (artery and/or vein)
RScA	right scapuloanterior (fetal position)
RScP	right scapuloposterior (fetal posiion)
RSCT	rostral spinocerebellar tract
RSD	reflex sympathetic dystrophy (post-traumatic dystrophy)
	relative standard deviation
	repetitive strain disorder
RSDS	reflex sympathetic dystrophy syndrome
RSDV	respiratory sialodacryoadenitis virus
RSE	reference standard endotoxin
RSEP	right somatosensory evoked potential
RSH	rectus sheath hematoma
RSI	repetitive strain injury
RSIVP	rapid-sequence intravenous pyelography
RSLN	retrosternal lymph node
Rsma	superior mesenteric artery resistance
RSMR	relative standard mortality rate
RSO	right salpingo-oophorectomy

RSNA	Radiological Society of North America
RSP	retrosternal pain
	rhinoseptoplasty
	right sacroposterior (fetal position)
RSR	regular sinus rhythm
RSR	renal systemic renin index
RSS	radiation sickness syndrome
	rectosigmoidoscopy
	recurrent *Salmonella* septicemia
RST	radiosensitivity test
	reagin screen test
	reticulospinal tract
	right sacrotransverse (fetal position)
	rubrospinal tract
RSV	respiratory syncytial virus
	right subclavian vein
	Rous sarcoma virus
RSVA	respiratory syncytial virus antibody
RSVI	respiratory syncytial virus infection
RSVP	*répondez s'il vous plaît* French] please reply
RSW	renal salt wasting
	right-sided weakness
RT	radiation therapy (local modality for treating cancer)
	radiologic technician
	radiologic technologist
	radiotelemetry
	radiotherapy
	radium therapy
	reaction time
	reading test
	reciprocating tachycardia
	recreational therapy
	rectal temperature
	registered technician
	registered technologist
	renal transplant
	reperfusion time (the mean time for restoring blood flow to the heart)

	respiratory therapy
	reverse transcriptase
	right
	Rinne test (of auditory function)
	Romberg's test (to assess the function of the posterior column of the spinal cord)
	room temperature
	rubella titer
R/T	rectal temperature
	related to
Rt	right
R/t	related to
rT	ribothymidine
rT₃	reverse triiodothyronine
rt	right
RTA	ready to administer
	renal tubular acidosis
	road traffic accident
RTAT	right anterior thigh
RTC	Rape Trauma Center
	renal tubular cell
	return to clinic
	round the clock
RTD	residency training director
	respiratory tract disease
	Rhus toxicodendron
Rtd	retarded
RTE	reverse tennis elbow
RTECS	registry of toxic effects of chemical substances
RTF	ready to feed
	resistance transfer factor
	respiratory tract fluid
RT+5-FU	radiation therapy with 5-fluorouracil
RTI	respiratory tract infection
	reverse transcriptase inhibitor
RTL	reactive (pupils) to light
RTM	registered trademark
	ruptured tympanic membrane (eardrum)
RTN	renal tubular necrosis
rtn	return
rTNF	recombinant tumor

necrosis factor

RT(NM) registered technologist in nuclear medicine

rTNM retreatment of tumor, nodes (lymph) and metastasis

RTO return to office

RTOG radiation therapy oncology group

RTP renal transplantation patient

reproductive-tract patency

rtPA recombinant tissue plasminogen activator

RT-PCR reverse transcription – polymerase chain reaction

RTR renal transplant rejection

RT(R) radiologic technician (registered)

recreational therapist (registered)

RTRR return to recovery room

RTS real time scan

return to sender

Revised Trauma Score

RTT radiation therapy technician

respiratory therapy technician

RTU relative time unit

RT₃U resin triiodothyronine uptake

RTW return to work

RTWD return to work decision

RTX resiniferatoxin

RTx radiation therapy

RT-ZCS rapid time-zone change syndrome (jet lag)

RU radial-ulnar

radioactive uptake

rat unit

rectourethral

recurrent ulceration

residual urine

retrograde ureterogram

retrograde urogram

roentgen unit

routine urinalysis

RU-1 human embryonic lung fibroblast

Ru ruthenium (rare metallic element)

RU 486 mifepristone (abortion agent)

ru radiation unit

RUA routine urinalysis

rub. *ruber* [Latin] red

RUE right upper extremity

RUG retrograde ureterogram

RUJ radioulnar joint

RUL right upper lid (eyelid)

right upper limb

right upper lobe (of lung)

RUO right ureteral orifice

RUOQ right upper outer quadrant (e.g., of the abdomen)

rupt ruptured

RUQ right upper quadrant (e.g., of the abdomen)

RUR resin-uptake ratio

RURTI recurrent upper respiratory tract infection

RUS radioulnar synostosis

RUSB right upper sternal border

RUV residual urine volume

RUX right upper extremity

RV Rauscher virus

rectovaginal

renal vein

residual volume

respiratory volume

retroversion

return visit

rheumatic vegetation

rheumatoid vasculitis

rhinoviruses

right ventricle

rubella vaccine

rubella virus

RVA rabies vaccine absorbed

reovirus antibody

right vertebral artery

RVAD right ventricular assist device

RVCF removable vena caval filter

RVD (used in local thrombolytic therapy)
relative vertebral density
restrictive ventilatory disorder
retinal vascular disease
rheumatic vascular disease
right ventricular dysplasia

RVDP right ventricular diastolic pressure

RVDV right ventricular diastolic volume

RVE right ventricular enlargement

RVEDP right ventricular end-diastolic pressure

RVEF right ventricular ejection fraction

RVESV right ventricular end-systolic volume

RVET right ventricular ejection time

RVF rectovaginal fistula
Rift Valley fever (an acute febrile infection caused by bunyavirus)
right ventricular failure

RVG radionuclide ventriculography

RV

right ventricle

RVH renovascular hypertension
retinal vascular hamartoma
right ventricular hypertrophy

RVHD rheumatic valvular heart disease

RVI relative value index
retavirus infection (leading cause of severe acute infantile gastroenteritis)

RVID right ventricular internal dimension

RVLG right ventral lateral gluteal (common muscle injection site)

RVLM rostral ventrolateral medulla

RVM rostral ventromedial medulla

RVO relaxed vaginal outlet
retinal vein occlusion
right ventricular outflow

RVOD renovascular occlusive disease

RVOT right ventricular outflow tract

RVOTO right ventricular outflow tract obstruction

RVOU retroversion of uterus

RVP Reality vaginal pouch (for collecting amniotic fluid)
resting venous pressure
right ventricular pressure

RVPFR right ventricular peak filling rate

RVR rapid ventricular response
reduced vascular response
renal vascular resistance
resistance to venous return

RVRA renal venous renin assay

RVRC renal vein renin concentration

RVS rectovaginal septum
rectovaginal space
relative value scale
retrovaginal space

RVs retroviruses

RVSO right ventricular

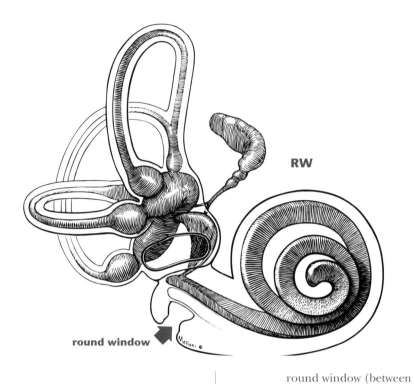

RW

round window

	stroke output
RVSP	right ventricular systolic pressure
RVSW	right ventricular stroke work
RVSWI	right ventricular stroke work index
RVT	renal vein thrombosis
	retinal vein thrombosis
RVTE	recurring venous thromboembolism
RV/TLC	residual volume/total lung capacity
RVU	relative value unit
	retroversion of uterus (abnormal position of uterus)
RVV	rubella virus vaccine
RVVL	rubella virus vaccine live
RVx	radical vulvectomy
RW	ragweed
	rapid walking
	recalcitrant warts
	ringworm (tinea)

	round window (between scala tympani of inner ear and chamber of middle ear)
	roundworm (*Ascaris lumbricoides*)
R/W	return to work
R wave	the first upward deflection of the QRS complex of the ECG cycle, due to apical left ventricular depolarization
RWOT	renal washout time
RWP	ragweed pollen
RWS	ragweed sensitivity
Rx	drug
	medication
	prescription
	recipe [Latin] take
	therapy
	treatment
RXLI	recessive X-linked ichthyosis
RXN	reaction
RXT	radiation therapy
R-Y	Roux-en-Y anastomosis

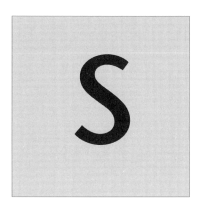

S   entropy
heart sound
sacral vertebra
(S1 through S5)
saline
Salmonella (a genus of
gram-negative, rod-
shaped, motile bacteria,
species of which cause
acute intestinal
inflammation)
saturated
scapula
Schistosoma (a genus of
blood flukes; some
species are parasitic in
man, causing debilitating
illnesses)
schizophrenia
seconds
section
sedimentation coefficient
selection coefficient
semilente (insulin)
senile
senility
sensitive
septum
serine (nonessential
amino acid)
serum
shingles (herpes zoster)
single
skeleton

skull
small
smooth
solid
soluble
somite
space
sperm
spermatozoon
spherical (lens)
Spirillum (a genus of
flagellated spiral or
corkscrew-shaped
bacteria which are
found in water and
putrid infusions)
spleen
Staphylococcus (a genus of
gram-positive, nonmotile,
usually pathogenic

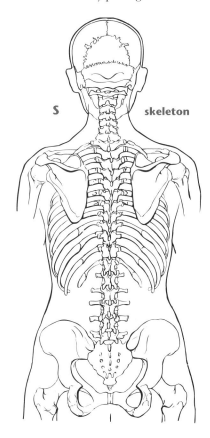

S   skeleton

bacteria which tend to aggregate in regular grapelike clusters)
stimulus
Streptococcus (a genus of gram-positive, round or ovoid bacteria, pathogenic and/or nonpathogenic in man, occurring in pairs or chains)
sternum
stomach
subject (patient involved in experiment)
subjective
substrate
succinylcholine
suction
sulfur
supervision
supine
surgery
susceptible
Svedberg unit (sedimentation coefficient)
syndrome (a set of signs and symptoms that coexist with reasonable consistency, more frequently than would be expected by chance)
systolic (the pressure when the heart muscle contracts)

S.   *signa* [Latin] signature; label

s   second
section
sedimentation coefficient
series
single

s.   *semis* [Latin] half

sine [Latin] without
sinister [Latin] left

S1   first sacral spinal nerve
first sacral vertebra

S2   second sacral spinal nerve
second sacral vertebra

S3   third sacral spinal nerve
third sacral vertebra

S4   fourth sacral spinal nerve
fourth sacral vertebra

S5   fifth sacral spinal nerve
fifth sacral vertebra

S_1   first heart sound
S_2   second heart sound
S_3   third heart sound (ventricular gallop)
S_4   fourth heart sound (atrial gallop)

S I   first heart sound
S II   second heart sound
S III   third heart sound (ventricular gallop)
S IV   fourth heart sound (atrial gallop)

SA   sacroanterior
salicylic acid
salt added
same as
sarcoma
Schizophrenics Anonymous
seasonal allergy
secondary amenorrhea
secondary anemia
self-analysis
semen albumin
semen analysis
sensory aphasia
separation anxiety
serum albumin
Sexaholics Anonymous
sinoatrial (node)
sinus arrest
sinus arrhythmia

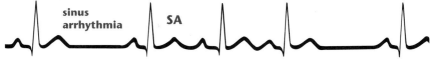

sinus arrhythmia   SA

skin absorption
sleep apnea
solitary adenomas
Spanish American
speech audiometry
spiking activity
spider angioma
spinal anesthesia
spontaneous abortion
spousal abuse
stable angina
Staphylcoccus aureus (a
  species containing the
  pigmented, coagulase-
  positive variety which
  causes boils, carbuncles,
  abscesses, and other
  suppurative
  inflammations)
sternal angle (angle of
  Louis, at junction of
  manubrium and body
  of sternum)
stranger anxiety
subarachnoid
substance abuse
Sudeck's atrophy (mottled
  osteopenia of involved
  distal extremity)
suicide alert
suicide attempt
surface action
surface antigen
surface area
sustained action

SA-   stretch-activated
    (channels)
S-A   sinoatrial
    sinoauricular
S & A   sugar and acetone
SAA   same as above
    serum amyloid A
    severe aplastic anemia
    Stokes-Adams attack
    subareolar abscess
SAARDs slow-acting antirheumatic
    drugs
SAAT   serum aspartate
    aminotransferase

SAB   serum albumin
    significant asymptomatic
     bacteriuria
    sinoatrial block
    sinoauricular block
    spontaneous abortion
    subacromial bursa
    subacromial bursitis
    subarachnoid bleed
    subarachnoid block
SA bolt subarachnoid bolt
    (technique)
SABP   spontaneous acute
    bacterial peritonitis
SAC   saccharine
    secretory adenocarcinoma
    serum aminoglycoside
     concentration
    short-arm cast (extends
     from palm to elbow)
    sound-absorption
     coefficient
    substance abuse counselor
sacch   saccharin
SACD   subacute combined
    degeneration
SACE   serum angiotensin-
    converting enzyme
SACH   solid ankle- cushioned heel
SACT   single-agent chemotherapy
    sinoatrial conduction time
SAD   seasonal affective disorder
    (winter depression)
    self-assessment depression
    (self-evaluation scale)
    separation anxiety disorder
    sexual ateliotic dwarfism
    (isolated growth
    hormone deficiency)
    small airway disease
    standard American diet
    subacute dialysis
SADD   standardized assessment of
    depressive disorders
    Students Against Driving
    Drunk (617) 481-3568
SADR   suspected adverse
    drug reaction
SADS   seasonal affective
    disorder syndrome

sudden arrhythmia
death syndrome

SAE specific action exercise
supported arm exercise

SAEB sinoatrial entrance block

SAED selected area electron
diffraction

SAEM Society for Academic
Emergency Medicine

SAF scrapie-associated fibril
self-articulating femoral
(total hip replacement)
serum accelerator factor
superior articular facet

SAFA soluble antigen fluorescent
antibody

sag sagittal

Sag D sagittal diameter

SAH subarachnoid hemorrhage
systemic arterial
hypertension

SAHOS senile ankylosing
hyperostosis of spine

SAHS sleep apnea/
hypersomnolence
syndrome
sleep apnea/hypopnea
syndrome

SAI secondary adrenal
insufficiency
(ACTH deficiency)
systemic active
immunotherapy

SAICAR succinyl aminoimidazole
carboxamide riboside

SAIDS sexually acquired
immunodeficiency
syndrome

SAL salicylate
saline
Salmonella (a genus of
gram-negative, rod-
shaped, motile bacteria,
some species of which
cause acute intestinal
inflammation)
suction-assisted lipectomy
(adipectomy)
surface-active layer

(surfactant)

SAL-12 sequential analysis of 12
chemical constituents

sal salicylate
saline
saliva
salt

salicyl salicylate

SAM self-administered
medication
serratus anterior muscle
sex arousal mechanism
small-amplitude murmur
smoking-attributable
mortality
Society for Adolescent
Medicine
sulfated acid
mucopolysaccharide
systolic anterior motion

SAMA Student American Medical
Association

SAMHSA Substance Abuse and
Mental Health Services
Administration

SAM splint
structural aluminum
malleable splint

SAMN subacute motor
neuropathy

SAN sinoatrial node
slept all night
solitary autonomus nodule
spinal accessory (11th
cranial) nerve
styrene-acrylonitrile

SANC short-arm navicular cast

sang sanguinous

sanit sanitary

S-A node
sinoatrial node

SANS autonomic nervous system
(sympathetic part)

SAO small airway obstruction

SaO₂ arterial oxygen saturation
(percentage)

SAP serum acid phosphatase
serum alkaline
phosphatase

serum amyloid P
standard assessment
  of personality
subacute axonal
  polyneuropathy
systemic arterial pressure
systolic arterial pressure

SAPD self-administration of
  psychotropic drugs

SAPHO synovitis, acne, pustulosis,
  hyperostosis,
  osteomyelitis (syndrome)

SAPS short arm plaster of
  Paris splint
simplified acute
  physiology score

SAPV superior articular process
  of vertebra

SAQC statistical analysis of
  quality control

SAR seasonal allergic rhinitis
seasonal allergy relief
severe allergic reaction
sexual attitude
  reassessment
structure-activity
  relationship

SARA system for anesthetic and
  respiratory analysis

sarc sarcoma

SART sinoatrial recovery time
standard acid reflux test

SAS scalenus anterior syndrome
self-rating anxiety scale
severe ankle sprain
short-arm splint
sleep apnea syndrome
sterile aqueous solution
subaortic stenosis
subarachnoid space
suicide and aggression
  survey
supravalvular aortic
  stenosis

SASA Sex Abuse Survivors
  Anonymous

SAT satellite
saturation
Saturday

Scholastic Achievement
  Test
Scholastic Aptitude Test
Senior Apperception Test
serum antitrypsin
speech awareness
  threshold
streptococcal antibody test
subacute thrombosis
subacute thyroiditis
  (giant cell)
systematic assertive therapy

SATB special aptitude test battery

SATC Substance Abuse
  Treatment Center

sat'd saturated

SATL surgical Achilles tendon
  lengthening

SATU substance abuse
  treatment unit

S. aureus *Staphylococcus aureus*
  (a species containing the
  pigmented, coagulase-
  positive variety which
  causes boils, carbuncles,
  abscesses, and other
  suppurative
  inflammations)

SAVD spontaneous assisted
  vaginal delivery

SAVF systemic arteriovenous
  fistula

SAVS subaortic valvular stenosis

SB safety belt
seat belt
seen by
selection bias
serum bilirubin
sesamoid bone
shortness of breath
sinus bradycardia
sitz bath
small bowel
smegma bacillus
spina bifida (spinal
  dysraphism)
stand-by
sternal border
stillbirth (fetal death)

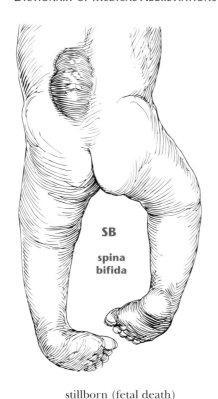

SB

spina bifida

stillborn (fetal death)
subarachnoid (saddle)
   block
sunburn
surface biopsy

SB+ was wearing seat belt
   during automobile
   accident
SB– was not wearing seat belt
   during automobile
   accident
Sb antimony (a metallic
   element)
   strabismus
SBA sideroblastic anemia
   saddle block anesthesia
   spina bifida aperta
   standby angioplasty
   standby assistance
SBAA Spina Bifida Association of
   America
SBC standard bicarbonate
   strict bed confinement
SBD senile brain disease

spinal bone density
sphincter of bile duct
spotted bone disease
   (osteopoikilosis)
straight bag drainage
SBDS social breakdown
   syndrome (due to long-
   term effects of
   institutionization of
   mental patients)
SBE self breast examination
   shortness of breath
   on exertion
   subacute bacterial
   endocarditis
sbep somatosensory brainstem
   evoked potential
SBF seat belt fracture (usually
   a thoracolumbar
   spine fracture)
   sesamoid bone fracture
SBFT small-bowel follow-through
   (radiologic study)
SBGM self blood glucose
   monitoring
SBH small bowel herniation
SBI serious bacterial infection
   silicone breast implant
   systemic bacterial infection
SBIT Stanford-Binet
   Intelligence Test
sBL sporadic Burkitt's
   lymphoma
SBN Seabright Bantam
   syndrome
   single-breath
   nitrogen (test)
SBO small bowel obstruction
   spina bifida occulta
SBOH State Board of Health
SBOT single-breath oxygen test
   (single inflation to total
   lung capacity with 100%
   oxygen)
SBP serotonin-binding protein
   spontaneous bacterial
   peritonitis
   steroid-binding protein
   subacute bacterial

peritonitis
systemic biopsy of prostate
systolic blood pressure
SBR strict bed rest
SBRN superficial branch of
radial nerve
SBS shaken baby syndrome
short bowel syndrome
sick building syndrome
small bowel series
straight back syndrome
(a skeletal deformity)
SBT serum bactericidal titer
single-blind trial
SBTT Simplate bleeding time test
small bowel transit time
SC sacrococcygeal
satiety center
Schwann cell
sciatic (nerve)
sclerocorneal
sebaceous cyst
secondary care
secretory component
self-care (self-help)
semicircular (canals and/
or ducts)
senile cataract
senior citizen
septal cartilage
serum creatinine
sex chromatin
sex chromosome
sickle cell

SC sickle cell

sigmoid colon
simian crease
(of the palm)
skin cancer

skin conductance
smoker's cough
smoking cessation
Snellen's chart
sodium citrate
soft cancer (medullary
carcinoma)
spermatocyte
spermatic cord
sperm count
spinal canal
(vertebral canal)
spinal column
spinal cord
squamous carcinoma
sternoclavicular (joint)
subclavian
subcutaneous
succinylcholine
suction curettage
sugar coated
superior colliculus
supracondylar
Sydenham's chorea
systemic candidiasis
S-C sickle cell
Sc scandium (rare
metallic element)
scapula
sc subcutaneous
SCA selective coronary
angiogram
semen collection
and analysis
serous cystadenoma
severe congenital anomaly
sickle-cell anemia
spur cell anemia
stem-cell assay
(clonogenic assay)
steroidal-cell antibody
subclavian artery
sudden cardiac arrest
sunscreening agent
superior cerebellar artery
SCA 1 spinocerebellar ataxia
type one
SCA 2 spinocerebellar ataxia
type two

SCABP single coronary artery
bypass
SCAN scintiscan
suspected child abuse and/
or neglect
SCAT sickle cell anemia test
SCB shallow coin biopsy
strictly confined to bed
SCBA self-contained breathing
apparatus
SCBC small-cell bronchogenic
carcinoma
SCBE single contrast barium
enema
SCBU special care baby unit
SCC semicircular canal
serum cholesterol
concentration
short-course chemotherapy
sickle cell crisis
small-cell carcinoma
Society for Children with
Craniosynostosis
soft cervical collar
(cervical othosis)
spinal cord compression
squamous cell carcinoma
surgical critical care
SCCa squamous cell carcinoma
SCCB small-cell carcinoma of
bronchus
SCCC squamous cell cervical
carcinoma
SCCD subacute corticoid
cerebellar degeneration
SCCL small-cell carcinoma
of lung
SCCM Society for Critical Care
Medicine
SCCS spinal cord compression
syndrome
SCCT severe cerebrocranial
trauma
SCD sequential compression
device
shepherd's crook
deformity
sickle cell disease
spinal cord disease

spondylocostal dysostosis
straight collecting duct
(of kidney)
subacute cerebellar
degeneration
subacute combined
degeneration
subacute coronary disease
sudden cardiac death
ScD Doctor of Science
ScDA *scapulodextra anterior*
[Latin] right
scapuloanterior
(fetal position)
ScDP *scapulodextra posterior*
[Latin] right
scapuloposterior
(fetal position)
SCDSC subacute combined
degeneration of
spinal cord
SCE secretory carcinoma of the
endometrium
simple columnar
epithelium

SCE
simple
columnar
epithelium

simple cuboidal epithelium
squamous cell epithelioma
subcutaneous emphysema
SCF Skin Cancer Foundation
stem cell factor
subcapital fracture
supracondylar fracture
SCFAs short-chain fatty acids
SCFE slipped capital
femoral epiphysis

SCG	sodium cromoglycate
	superior cervical ganglion
SCH	sole community hospital
	squamous cell hyperplasia
	supracervical hysterectomy
SCh	succinylcholine chloride
SChE	serum cholinesterase
sched	schedule
SCHI	severe closed-head injury
SCHIZ	schizophrenia
schiz	schizophrenia
SCHL	subcapsular hematoma of liver
SCI	spinal cord injury
	staphylococcal infection
	streptococcal infection
sci	science
SCID	severe combined immunodeficiency disease
	severe combined immunodeficiency disorder
SCIH	Spinal Cord Injury Hotline (800) 526-3456
SCIPP	sacrococcygeal to inferior pubic point
SCIR	Society of Cardiovascular and Interventional Radiology
SCIU	spinal cord injury unit
SCIwoRA	
	spinal cord injury without radiographic abnormalities
SCJ	sclerocorneal junction
	squamocolumnar junction
	sternoclavicular joint
	sternocostal joint
SCJD	sternoclavicular joint dislocation
SCK	serum creatinine kinase
SCL	sacrococcygeal ligament
	serum creatinine level
	soft contact lens
	symptoms checklist
ScLA	*scapulolaeva anterior* [Latin] left scapuloanterior (fetal position)

SCLC	small cell lung cancer
SCLD	severe chronic liver disease
SCLE	subacute cutaneous lupus erythematosus
scler	sclerosis
SCLN	subclavian lymph node
	supraclavicular lymph node
ScLP	*scapulolaeva posterior* [Latin] left scapuloposterior (fetal position)
SCM	Schwann cell membrane
	sensation, circulation, and motion
	sex-chromatin mass (Barr body)
	Society of Computer Medicine
	spondylitic caudal myelopathy
	State Certified Midwife
	sternocleidomastoid (muscle)
	subcutaneous mastectomy
SCMM	sternocleidomastoid muscle
SCMP	superior constrictor muscle of pharynx
SCN	sickle cell nephropathy
	subcostal nerve
	suprachiasmatic nuclei
SCOP	scopolamine (hyoscine; an anticholinergic alkaloid)
Scope	microscope
S. cordifolia	
	Sida cordifolia (plant containing ephedrine alkaloids)
SCORE	Service Corps of Retired Executives
SCP	sodium cellulose phosphate
	standard care plan
	Streptococcus pyogenes (a species that is the cause of several acute pus-forming infections in man, such as scarlet fever,

erysipelas and
sore throat)
subacute cor pulmonale
subcostal plane
SCPK serum creatine
phosphokinase
SCPPB subcutaneous prepatellar
bursa
SCR skin conductance response
spondylitic caudal
radioculopathy
SCr serum creatinine
scRNA small cytoplasmic RNA
SCS Schwann cell sheath
shaken child syndrome
small-capacity syndrome
Society of Clinical Surgery
Spinal Cord Society
spinal cord stimulation
spinal cord syndrome
splenocaval shunt
spur-cell syndrome
SCs Schwann cells
sex chromosomes
SCT Sertoli cell tumor
sex chromatin test
sickle-cell trait
sperm cytotoxicity
subcutaneous tissue
sugar-coated tablet
sweat chloride test
SCTAT sex cord tumor with
annular tubules
SCTC superior cornu of
thyroid cartilage
SCTx spinal cervical traction
SCU self-care unit
special care unit
SCUBA self-contained underwater
breathing apparatus
SCUCP small cell undifferentiated
carcinoma of prostate
SCUD septicemia cutaneous
ulcerative disease
SCUF slow continuous
ultrafiltration
(hemodialysis)
scuPA single chain urokinase-type
plasminogen activator

SCUT schizophrenic, chronic
undifferentiated type
SCV small cardiac vein
squamous cancer of vagina
subclavian vein
subcutaneous vaginal
(anesthetic block)
SD salt deficiency
Sandhoff's disease
Saunder's disease
Schamberg's disease
Scheuermann's disease
Schilder's disease
Schmorl's disease
Schroeder's disease
scleroderma (systemic
disease marked by
hardening of
connective tissue)
schistosome dermatitis
(swimmer's itch)
Scotch douche
seborrheic dermatitis
secondary disease
secretory diarrhea
selective decontamination
senile dementia
septal defect
septic disease
sequence deletion
serologically defined
serum disease
severely disabled
sex drive
sexual dysfunction
short dialysis
shoulder disarticulation
shoulder dislocation
shuttlemaker's disease
single dose
sixth disease
skin dose
sleep deprivation
sleep disorder
slipped disk (herniated
nucleus pulposus of
intervertebral disk)
soma-dendritic
(EEG spikes)

somatoform disorder
speech defect
sphincter dilatation
spontaneous delivery
stable disease
standard deviation
 (of observed sample)
standard diet
Stargardt's disease
sterile dressing
Still's disease (juvenile
 rheumatoid arthritis)
storage disease
Streeter dysplasia
streptodornase
streptozocin and
 doxorubicin
 (combination
 chemotherapy)
Strumpell's disease
Stuttgart disease
substance dependence
sudden death
Sudeck's disease
surgical drain
swallowing disorder

S-D suicide-depression
S & D stomach and duodenum
SDA *sacrodextra anterior* [Latin]
 right sacroanterior
 (fetal position)
 same day admission
 sialodacryoadenitis
 specific dynamic action
 specific dynamic activity
 steroid-dependent
 asthmatic
 subdiaphragmatic abscess
SDAP single donor apheresis
 platelets
SDAT senile dementia of the
 Alzheimer type
SDB second-degree burn
 self-destructive behavior
 subdeltoid bursa
 subdeltoid bursitis
SDBP supine diastolic
 blood pressure
SDC serum digoxin
 concentration

Sleep Disorder Center
sodium deoxycholate
SD & C suction, dilatation and
 curettage
SDD sclerodermoid dermatitis
 selective decontamination
 of digestive tract
 selective digestive
 decontamination
 sterile dry dressing
SDDD spinal degenerative disk
 disease
SDDS striated dopamine-
 deficiency syndrome
 (Parkinsonism)
SDE specific dynamic effect
 subdural empyema (pus
 between the dura mater
 and arachnoid
 membranes)
SDH sorbitol dehydrogenase
 spinal dorsal horn
 subdural hematoma
 succinic acid
 dehydrogenase
SDHD sudden death heart
 disorder
SDI standard deviation index
 State Disability Insurance
SDIHD sudden death ischemic
 heart disorder
SDL serous demilunes
 serum drug level
 speech discrimination level
SDLN subdiaphragmatic
 lymph node
SDM standard deviation of mean
SDMS Society of Diagnostic
 Medical Sonographers
SDMT symbol digital
 modalities test
SDP *sacrodextra posterior* [Latin]
 right sacroposterior
 (fetal position)
 single-donor platelets
 subacute demyelinating
 polyneuropathy
SDPD self-defeating personality
 disorder

SDR spontaneous discharge rate
surgical dressing room
SDRSC single-dose radiation
survival curve
SDS salivary duct strictures
same-day surgery
Self-Rating Depression
Scale
sensory deprivation
syndrome
Shy-Drager syndrome
(progressive disorder of
unknown cause)
sodium dodecyl sulfate
speech discrimination
score
standard deviation score
subdural space
sudden death syndrome
surfactant deficiency
syndrome
SDS-agarose
sodium dodecyl
sulfate-agarose
SD-SK streptodornase-
streptokinase
SDSPAGE sodium dodecylsulfate–
polyacrylamide gel
electrophoresis
SDT *sacrodextra transversa*
[Latin] right
sacrotransverse
(fetal position)
sensory decision theory
single-donor transfusion
speech-detection threshold
synchronizing drug
therapies (with body
rhythms)
SDU standard deviation unit
SDW safe drinking water
SDWA Safe Drinking Water Act
SE saline enema
Salmonella enteritides
(species that is the
causative agent of
paratyphoid fever,
septicemia, and
gastroenteritis)
sex education
side effect
smoke exposure
sphenoethmoidal suture
spin-echo
stage of exhaustion
standard error (of estimate
of mean value)
staphylococcal endotoxin
status epilepticus
Se selenium (nonmetallic
element)
SEA staphylococcus
enterotoxin A
subendocardial abscess
subepicardial abscess
SEB staphylococcus
enterotoxin B
SEBA staphylococcal enterotoxin
B antiserum
SEC Singapore epidemic
conjunctivitis
Snellen eye chart
spurious erythrocytosis
stress erythrocytosis
sec second(s)
secondary
section
sECG stress electrocardiography
SECP subacute effusive
constrictive pericarditis
SECPR standard external
cardiopulmonary
resuscitation
sect section
SED sedimentation (rate)
seriously emotionally
disturbed
side effects of drugs
skin erythema dose
(radiotherapy)
socially and emotionally
disturbed
spondyloepiphyseal
dysplasia
standard error of the
deviation
staphylococcal
enterotoxin D

sed.   *sedes* [Latin] stool
SEDA   spinal epidural abscess
sed rate   sedimentation rate
     (of blood)
SEE   standard error of the
     estimate
SEF   staphylococcal
     enterotoxin F
SEG   segment
     segmented
     sonoencephalogram
SEG-CES   segmental cement
     extraction system
segm   segment
SEH   spinal epidural hematoma
     subependymal
     hemorrhage
SEI   substance-exposed infant
SEM   sample evaluation method
     scanning electron
     microscopy
     semen
     standard error of the mean
     subacute
     encephalomyelopathy
     systolic ejection murmur
sem   semen
sem.   *semi* [Latin] one half
semel in d.
     semel in die [Latin] once
     a day
semf   seminal fluid
SEMI   subendocardial myocardial
     infarction
semih.   *semihora* [Latin] half
     an hour
SEMs   slow eye movements
sem ves   seminal vesicle
SEN   substance-exposed
     newborn
Sen   sensitive
Sens   sensitivity
S. enteritidis
     Salmonella enteritidis
     (species that is the
     causative agent of
     paratyphoid fever,
     septicemia, and
     gastroenteritis)

SEO   shoulder-elbow orthosis
SEP   sensory-evoked potential
     serum electrophoresis
     somatosensory-evoked
     potential
     sperm entry point
     stimulus-evoked pain
     surface epithelium
     systolic ejection period
sep   separate
     separated
sept   septum
seq.   *sequela* [Latin] that
     which follows
seq.luce   *sequenti luce* [Latin] the
     following day
SER   sebum excretion rate
     sensory evoked response
     smooth endoplasmic
     reticulum
     somatosensory evoked
     response
     supination external-
     rotation
     systolic ejection rate
sER   smooth endoplasmic
     reticulum
SER IV   supination external-
     rotation, type four
     fracture
Ser   serine (nonessential
     amino acid)
SERHOLD
     serials holding database
SERLINE
     serials (journals) online
sero   serology
serv.   *serva* [Latin] keep
SES   sick euthyroid syndrome
     socioeconomic status
     standard electrolyte
     solution
sesquih.   *sesquihora* [Latin] an hour
     and a half
SET   systolic ejection time
SF   sacral foramen
     safety factor
     salt free
     saturated fat

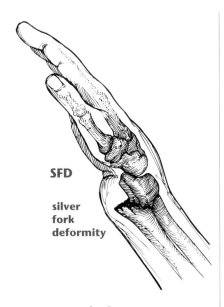

SFD

silver fork deformity

scapular fracture
scarlet fever (acute
    contagious streptococcal
    infection)
Segond fracture
seminal fluid
serum fibrinogen
sex factors
shortening fraction
simple fracture
skeletal fluorosis
skin fibroblast
skull fracture
slice fracture
spinal fluid
spinal fusion (of
    contiguous vertebrae)
splayfoot
spontaneous fracture
    (pathologic fracture)
straddle fracture
stress fracture
sugar-free
superior facet
swine fever
symptom-free
synovial fluid
S & F structure and function
Sf Svedberg flotation unit

SFA seminal fluid assay
serum folic acid
Stuttering Foundation
    of America
synovial fluid aspiration
SFAs saturated fatty acids
SFC spinal fluid count
SFD seal-fin deformity (ulnar
    deviation of the fingers in
    rheumatoid arthritis)
silver fork deformity (seen
    in Colles' fracture)
skin-film distance
small-for-dates
SFEMG single fiber
    electromyography
SFFA serum free fatty acid
SFG subglottic foreign body
SFH serum-free hemoglobin
stroma-free hemoglobin
SFI saline-filled implants
SFL serum folate level
synovial fluid lymphocyte
SFM spectrofluorometer
SFP simultaneous foveal
    perception
spinal-fluid pressure
SFR spot-film radiography
stroke with full recovery
SFS splenic flexure syndrome
SFTT skin-fold-thickness test
SFU surgical follow-up
SFV Semliki Forest virus
    (togavirus)
SFW shell-fragment wound
slow-filling wave
SG salivary gland
sebaceous gland
serum globulin
serum glucose
severe gingivitis
shoulder girdle
signs
simple goiter (nontoxic)
skin graft
specific gravity
spinal ganglia
suppressor gene
Surgeon General

	sympathetic ganglia
S/G	Swan-Ganz (catheter)
sg	specific gravity
SGA	small for gestational age (infant)
	sweat gland adenoma
SGAH	second-generation antihistamine
SGBI	silicone gel breast implant
SGC	spiral ganglion of cochlea
	Swan-Ganz catheter
SGD	single gene defect
	straight gravity drainage
SGE	significant glandular enlargement
SGF	skeletal growth factor
SGH	subgluteal hematoma
SGL	secretory gland lobules
SGM	Society of General Microbiology
	styloglossal muscle
SGML	sandard generalized markup language
SGO	Society of Gynecologic Oncology
	Surgeon General's Office
SGOT	serum glutamic-oxaloacetic transaminase (preferred: AST, aspartate aminotransferase; aspartate transaminase)
SGP	salivary gland pain
	serine glycerophosphatide
	sialoglycoprotein
	stress-generated potentials
SGPT	serum glutamic-pyruvic

	transaminase (preferred: ALT, alanine aminotransferase)
SGRM	Stimson gravity reduction maneuver
SGS	subglottic stenosis
SGT	somatic gene therapy
	stool guaiac test
SGTT	standard glucose tolerance test
SGV	salivary gland virus (cytomegalovirus)
SGVHD	syngeneic graft-versus-host disease
SH	self-help
	self-hypnosis
	sentinel headache
	serum hepatitis
	sex hormone
	sexual harassment
	sexual history
	short
	shoulder
	shower
	social history
	somatotropic hormone
	spinal headache (lumbar puncture headache)
	state hospital
	strawberry hemangioma

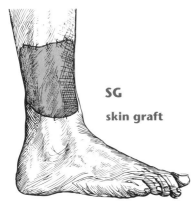

SG

skin graft

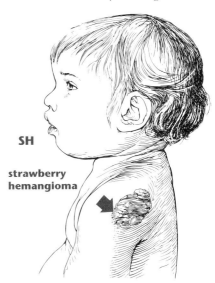

SH

strawberry hemangioma

sulfhydryl

surgical history

symptomatic hypoglycemia

S & H speech and hearing

sh shoulder

SHA simple hyperopic
astigmatism (one
meridian is emmetropic
and the other is
hyperopic)

super-heated aerosol

superior hypophyseal
artery

SHAA Society of Hearing Aid
Audiologists

SHARE Supporting Hospitals
Abroad with Resources
and Equipment

SHb sickle hemoglobin (screen)

SHBD serum alpha
hydroxybutyric
dehydrogenase

SHBG serum hormone-binding
globulin

sex hormone-binding
globulin (testosterone
binding globulin)

SHCS second hand
cigarette smoke

SHD syphilitic heart disease

SHEA Society for Healthcare
Epidemiology of America

SHF subfulminant
hepatic failure

SHG sonic hedgehog gene

sonohysterography

synthetic human gastrin

SHHH Self-Help for Hard of
Hearing People

SHI severe head injury

SHL sensorineural hearing loss

stylohyoid ligament

sudden hearing loss

SHLA soluble human
lymphocyte antigen

SHLN suprahyoid lymph node

SHM self-help method

sternohyoid muscle

stylohyoid muscle

SHN spontaneous hemorrhagic
necrosis

subacute hepatic necrosis

SHO secondary hypertrophic
osteoarthropathy

Student Health
Organization

SHP scapulohumeral
periarthritis

Schönlein-Henoch
purpura

SHS Sayre head sling

second-hand smoke

shoulder-hand syndrome

staghorn stone (large
renal stone with
many branches)

SHTS second hand tobacco
smoke

SHV superior hemiazygos vein

SI sacroiliac (joint)

saline injection

self-inflicted injury

septic inflammation

seriously ill

serum iron

sexual infantilism

sexual intercourse (coitus)

small intestine

stimulation index

straddle injury

SHL

**stylohyoid
ligament**

streptococcal infection
stress incontinence
stroke index
suicidal ideation
swimmer's itch
Système International d'Unités
[French] (International
System of Units,
designating meter (m)
for length, kilogram (kg)
for mass, second(s) for
time, and Celsius (C) for
temperature)
system inventory (review
of systems)

S & I suction and irrigation
Si silicon (a nonmetallic
element)
silicone (organic
compound in which the
carbon is replaced
with silicon)

SIA stress-induced anesthesia
sulfite-induced asthma
subacute infectious
arthritis

SIADH syndrome of inappropriate
antidiuretic hormone
secretion (vasopressin)
syndrome of inappropriate
secretion of antidiuretic
hormone (vasopressin)

SIB self-injurious behavior
SIBC serum iron-binding
capacity
sib sibling
sibs siblings
SIC self intermittent
catheterization
serum insulin
concentration
sic *siccus* [Latin] to be read
as it stands
siccus [Latin] dry
SICB sodium ion channel
blocker
SICT selective intracoronary
thrombolysis
SICU surgical intensive care unit

SID sensory integration
dysfunction
severe iron deficiency
small-intestinal diverticula
Society for Investigative
Dermatology
sudden inexplicable death
sudden infant death
(syndrome)
surgically implanted
defibrillator
systemic inflammatory
disease
s.i.d. *semel in die* [Latin] once
a day
SIDS sudden infant death
syndrome
SIECUS Sex Information and
Education Council of the
United States
SIELs squamous intraepithelial
lesions
SIF serum inhibition factor
SIG sigmoidoscopy
special intervention group
SIg serum immunoglobulin
significant
surface immunoglobulin
Sig. *signetur* [Latin] let it be
labeled (directions)
sig. *signetur* [Latin] let it be
labeled (directions)
sigmo sigmoidoscopy
sig. n. pro. *signa nomine proprio* [Latin]
label with proper name
SIH stress-induced
hyperthermia
sulfonylurea-induced
hypoglycemia
SIJ sacroiliac joint
S-I joint sacroiliac joint
SIL soluble interleukin
speech-interference level
squamous intraepithelial
lesion
SILN subinguinal lymph node
superficial inguinal
lymph node
SIM selected ion monitoring

	Society of Industrial Microbiology
simp	simple
SIMS	secondary ion mass spectrometry
simul	simultaneously (at the same time)
SIMV	spontaneous intermittent mandatory ventilation
	synchronized intermittent mandatory ventilation
SIN	salpingitis isthmica nodosa
	spinal interneuron
si n. val.	*si non valet* [Latin] if it is not enough
SIO	sacroiliac orthosis
si op. sit	*si opus sit* [Latin] if needed
SIP	sickness impact profile
	stroke in progression
	surface inductive plethysmography
	sutured in place
SIR	secondary immune response
	specific immune release
	standardized incidence ratio
	subcutaneous inguinal ring
SIRF	severely impaired renal function
SIRS	soluble immune response suppressor
	systemic inflammatory response syndrome
SIS	second impact syndrome
	shaken impact syndrome
	sister
	sterile injectable suspension
	structured interview for schizotypy
SISI	short increment sensitivity index
SISS	severe-invasion streptococcal syndrome
SIT	saline infusion test
	serum inhibiting titer
	sperm immobilization test
SiTr	silent treatment

SIU	*Système International d'Unités* (SI units)
SI units	*Système International d'Unités* (SI units)
SIV	simian immuno-deficiency virus
SIVC	Silastic intravenous catheter
si vir. perm.	
	si vires permitant [Latin] if the health will permit
SIW	self-inflicted wound
SIWIS	self-induced water intoxification and schizophrenia
SJ	saddle joint (diarthrosis)
	Society of Jesus
	synovial joint
sJCA	systemic onset juvenile chronic arthritis
SJS	Stevens-Johnson syndrome (an occasional fatal form of erythema multiforme)
	stiff joint syndrome
	Swyer-James syndrome (Macleod syndrome)
SK	seborrheic keratosis
	senile keratosis
	skin
	solar keratosis
	streptokinase (Streptase)
	striae keratoplasty
Sk	skin
SKAO	supracondylar knee-ankle orthosis
skel	skeletal
	skeleton
SKI	Sloan-Kettering Institute
SKSD	streptokinase-streptodornase (test)
SKT	skin-fold test
sk trx	skeletal traction
SL	salt loss
	sarcolemma
	secondary leukemia
	senile lentigens
	sensation level (hearing)
	serious list
	shock lung

short leg (cast)
sign language
silk laser
simian line
slight
slit lamp
small lymphocyte
solar lentigens
sound level
sporadic listeriosis
streptolysin
sublingual

s.l. *secundum legem* [Latin]
according to the law
sensu lato [Latin] in the
broad sense

SLA *sacrolaeva anterior* [Latin]
left sacroanterior (fetal
position)
superior laryngeal artery
surfactant-like activity

SLAC scapholunate advanced
collapse

SLAM Society's League Against
Molestation

SLAP superior labrum anterior
to posterior (of shoulder)

SLB short leg brace
slit lamp biomicroscopy
suspensory ligament
of breast

SLC short-leg cast (extends
from below the knee
to the toes)

SLCT Sertoli-Leydig cell tumor
second-line chemotherapy

SLD serum lactic
dehydrogenase
specific learning disability

SLDH serum lactic
dehydrogenase

SLDH1 serum lactic
dehydrogenase,
isoenzyme1

SLDH5 serum lactic
dehydrogenase,
isoenzyme 5

SLE slit lamp examination

St. Louis encephalitis
systemic lupus
erythematosus

SLEP short latent evoked
potential

SLEV St. Louis encephalitis virus

SLEX slit lamp examination

SLF sublingual fossa

SLFC semilunar folds of colon

SLG sublingual gland

SLH subluxation of humerus

SLI selective lymphoid
irradiation
sex-linked inheritance

SLJD Sinding-Larsen-Johansson
disease

SLJS Sinding-Larsen-Johansson
syndrome

SLKC superior limbic
keratoconjunctivitis

SLL second-look laparotomy
small lymphocytic
lymphoma
subluxation of lens

SLM sound level monitor

SLMP since last menstrual period

SLN salt-losing nephritis
subclavian lymph node
superior laryngeal nerve

superior
laryngeal
nerve

SLN

SLNs	sentinel lymph nodes		skim milk
SLNWC	short-leg nonwalking cast		small
SLO	second-look operation		smoker
	Stein-Leventhal ovaries		smooth muscle
	streptolysin O (test)		somatomedins
SLOC	suspensory ligaments		(somatotropin-mediating
	of Cooper		hormones)
SLOS	Smith-Lemli-Opitz		space maintainer
	syndrome (hereditary		sperm motility
	syndrome marked by		sphingomyelin
	multiple congenital		sports medicine
	anomalies)		streptomycin
SLP	*sacrolaeva posterior* [Latin]		stress management
	left sacroposterior		stretch mark
	(fetal position)		striated muscle
SLPP	serum lipophosphoprotein		subcutaneous mastectomy
SLR	stapled lung reduction		submandibular
	straight-leg-raising (test)		submucous
SLRT	straight-leg-raising test		substitute for morphine
SLS	salt-losing syndrome		sustained medication
	short-leg splint		Swedish massage
	Sjögren-Larsson syndrome		synaptic membrane
	Stein-Leventhal syndrome		synovial membrae
	stiff lung syndrome		syringomyelia
	streptolysin S		systolic mean
SLT	*sacrolaeva transversa* [Latin]		systolic murmur
	left sacrotransverse	**Sm**	samarium (rare
	(fetal position)		metallic element)
	single lung transplant		small
SlTr	slight trace		smear
SLV	selective lung ventilation	**SMA**	sequential multichannel
	semilunar valve		autoanalyzer
	since last visit		sequential multiple analysis
	superior labial vein		sequential multiple
SLVI	semilunar-valve		analyzer
	insufficiency		smooth-muscle antibody
SLWC	short-leg walking cast		spinal muscular atrophy
	(extends from below the		superior mesenteric artery
	knee to the toes with a	**SM-A**	somatomedin A
	rubber sole walker)	**SMA I**	infantile spinal muscular
SLX	slit lamp examination		atrophy (Werdnig-
SM	sadomasochism		Hoffmann disease)
	scientific misconduct	**SMA II**	chronic childhood spinal
	segmental mastectomy		muscular atrophy
	(lumpectomy)	**SMA-III**	juvenile spinal muscular
	self-medication		atrophy (Wohfart-
	self-monitoring		Kugelberg-Welander
	simple mastectomy		disease)
	skeletal muscle		

SMA 6/60
> sequential multiple analyzer (a panel of laboratory tests that determine the concentration of six substances in serum in 60 minutes, including creatinine (or glucose), potassium, sodium, chloride, blood urea nitrogen (BUN) and carbon dioxide)

SMA 12/60
> sequential multiple analyzer (a panel of laboratory tests that determine the concentration of twelve substances in serum in 60 minutes, including glucose, calcium, blood urea nitrogen (BUN), uric acid, cholesterol, albumin, alkaline phosphatase, phosphorus, total protein, total bilirubin, serum glutamic oxaloacetic transaminase (SGOT), and lactate dehydrogenase (LDH))

SMAC sequential multiple analyzer computer

SMAE superior mesenteric artery embolism

SMAF specific macrophage arming factor

SMAL serum methyl alcohol level

SMAO superior mesenteric artery occlusion

S. marcescens
> *Serratia marcescens* (causative agent of hospital acquired infection, especially in patients with impaired immunity)

SMAS superficial muscular

aponeurotic system
superior mesenteric artery syndrome

SMB selected mucosal biopsy

SMC Scientific Manpower Commission
scientific misconduct
selenomethylnorcholesterol
smooth muscle cell
systemic mastocytosis

SM-C somatomedin C

SMCD senile macular chorioretinal degeneration
systemic mast cell disease

SMD senile macular degeneration
suspensory muscle of duodenum

SMDA Safe Medical Device Act

SMDM Society for Medical Decision Making

SMDS secondary myelodysplastic syndrome

SME severe myoclonic epilepsy

SMEI severe myoclonic epilepsy of infancy

SMF streptozocin + mitomycin + 5-fluorouracil (combination chemotherapy)
stylomastoid foramen
submandibular fossa

SMG submandibular ganglion
submandibular gland

SMHPA sphincter muscle of hepatopancreatic ampulla

SMI senior medical investigator
severely mentally impaired
supplemental medical insurance
sustained maximal inspiration

SMIPG seromuscular intestinal patch graft

SMJN Sister Mary Joseph's nodule (hard periumbilical nodule)

SML	sphenomandibular ligament
	stylomandibular ligament
SMLN	sternomastoid lymph node
	submandibular lymph node
	superior mesenteric lymph node
SMN	second malignant neoplasm
	sensorimotor neuropathy
	subacute motor neuronopathy
SMON	subacute myelo-optic neuropathy
SMP	sadomasochistic pornography
	slow-moving protease
	sulfamethoxypyrazine
	sympathetically maintained pain
	sympathetic mediated pain
SMPS	sympathetically maintained pain syndrome
SMR	senior medical resident (chief medical resident)
	severe mental retardation
	skeletal muscle relaxant
	standardized morbidity ratio
	standardized mortality ratio
	submucous resection
SMRR	submucous resection and rhinoplasty
SMRs	sexual maturity ratings
SMS	scalded mouth syndrome
	self-mutilation syndrome
	serial motor seizures
	sperm motility study
	Stewart-Morel syndrome (hyperostosis frontalis interna)
	stiff man syndrome (progressive fluctuating rigidity and spasm of muscles)
SMSD	sphingomyelin storage disease

SMT	spinal manipulative therapy
SMV	submentovertex (radiologic view)
	superior mesenteric vein
SMX	sulfamethoxazole
SMX/TMP	sulfamethoxazole and trimethoprim
SMZ	sulfamethazine (sulfadimidine; a sulfonamide antibacterial agent)
	sulfamethozole (a sulfonamide anti-bacterial agent)
SN	saddle nose
	Schmorl node (an irregular bone defect in the vertebral body)
	sciatic notch
	scrub nurse
	signal node (an enlarged , palpable, supraclavicular lymph node that is often the first sign of an abdominal neoplasm)
	singer's node (teacher's node; trachoma of the vocal bands)
	sinus node
	splanchnic nerve
	staff nurse
	subnormal
	supernatant
	suprasternal notch (jugular notch)
	student nurse
	sympathetic nerve
Sn	*stannum* [Latin] tin
SNA	specimen not available
	standard nomenclature of anatomy (*Nomina Anatomica*)
	Student Nurses' Association
SNagg	serum normal agglutinator
SNAI	standard nomenclature of athletic injuries

SNAP score of neonatal acute
physiology
sensory nerve action
potential
SNB sacral nerve block
scalene node biopsy
Silverman needle biopsy
spinal nerve block
SNC swan-neck catheter
SNCL sinus node cycle length
SNCV sensory nerve
conduction velocity
SND saddle-nose deformity
sinus node dysfunction
swan-neck deformity
SNDA supplemental new drug
application
SNE subacute necrotizing
encephalomyelopathy
(Leigh disease)
SNEG simple nonendemic goiter
SNES suprascapular nerve
entrapment syndrome
SNF skilled nursing facility
SNGFR single-nephron glomerular
filtration rate
SNHL sensorineural hearing loss
SNIVT Society of Non-Invasive
Vascular Technology
SNJ severe neonatal jaundice
SNM Society of Nuclear
Medicine
sulfanilamide
SNMG supernumerary
mammary gland
SNMJ skeletal neuromuscular
junction
SNODERM
Systematized
Nomenclature of
Dermatology
SNODO Standard Nomenclature of
Diseases and Operations
Systematized
Nomenclature of Diseases
and Operations
SNO MED Systematized
Nomenclature
of Medicine

SNOP Standard Nomenclature
of Pathology
Systematized
Nomenclature of
Pathology
SNP severe necrotizing
pancreatitis
sinus node potential
sodium nitroprusside
SNR signal-to-noise ratio
spinal nerve root
supernumerary rib
SNr substantia nigra reticulata
snRNA small nuclear RNA
snRNP small nuclear
ribonucleoprotein
SNRT sinus node recovery time
SNS sterile normal saline
sympathic nervous system
(thoracolumbar)
SNT sinuses, nose, and throat
SNU skilled nursing unit
SNV spleen necrosis virus
systemic necrotizing
vasculitis
SNW slow negative wave
SO salpingo-oophorectomy
saphenous opening
(fossa ovalis)
second opinion
severe obesity
sex offender
sexual orientation
shoulder orthosis
sphincter of Oddi
standing order
superior oblique
(eye muscle)
supraoptic
sutures out
sympathetic ophthalmia
SO₂ oxygen saturation
sulfur dioxide
SOA spinal opioid analgesia
swelling of ankles
SOAA signed out against advice
SOAD sleep onset
association disorder
SOAMA signed out against

medical advice

SOAP subjective, objective, assessment and plan (format for clinical, hospital and physician notes in problem-oriented medical record keeping)

SOAPA signed out against physician's advice

SOAPIE subjective, objective, assessment, plan, intervention and evaluation (problem-oriented record)

SOB shortness of breath
short of breath

SOBE short of breath on exertion

SOC sequential-type contraceptive
society
spiral organ of Corti (organ of Hearing)
standard of care
state of consciousness

S & OC signed and on chart (permit)

SOD sphincter of Oddi dysfunction
superoxide dismutase

Sod sodomy

sod bicarb
sodium bicarbonate

SODH sorbitol dehydrogenase

SOF superior orbital fissure

SOFT Support Organization for Trisomy

SOH sympathetic orthostatic hypotension

SOHN supraoptic hypothalamic nucleus

SOI syrup of ipecac

SOJA systemic onset juvenile arthritis

SOJCA systemic onset juvenile chronic arthritis

sol soluble
solution

soln solution

solv. *solve* [Latin] dissolve

SOM serous otitis media
somatotropin (growth hormone)
superior oblique muscle
suppurative otitis media

SOMA Special Operations Medical Association
Student Osteopathic Medical Association

somat somatic

SOMI sternal-occipital-mandibular immobilizer (orthosis)

SOMR source-oriented medical record

SON supraoptic nucleus

sono sonogram

SOO sphincter of Oddi

SOOC spiral organ of Corti (organ of hearing)

SOOL spontaneous onset of labor

SOP standard of proof
standard operating procedure

SOPA syndrome of primary aldosteronism

SOPH &V
sudden onset of progressive hirsutism and virilization

SOR supraorbital rhytidoplasty
supraorbital ridge

Sorb sorbitol

SOREMP sleep-onset REM period

SOS self obtained smear
suboptimal surgery
supplemental oxygen system

s.o.s. *si opus sit* [Latin] if needed

SOSF single organ system failure

SOT systemic oxygen transport

SOU sphincter of urethra

SP salicylate poisoning
schizotypal personality
semi-private (hospital room)
senile purpura
septum pellucidum

sexual perversion
sexual precocity
skin patch
sleep deprivation
smallpox (variola major)
sodium pentothal
soft palate
spastic paralysis
speech pathologist
speech pathology
spermatid
spine
standard procedure
Steinmann pin (used for internal fixation of bones)
steroid psychosis
Streptococcus pneumoniae (the causative agent of lobar pneumonia and other acute pus-forming conditions such as middle ear infections and meningitis)
Streptococcus pyogenes
strychnine poisoning
styloid process
substance P
suicide precautions
suprapubic
surfactant protein
surgery performed
symphysis pubis (pubic sysphysis)
systolic pressure

SP 1	suicide precautions level 1
SP 2	suicide precautions level 2
S/P	semiprivate (hospital room)
	status post
S & P	staging and prognosis
sp	space
	species
	specific
	sperm
sp.	*spiritus* [Latin] spirit
SPA	serum prothrombin activity
	single-photon absorptionmetry

sperm penetration assay (hamster egg assay)
sphenopalatine artery
spinal progressive amyotrophy
spontaneous platelet aggregation
staphylococcal protein A
stimulation produced analgesis
superior pelvic aperture
suprapubic aspiration
synovial pseudoarthrosis

SpA	staphylococcal protein A
SP-A	surfactant protein A
SPAB	Society of Psychologists in Addictive Behaviors
SPAC	satisfactory post-anesthesia course
sp act	specific activity
SPAG	small particle aerosol generator
SPAI	steroid protein activity index
sp an	spinal anesthesia
SPAS	sleep phase advance syndrome
SPAT	slow paroxysmal atrial tachycardia
SPB	suprapatella bursa
SPBI	serum protein bound iodine
SPBM	spherophakia brachymorphia (Marchesani syndrome)
SPBT	suprapubic bladder tap
SPC	salicyamide, phenacetin and caffeine
	seropapillary cystadenoma
	single palmar crease
	standard platelet count
	suprapubic catheter
SpC	spinal cord
SPCA	serum prothrombin conversion accelerator (proconvertin, clotting factor VII)
	Society for the Prevention of Cruelty to Animals

SPCD syndrome of primary
ciliary dyskinesia
sp cd spinal cord
SPD sadistic personality
disorder
schizophrenic disorder
schizophreniform disorder
sociopathic personality
disorder
storage pool deficit
storage pool disease
subcorneal pustular
dermatosis
SPDI subperiosteal dental
implant
SPDS sleep phase delay
syndrome
SPE septic pulmonary edema
serum protein
electrophoresis
streptococcal pyogenic
exotoxin
sucrose polyester
superficial punctate
erosions
spec specification
specimen
speculum
spec ed special education
spec grav
specific gravity
SPECT single photon emission
computerized
tomography
SPEEP spontaneous positive end
expiratory pressure
SPEP serum protein
electrophoresis
SPET single photon emission
tomography
SPF skin protection factor
specific-pathogen free
(breeding colonies)
sphenopalatine foramen
split products of fibrin
standard perfusion fluid
sun-protection factor
SpF spinal fusion (stimulator)
sp fl spinal fluid

SPG sphenopalatine ganglion
sucrose, phosphate, and
glutamate
swimming pool granuloma
(mycobacterial infection
acquired from swimming
pools)
SpG specific gravity
spg sponge
sp gr specific gravity
(relative density)
SPH secondary pulmonary
hemosiderosis
severely and profoundly
handicapped
sighs per hour
Sph spherical (lens)
sphingosine (aliphatic
amino alcohol)
S-phase the mean duration of the
DNA synthesis time
sp ht specific heat
SPI serum precipitable iodine
short process of incus
surgical peripheral
iridectomy
SPIA solid phase
immunoabsorbent assay
SPIF solid-phase immunoassay
fluorescence
S-pin Steinmann pin (for
internal fixation
of fractures)
SPIP sodium-potassium
ion pump
spir. *spiritus* [Latin] spirit
SPK superficial punctate
keratitis
SPL Scientific Protein
Laboratories
sound pressure level
SPLATT split anterior tibial tendon
transfer
sPLM sleep-related periodic leg
movements
SPLN subparotid lymph node
SPM spectrophotometer
stylopharyngeus muscle
synchronous pacemaker

SPMA spinal progressive muscle atrophy

SPMS solid-phase minisequencing

S. pneumoniae
Streptococcus pneumoniae (causative agent of lobar pneumonia and other acute pus-forming conditions such as middle ear infections and meningitis)

SPNH spinal cord neuron hyperexcitability

SPN solitary pulmonary nodule
supplemental parental nutrition

SPO status postoperative

SpO₂ oxygen saturation determined by pulse oximetry

spont spontaneous

SPP spontaneous paroxysmal pain
stump/phantom pain
super packed platelets
suprapubic prostatectomy

SPR solid phase radioimmunoassay

spr sprain

SPRIA solid phase radioimmunoassay

SPRINT special psychiatric rapid intervention team

SPROM spontaneous premature rupture of membranes (not in labor)

SPS shoulder pain and stiffness
sleep-promoting substance
slow-progressive schizophrenia
social-problem-solving
sodium polyethanol sulfonate
suicide probability scale
sulfite polymyxin sulfadiazine
systemic progressive sclerosis

SPSAL serum prostate-specific antigen level

SPT skin prick test
spontaneous pneumothorax

sp tap spinal tap

SPTB styloid process of temporal bone

SPTS subjective post-traumatic syndrome

SPTx static pelvic traction

SPU Society of Pediatric Urology

sput sputum

SPV Shope papilloma virus
systolic pressure variation

SPVR systemic peripheral vascular resistance

S. pyogenes
Streptococcus pyogenes (the causative agent of several acute pus-forming infections in man, such as scarlet fever, erysipelas, and sore throat)

SQ status quo (existing condition)
subcutaneous

Sq subcutaneous

sq squamous
square

Sq C Ca squamous cell carcinoma

sq cm square centimeter (cm²)

SQE subcutaneous emphysema

sqq. *sequentia* [Latin] and following

squ squamous

SR sarcoplasmic reticulum
scatter radiation
secreting rate
sedimentation rate
seizure resistant
senior
sensitivity response
side rails (of bed)
sinus rhythm
slow release
spontaneous respiration
stimulation ratio

stomach rumble
stress related
stretch receptors
superior rectus
  (eye muscle)
sustained release
suture removed
systemic resistance
systems review

Sr strontium (easily oxidized
  metallic element)

s-r stimulus-response
  (psychology)

SRA sleep-related asthma
Society for Risk Analysis

SRBC sickle red blood cells

SRBD sleep-related breathing
  disorders

SRBOW spontaneous rupture of
  bag of waters

SRC sedimented red ells
small retinal coloboma
social rehabilitation center
suicide risk classification
  (from S^{-1} to S^{-4})

SRD severe renal dysfunction
smoking-related diseases
Society for Relief of
  Distress
sodium restricted diet
specific reading disability

SRDS severe respiratory
  distress syndrome

SRDT single radial diffusion test

SRE sleep-related enuresis
sleep-related erection

SRF severe renal failure
skin reactive factor
somatotropin-releasing
  factor
subretinal fluid
synchrotron radiation
  facility

SRF-A slow releasing factor
  of anaphylaxis

SRG suprarenal gland
  (adrenal gland)

SRH somatotropin-releasing
  hormone

stigmata of recent
  hemorrhage
suprarenal hyperplasia

SRI sacral root injury
Scripps Research Institute
  (La Jolla, California)
serotonin reuptake
  inhibitor
severe renal insufficiency

SRID single radial
  immunodiffusion

SRIF somatotropin release-
  inhibiting factor
  (somatostatin)

SRM specific single residue
  method
spontaneous rupture of
  membranes
superior rectus muscle
sustained-release
  medication

SRMD stress-related mucosal
  disease

SRN subretinal
  neovascularization

sRNA soluble ribonucleic acid
  (RNA)

SRNG sustained release
  nitroglycerin

SRNS steroid-responsive
  nephrotic syndrome

SRNVM senile retinal neovascular
  membrane

SRO single room occupancy

SROM spontaneous rupture of
  membranes (fetal)

SRP signal recognition particle
Society for Radiological
  Protection
stapes replacement
  prosthesis

SRPS short rib-polydactyly
  syndrome

SRR standardized rate ratio

SRRD sleep-related respiratory
  disturbance

SRS schizophrenic
  residual state
slow-reacting substance

splenorenal shunt

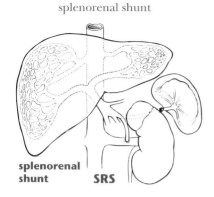

splenorenal shunt **SRS**

    sweat retention syndrome (skin condition due to occlusion of sweat ducts)

SRS-A slow-reacting substance of anaphylaxis (principal autacoid responsible for allergic bronchoconstriction)

SRSO Scoliosis Research Society

SRSTs sun-reactive skin types

SRSVs small round structured viruses

SRT sedimentation rate test
    simple reaction time
    speech reception threshold
    stroke rehabilitation technician
    surfactant replacement therapy
    sustained release tablet

SRU side rails up
    solitary rectal ulcer

SRUx2 both side rails up

SRUS solitary rectal ulcer syndrome

SRY sex determining region of Y chromosome (short arm of Y sex chromosome)

SS sacrosciatic
    saline soak
    saline solution
    saliva sample
    salt sensitive
    salt substitute

Sanfilippo syndrome (mucopolysacch-aridosis III)
Sarcoptes scabiei (human itch mite that infests millions of people)
saturated solution
Scheie's syndrome (mucopolysacch-aridosis IS)
schizophrenia spectrum
Schnitzler's syndrome
secondary syphilis
septic shock
serum sickness (anaphylactic reaction following serum therapy)
severe sepsis
Sézary syndrome (a form of T cell lymphoma)
Sheehan's syndrome (postpartum pituitary necrosis)
Shigella sonnei
shin splints (medial tibial stress syndrome, an exercise-induced leg pain)
short stay
shunt scintigraphy
siblings
sicca syndrome (Sjögren's syndrome without a connective tissue disorder)
signs and symptoms
Silver's syndrome (Russell-Silver short stature)
single-stranded
Sipple's syndrome (a type of multiple endocrine neoplasia)
Sjögren's syndrome (marked by the triad of keratoconjunctivitis sicca, xerostomia and a connective tissue disorder)
sleeping sickness (African trypanosomiasis)

Sly syndrome
(mucopolysacch-
aridosis VII)
soap suds
Social Security
social service
social snoring
(habitual snoring)
sodium salicylate
somatostatin
somnolence syndrome
(transient lethargy and
irritability seen in
children after irradiation
of the head)
special senses
Sphrintzen syndrome
(velocardiofacial
syndrome)
spinal stenosis
Spurway syndrome
(osteogenesis imperfecta
associated with blue
sclerae)
staccato syndrome
standard score
statistically significant
statistical significance
sterile solution
Stickler syndrome
stroke syndrome (sudden
onset condition due to
cerebral hemorrhage,
embolism, thrombosis, or
rupturing aneurysm;
commonly called stroke
and cerebrovascular
accident)
Strongyloidiasis stercoralis
(Anguillula intestinalis)
struvite stones
($MgNH_4PO_4$)
subaortic stenosis
substernal
supersaturated
Sweet's syndrome (acute
febrile neutrophilic
dermatosis)
sylvian syndrome

	(nystagmus refractorius)
	syringomelic syndrome
	(syringomelia)
SS#	Social Security number
S/S	salt substitute
	signs and symptoms
SS 14	somatostatin 14
S & S	screeening and
	surveillance
	sedation and sleep
	sensitivity and specificity
	signs and symptoms
	sling and swathe
	sprains and strains
	swish and swallow
	synthesis and secretion
ss.	*semis* [Latin] one-half
SSA	salicylsalicylic acid
	(salsalate)
	skin-sensitizing antibody
	Social Security
	Administration
	sperm-specific antiserum
	sulfosalicylic acid (test for
	protein in urine and
	CSF)
	sunscreening agent
	systems safety analysis
SS-A	Sanfilippo syndrome,
	type A
	Sjögren syndrome, type A
SSB	short spike burst
SS-B	Sanfilippo syndrome,
	type B
	Sjögren syndrome, type B
SSBG	sex steroid-binding
	globulin
SSC	secondary sex
	characteristics
	secondary spermatocyte
SSc	systemic scleroderma
	systemic sclerosis
SSCA	single-shoulder contrast
	arthrography
SSCG	solid state carcinogenesis
SSCP	single-strand confirmation
	polymorphism
	substernal chest pain
SSCs	secondary sex

characteristics

SSCU special surgical care unit

SSCx somatosensory cortex

SSD sickle cell disease

social security disability

source-surface distance

sudden sniffing death

syndrome of sudden death

systemic scleroderma

SSDE spinal subdural empyema

SSDI social security disability income

ssDNA single-stranded DNA

SSE saline solution enema

skin self-examination

soapsuds enema

systemic side effects

SSEC subacute spongiform encephalopathy

SSEP somatosensory-evoked potential

SSER somatosensory-evoked response

SSG substernal goiter

SSH sensitive sexual history

SSHL severe sensorineural hearing loss

SSI segmental sequential irradiation

subshock insulin

segmental spinal instrumentation

SSKI saturated solution of potassium iodide

SSL sacrospinous ligament

(connects the spine of the ischium to the lateral margins of the sacrum)

supraspinous ligament (connects the dorsal tips of the spinous processes of individual vertebra)

S sleep non-rapid-eye movement sleep

SSLI serum sickness-like illness

SSM sacrospinal muscle

Schistosoma mansoni (species of blood flukes that are pathogenic in man and reside within veins of the large intestine)

superficial spreading melanoma

SSN social security number

subacute sensory neuropathy

suprascapular notch

suprasternal notch

SSNS steroid-sensitive nephrotic syndrome

SSO Society of Surgical Oncology

S. sonnei

Shigella sonnei (implicated in contaminated drinking water)

SSP supersensitivity perception

SSPE subacute sclerosing panencephalitis

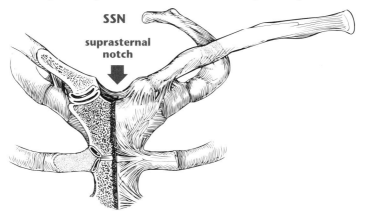

SSN

suprasternal notch

SSPG	steady state plasma glucose
SSPI	steady state plasma insulin
SSPL	saturation sound pressure level
SSR	somatostatin receptor
	somatostatin response
	surgical supply room
SSRI	selective serotonin reuptake inhibitor
	serotonin-specific reuptake inhibitor
ssRNA	single-stranded RNA
SSRO	sagittal split ramus osteotomy
SSRS	Social Security Reporting Service
SSS	scalded skin syndrome
	sepsis severity score
	sickle cell syndrome
	sick sinus syndrome
	Simvastatin Survival Study
	soluble specific substance
	specific soluble substance
	sterile saline soaks
	strong soap solution
	subclavian steal syndrome

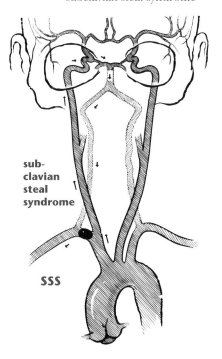

**sub-
clavian
steal
syndrome**

SSS

	superior sagittal sinus
	systemic sicca syndrome
s.s.s.	*stratum super stratum* [Latin] layer upon layer
SSSS	staphylcoccal scalded skin syndrome
SSST	superior sagittal sinus thrombosis
SST	sciatic stress test
	solid state transducer
	somatostatin
	streptococcal sore throat
s. str.	*sensu stricto* [Latin] in the strict sense
S. stercoralis	
	Strongyloides stercoralis (parasitic threadworm)
SSU	sterile supply unit
SSV	simian sarcoma virus
s.s.v.	*sub signo veneni* [Latin] under a poison label
SSX	sulfisoxazole (sulfa drug)
S & Sx	signs and symptoms
SSZ	sulfasalazine (an antibacterial sulfonamide derivative)
ST	heat-stable
	scala tympani
	Scarpa's triangle (femoral triangle)
	scar tissue
	sclerotherapy
	scratch test
	scrub typhus
	sedimentation time
	sella turcica
	seminiferous tubules
	sinus tachycardia
	skin test
	sleep talking (somnilloquy)
	slight trace
	slow twitch
	smokeless tobacco
	sore throat
	speech therapist
	sphincter tone
	sternothyroid
	stable toxin
	Stamey test

standardized test
sternothyroid
steroid therapy
stimulus
stomach
straight
stress test
stretcher
subtotal
superior turbinate
(concha)
survival time

STA serum thrombotic
accelerator
standard tube
agglutination (test)
superficial temporal artery

STAG split thickness
autogenous graft

staph *Staphylococcus*
(usually implies
Staphylococcus aureus)

STAT Stop Teenage Addiction
to Tobacco

stat. *statim* [Latin] at once

stats statistics

Stb stillbirth

ST BY stand by

STC slow-transit constipation
soft tissue calcification
straight collecting duct
subtotal colectomy

STD sclerosing tubular
degeneration
seminiferous tubular
dysgenesis
sexually transmitted
disease
skin test dose
skin-to-tumor distance
standard test dose

std standard

STDH skin test for delayed
hypersensitivity

STEI sexually transmitted
enteric infections

STEL short-term exposure limit

STEM scanning transmission
electron microscopy

sten stenosis

stet *stet* [Latin] to nullify a
correction; let it stand

steth stethoscope

STF slow-twitch fiber
special tube feeding

STFR superior transverse fold
of rectum

STG split-thickness graft

STH soft tissue hematoma
somatotropic homone
(growth hormone)
subtotal hysterectomy

STHRF somatotropic hormone
releasing factor

STI short-term insomnia
soft tissue injury
systolic time index
systolic time interval

stillb stillbirth

stim stimulation

S-T interval
the combination of the S-T
segment and the T wave
of the ECG cycle

STIR short tau inversion
recovery

STJ subtalar joint

STK streptokinase (antibiotic)

STL sacrotuberous ligament
sent to lab

STLE St. Louis encephalitis

STLI subtotal lymphoid
irradiation

STLM swelling + tenderness +
limited motion

STM secondary tympanic
membrane
short-term memory (for
just a few minutes)
sternothyroid muscle
streptomycin

STN solitary tract nucleus
subthalamus nucleus
supratrochlear nerve

STNI sub-total nerve injury

STNR symmetrical tonic
neck reflex

STNV satellite tobacco
necrosis virus

stom   stomach
STOP   segmental transplantation
of pancreas

segmental transplantation of pancreas

STOP

sensitive, timely and
organized programs
(for abused spouses)
STORCH syphilis, toxoplasmosis,
other agents, rubella,
cytomegalovirus
and herpes
STP   short-term plan
sodium thiopental
standard temperature
and pressure
supracondylar tibial
prosthesis
STR   scar-tissue replacement
short tandem repeat
Society of Thoracic
Radiology
stretcher
Strab   strabismus
strep   streptococcus (any
member of the genus
Streptococcus)
Streptococcus (a genus of
gram-positive, ovoid
bacteria, pathogenic
and/or nonpathogenic in
man, occurring in pairs
or chains)
STS   sequence-tagged sites
serologic test for syphilis
short-term survivors
sinus tarsus syndrome
sodium thiosulfate

soft tissue sarcoma
soft tissue shaving
sugar tong splint
(coaptation splint)
synaptic transmitter
substance
STs   sleep terrors
STSA   Southern Thoracic
Surgical Association
STSE   split-thickness skin excision
S-T segment
the part of the ECG cycle
that measures from the
end of the downward
deflection of the S wave
to the beginning of the
upward deflection of
the T wave
STSG   split-thickness skin graft
STSS   staphylococcal toxic shock
syndrome
STT   Schirmer tear test
serial thrombin time
skin temperature test
speaking tracheostomy
tube
spinothalamic tract
subtotal thyroidectomy
STU   shock trauma unit
skin test unit
STUMP   smooth-muscle tumor of
undetermined malignant
potential
STVA   subtotal villose atrophy
STVS   short-term visual storage
STX   saxitoxin (a neurotoxin
that may cause a severe
toxic reaction upon
ingestion of
contaminated shellfish)
S. typhimurium
Salmonella typhimurium
(causative agent of food
poisoning in man)
STZ   streptozocin (an
antineoplastic antibiotic)
SU   solar urticaria
stasis ulcer
status uncertain

	stomach ulcer
	stress ulcer
	stroke unit
	strontium unit
	subunit
su.	*sumat* [Latin] let the individual take
SUA	serum uric acid
subcu	subcutaneous (injection)
subl	sublingual
submand	submandibular
Sub P	substance P (group of polypeptides with potent effects on gastrointestinal smooth muscle)
Sub-Q	subcutaneous
sub q	subcutaneous
substd	substandard
SUC	severe ulcerative colitis
SUCs	sodium urate crystals (as seen in gout)
SUD	sudden unexpected death
	sudden unexplained death
SUDS	sudden unexplained death syndrome
SUF	slow continuous ultrafiltration

SUH	subungual hematoma
	subungual hemorrhage
SUI	stress urinary incontinence
SUID	sudden unexpected infant death
	sudden unexplained infant death
SUL	sacrouterine ligament
	subserous uterine leiomyomas
sulf	sulfur
sulfa	sulfonamide
sum.	*sumantur* [Latin] take *sumendum* [Latin] to be taken
SUMIT	streptokinase-urokinase myocardial infarct test
SUN	serum urea nitrogen (blood urea nitrogen)
SUO	syncope of unknown origin
SUP	stress ulcer prophylaxis
	superior
	supination
	symptomatic uterine prolapse
sup	superior
	supination

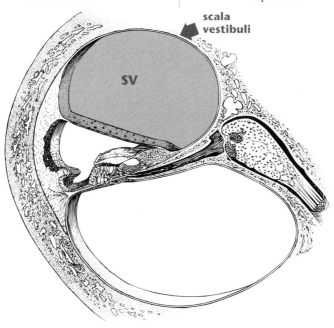

scala vestibuli

SV

	supinator
	supine
supin	supination
	supine
supp	suppository
suppl	supplement
SUPPORT	study to understand prognoses and preferences for outcomes and risks of treatment
suppos	suppository
SUR	Society of Uroradiology
Surf	surfactant
surg	surgery
	surgical
SURS	solitary ulcer of rectum syndrome
SUS	solitary ulcer syndrome
susp	suspension
SUTI	symptomatic urinary tract infection
SUUD	sudden unexpected, unexplained death
SUX	succinylcholine
SUZI	subzonal insertion of sperm microinjection subzonal insemination suction
SV	saphenous vein
	sarcoma virus
	satellite virus (a strain of virus that cannot replicate without the presence of a helper virus)
	scala vestibuli
	selective vagotomy
	seminal vesicle
	seminal vesiculitis
	Sendai virus (a parainfluenza 1 virus related to the mumps virus)
	senile vaginitis
	severe
	simian virus
	sinus venosus (the structure in the embryo

midheart that receives the umbilical, vitelline and the common cardinal veins)

slow virus (a virus causing degenerative diseases marked by a long incubation period and a gradual progression of symptoms and pathology)

snake venom

splenic vein

spoken voice

street virus (rabies virus)

stroke volume

subclavian vein

supraventricular

synaptic vesicle

Sv	Sievert, the unit of radiation dose (replaces rem which = 10^{-2} Sv
SVA	selective vagotomy and antrectomy
	subtotal villous atrophy
	supraventricular activity
	supraventricular arrhythmia

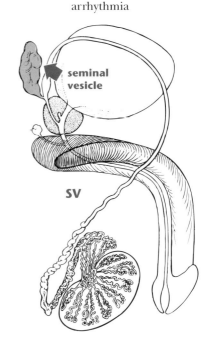

seminal vesicle

SV

SVAS	supravalvular aortic stenosis
SVBP	saphenous vein bypass
SVBPG	saphenous vein bypass graft
SVC	satellite videoconference
	segmental venous capacitance
	slow vital capacity
	subclavian vein compression
	superior vena cava

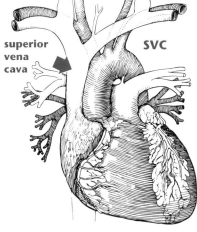

superior vena cava   SVC

SVCCS	superior vena cava compression syndrome
SVCB	superior vena caval branch (of right coronary artery) (nodal artery)
SVCL	spatial vectorcardio-graphic loop
SVCO	superior vena cava obstruction
SVCOG	saphenous vein cross-over graft
SVC-RPA	
	shunt between superior vena cava and right pulmonary artery
SVCS	superior vena cava syndrome
SVD	small vessel disease
	spontaneous vaginal delivery
	spontaneous vertex delivery
	St. Vitus' dance (chorea)
	sudden vaginal delivery
	swine vesicular disease
SVE	slow volume encephalography
	sterile vaginal examination
SVG	saphenous-vein graft
SVI	stroke volume index
SVIG	saphenous vein interposition graft
SVL	severe visual loss
SVN	small volume nebulizer
	superior vertebral notch
SVO$_2$	saturated venous oxygen content
SVP	sexually violent predator
	spontaneous venous pressure
	standing venous pressure
SVPB	supraventricular premature beat
SVR	slow ventricular response
	systemic vascular resistance
SVRI	systemic vascular resistance index
SVS	scleral venous sinus (canal of Schlemm)
	Society for Vascular Surgery
SVT	subclavian vein thrombosis
	superficial venous thrombosis
	supraventricular tachycardia
SW	seriously wounded
	social worker
	spike wave
	stab wound
	sterile water
	surgical waste
S & W	soap and water
S wave	the first downward deflection following the R wave of the ECG cycle, due to depolarization of the posterior basal region

of the left ventricle
SWD short-wave diathermy
substance withdrawal (syndrome)
SWDS substance withdrawal syndrome
SWDHT shortwave diathermy heat treatment
SWE slow wave encephalography
SWG standard wire gauge
SWI solar warning index (an index measuring the likely exposure to skin cancer-promoting ultraviolet light; taken daily at noon at specific locations)
stroke work index
surgical wound infection
SWIM sperm-washing insemination method
SWL shock wave lithotripsy
SWMS synergistic wrist motion splint
SWR serum Wassermann reaction
SWRs surgical waiting rooms
SWS slow-wave sleep (non-rapid eye movement sleep)
steroid-wasting syndrome
Sturge-Weber syndrome

Swt sweat
SX syndrome X
Sx signs
symptoms
sx sign
surgery
symptom
SXR skull x-ray
sym symmetrical
symptom
symph symphysis
sympt symptom
SYN synovitis
syn synovial
synd syndrome
syn fl synovial fluid
synth synthetic
Syph syphilis
syr syringe
syr. *syrupus* [Latin] syrup
syst system
systolic
syst bp systolic blood pressure
syst m systolic murmur
SZ schizophrenic
seizure
spermatozoa
Sz seizure
SZN streptozocin (Zanosar; an antineoplastic antibiotic)
SZP schizophrenia

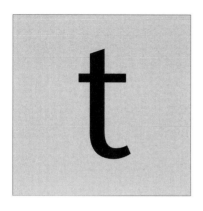

T
absolute temperature
intraocular tension
tablespoon (approximately
  15 mL)
Taenia
talus
tarsus
temperature
tension
term
terminal
tesla
testis
testosterone
therapy
thoracic vertebra
thorax
threonine (an essential
  amino acid)
thrombosis
thrombus
thymine (one of the
  pyrimidine bases
  commonly found in
  deoxyribonucleic acid)
thymus
tibia
time
tissue
tocopherol (vitamin E)
tongue
tonsil
torque (force that acts to
  produce rotation)
total
toxicity
trace
transmittance
transcription
translating
transplantation
trend (long-term
  movement in an
  ordered series)
Treponema (a genus of
  spiral bacteria, several
  species of which are
  pathogenic)
triage (the sorting of
  patients (as in an
  emergency room or
  battlefield) to determine
  their priority for
  treatment)
tritium (hydrogen-3)
trochlea
tumor
type

T+
increased intraocular
  tension (followed by a
  staging numeral)

T–
decreased intraocular
  tension (followed by a
  staging numeral)

$T_{1/2}$
biologic half-life
half-time

T1
first thoracic spinal nerve
first thoracic vertebra

T_1
tricuspid valve closure
  (tricuspid first sound)

T-1
1st stage of decreased
  intraocular tension (of
  anterior chamber of eye)

T+1
1st stage of increased
  intraocular tension (of
  anterior chamber of eye)

T2
second thoracic
  spinal nerve
second thoracic vertebra

T-2
2nd stage of decreased
  intraocular tension (of
  anterior chamber of eye)

T+2
2nd stage of increased

intraocular tension (of anterior chamber of eye)

T-2 dactinomycin + doxorubicin + vincristine + cyclophosphamide (combination chemotherapy with radiotherapy)

T3 third thoracic spinal nerve
third thoracic vertebra
Tylenol number 3 (with codeine)

T$_3$ serum triiodothyronine (inhibits TSH production)

T-3 3rd stage of decreased intraocular tension (of anterior chamber of eye)

T+3 3rd stage of increased intraocular tension (of anterior chamber of eye)

T4 fourth thoracic spinal nerve
fourth thoracic vertebra

T$_4$ levothyroxine
serum thyroxine (inhibits TSH production)

T5 fifth thoracic spinal nerve
fifth thoracic vertebra

T6 sixth thoracic spinal nerve
sixth thoracic vertebra

T7 seventh thoracic spinal nerve
seventh thoracic vertebra

T8 eight thoracic spinal nerve
eight thoracic vertebra

T9 ninth thoracic spinal nerve
ninth thoracic vertebra

T10 tenth thoracic spinal nerve
tenth thoracic vertebra

T11 eleventh thoracic spinal nerve
eleventh thoracic vertebra

T12 twelfth thoracic spinal nerve
twelfth thoracic vertebra

t teaspoon (approximately 5 mL)
temperature

temporal
terminal
tertiary
tesla
thymine (one of the pyrimidine bases commonly found in deoxyribonucleic acid)
thymidine (a condensation product of thymine with deoxyribose; a nucleoside in DNA)
time
tissue
tocopherol (vitamin E)
translocation
transmittance

t. *ter* [Latin] three times

TA Takayasu's arteritis (aortic arch syndrome)
tannic acid
tarsus
temporal arteritis (giant cell arteries; a chronic inflammation of the extracranial branches of the carotid artery)
test of articulation
therapeutic abortion
threatened abortion
thyroid adenoma
thyroid antibody
thyroid autoimmunity
tidal air
titratable acid
tobacco addiction
tonometry applanation
toothache
topical anesthesia
toxic adenoma
toxin-antitoxin
traffic accident
transaldolase
transplantation antigen
tricuspid atresia
truncus arteriosus
tumor-associated

T(A) temperature at axilla

T/A tonsillectomy/

T&A adenoidectomy
tonsillectomy and
adenoidectomy
tonsils (palatine tonsils)
and adenoids
(pharyngeal tonsils)

TAA thoracic aortic aneurysm
tobacco-alcohol amblyopia
total ankle arthroplasty
tumor-associated
antibodies
tumor-associated antigens

TA-AIDS transfusion-associated
AIDS

TAB tablet
Tachdjian abduction brace
therapeutic abortion
total autonomic blockage
triple antibiotic
typhoid + paratyphoid A +
paratyphoid B (vaccine)

TAb therapeutic abortion

tab tablet

TABC typhoid + paratyphoid A +
paratyphoid B +
paratyphoid C (vaccine)

tabs tablets

TABP type A behavior pattern

TAC Technology Assessment
Conference (at NIH)
terminal atrial contraction
tetracaine, Adrenalin
(epinephrine) and
cocaine
total abdominal colectomy
total allergen content
tricarboxylic acid cycle

Tac T cell activation receptor

tachy tachycardia

TACWBC technetium 99m albumin
colloid white blood cell

TAD test of auditory
discrimination
thoracic aortic dissection
thoracic asphyxiant
dystrophy
transient
acantholytic dermatosis

TADAC therapeutic abortion,
dilatation, aspiration,
curettage

TAE total abdominal
eventration
transcatheter arterial
embolization

TAF tissue-angiogenic factor
tumor-angiogenic factor
(stimulates rapid
formation of new
blood vessels)

TAG technical advisory group
Thalassemia Action Group

TAGVHD transfusion-associated graft
versus host disease

TAH total abdominal
hysterectomy

TAH/BSO total abdominal
hysterectomy with
bilateral salpingo-
oophorectomy

TAHL thick ascending limb of
Henle's loop

TAL tendon Achilles
lengthening
(lengthening of tendo
calcaneus)
transverse acetabular
ligament

talc talcum

TALL T cell acute lymphoblastic
leukemia

TAM tamoxifen (nonsteroidal
oral antiestrogen)
teen-age mother
total active motion
toxoid-antitoxoid mixture
transient abnormal
myelopoiesis
tumor-associated
macrophages

TAME toluenesulfonyl-L-arginine
methyl ester

TAN tricyclic antidepressant
nortriptyline

TANI total axial lymph node
irradiation

tan tangent

TANI total axial lymph-node

irradiation

TAO thromboangiitis obliterans (Buerger's disease)
tumor-associated osteomalacia

TAP therapy-associated pain
titanium acetabular prosthesis
tracheal antimicrobial peptide

TAPG tracheal antimicrobial peptide gene

TAR thoracic aortic rupture
thrombocytopenia and absent radius (syndrome)
total ankle replacement
transactivating response
Treatment Authorization Request

TARA total articular replacement arthroplasty (trademark)
tumor-associated rejection antigen

TAS tetanus antitoxin serum
total allergy syndrome
traumatic apallic syndrome

TASA tumor-associated surface antigen

TASH The Association for Persons with Severe Handicaps

TAT tetanus antitoxin
thematic apperception test
thromboplastin activation time
till all taken
toxin-antitoxin
transaxial tomography
turnabout time
turnaround time

TATA tumor-associated transplantation antigen

TATST tetanus antitoxin skin test

TAU transabdominal ultrasound

TB taste bud
Taussig-Bing syndrome (rare congenital malformation of the heart)

term birth
terminal bronchiole
testicular biopsy
tissue bank
tissue biopsy
Toronto brace
total bilirubin
total body
tracheobronchitis
trapezoid body
tub bath
tubercle bacillus
tuberculin
tuberculosis

T & B tendonitis and bursitis

Tb terbium (rare metallic element)
tubercle bacillus

TBA testosterone-binding affinity
thiobarbituric acid
to be added
to be admitted
total bile acids
tubercle bacillus

TBAN transbronchial aspiration needle

TBB transbronchial biopsy

TBC to be cancelled
total blood cholesterol
total body calcium
total body clearance

Tbc tubercle bacillus

TBD tick-borne disease
to be determined
total body density

TBE tick-borne encephalitis

TBEV tick-borne encephalitis virus

TBF total body fat

TBFB tracheobronchial foreign body

TBG testosterone-binding globulin
thyroid-binding globulin
thyroxine-binding globulin (interalpha globulin, a carrierr of thyroxin in the blood stream)

TBH	total body hematocrit		total burn surface area
TBHT	total body hyperthermia	**tbsp**	tablespoon (holds
	total body hypothermia		approximately 15mL
TBI	thyroxine-binding index		of fluid)
	total body irradiation	**TBT**	tolbutamine test
	traumatic brain injury		tracheobronchial tree
	(major causes include		transbuccal trocar
	motor-vehicle accidents,	**TBTI**	term birth, triving infant
	assaults and sports	**TBV**	total blood volume
	activities)		transluminal balloon
TBII	thyroid-binding inhibitory		valvuloplasty
	immunoglobulin	**TBW**	total body water
	TSH-binding inhibitory	**TBX**	thromboxane
	immunoglobulin		total body irradiation
T bili	total bilirubin	**TC**	tachycardia
TBK	total body potassium		target cell
TBL	tracheobronchial lavage		terminal cancer
tbl	tablet		terminal care
TBLB	trans-bronchial lung biopsy		testicular cancer
TBLC	term birth, living child		tetracycline
TBLI	term birth, living infant		thoracic cage
TBLN	tracheobronchial		thoracic circumference
	lymph node		throat culture
TBM	tracheobronchomalacia		thrombocythemia
	tuberculous meningitis		thrombocytosis
	tubular basement		thyrocalcitonin
	membrane		tissue culture
TBMN	thin basement membrane		torticollis (wryneck)
	nephropathy		total calcium
TBN	total body nitrogen		total cholesterol
TBNA	trans-bronchial needle		total complement
	aspiration		transcobalamin
	treated but not admitted		transverse colon
TBNAA	total-body neutron		trauma center
	activation analysis		traumatic cataract
TBP	testosterone-binding		treatment completed
	protein		true conjugate
	thyroxine-binding protein		tumor cell
	tuberculous peritonitis		tympanic cavity
TBPA	thyroxine-binding	**T/C**	to consider
	prealbumin (T4-binding	**T & C**	turn and cough
	protein)		type and cross-match
TBR	total bed rest		(blood)
	total bilirubin	**TC#3**	Tylenol with 30 mg
TBS	total body scanning		codeine
	total body solute	**TC II**	transcobalamin II
	total body surface	**3TC**	Epivir
	tracheobronchoscopy	**TC99**	technetium 99
TBSA	total body surface area		(radionuclide)

Tc	technetium
	tetracycline
T$_c$	cytotoxic T cell
tc	transcutaneous
TCA	total circulating albumin
	total circulatory arrest
	transluminal coronary angioplasty
	trichloroacetic acid
	tricuspid atresia
	tricyclic antidepressant
	tumor chemosensitivity assay
TCa	terminal cancer
TCAB	tetrachloroazobenzene
	triple coronary artery bypass
TCABG	triple coronary artery bypass graft
TCA cycle	
	tricarboxylic acid cycle
TCAD	tricyclic antidepressant
TCAR	T cell antigen receptor
TCB	tetrachlorobiphenyl
	total cardiopulmonary bypass
TCBi	transcutaneous bilirubin index
TCC	T'ai Chi Ch'uan (Chinese system of exercise)
	terminal complement complex
	tertiary care center
	transitional cell carcinoma
	trichlorocarbanilide
TCCA	transitional cell carcinoma-associated (virus)
TCCB	transitional cell carcinoma of (urinary) bladder
TCD	thiocyclodine
	tissue culture dose
	transcranial Doppler (sonography)
	transcranial Doppler (ultrasonography)
	transverse cardiac diameter
TCD50	median tissue culture dose
TC & DB	turn, cough and deep breath

TCDD	tetrachlorodibenzo-*p*-dioxin (presence in the environment poses a potential human health hazard)
TCDUS	transcranial Doppler ultrasonography
TCE	T cell enriched
	time course of exposue
	trichloroethylene
T cells	thymus-derived lymphocytes (lymphocytes originating in the thymus gland)
TCF	total coronary flow
TCFC	T-colony forming cell
TCFU	tumor colony-forming unit
TCGF	T cell growth factor
TCH	total circulating hemoglobin
	twin-coil hemodialyzer
TChE	total cholinesterase
TCI	transient cerebral ischemia
TCIA	transient cerebral ischemic attack
TCID	tissue-culture infectious dose
TCID50	median tissue culture infective dose
TCIE	transient cerebral ischemic episode
TCL	tibial (medial) collateral ligament (of knee)
	tibio-calcaneal ligament
	total capacity of lung
	transverse carpal ligament
T-CLL	T cell chronic lymphatic leukemia
TClow	toxic concentration low
TCM	tissue culture media
	transcutaneous monitor
T & CM	type and cross-match
TCMA	transcortical motor aphasia
TCMH	tumor-direct cell-mediated hypersensitivity
TCMI	T cell-mediated immunity
TCMZ	trichloro-methiazide (diuretic)
TCN	tetracycline (antibiotic)
TcNM	tumor with lymph node

metastases

TCNS transcutaneous nerve
stimulator

T$_{CO_2}$ total carbon dioxide

TCOM transcutaneous oxygen
monitor

TCP therapeutic continuous
penicillin
thrombocytopenia
titanium cervical plate
tranylcypromine
(monoamine oxidase
inhibitor)
tricalcium phosphate
trichlorophenol

Tcp toxin-coregulated pilus

TcPO$_2$ transcutaneous partial
pressure of oxygen

TCR T-cell reactivity
T cell receptor
(antigen receptor)

total cytoplasmic ribosome

TCRI Toxic Chemical Release
Inventory

tcRNA translation control
ribonucleic acid

T. cruzi *Trypanosoma cruzi*
(etiologic agent
of Chagas' disease
in humans)

TCS tethered cord syndrome
(abnormally low cone-
shaped distal end of the
spinal cord tethered by
any of various cordlike
intradural abnormalities)
tibial (medial) collateral
sprain
Treacher Collins syndrome
(Franceshetti syndrome;
mandibulofacial
dysostosis)

TCSF T-colony-stimulating factor

TCT thrombin-clotting time
thyrocalcitonin
total cholesterol test
triple chemotherapy

Tct tincture

TCU transitional care unit

TCVA thromboembolic
cerebrovascular accident

TCZ thermal comfort zone

TD tabes dorsalis
(Duchenne's disease)
Tangier disease
tardive dyskinesia
T-cell dependent
temporary disability
testicular deficiency
therapy discontinued
thoracic duct
threshold of discomfort
thymus-dependent
tic douloureux (trigeminal
neuralgia)
tissue donor
tocopherol deficiency
torsion dystonia
total disability
total dose

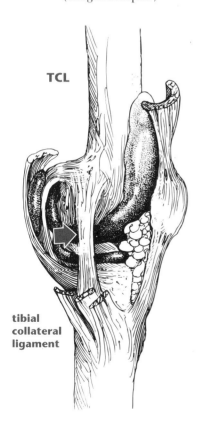

TCL

tibial
collateral
ligament

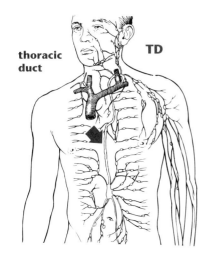

thoracic duct

TD

	toxic dose
	transverse diameter
	traveler's diarrhea (caused by a variety of infectious agents)
	treatment discontinued
	typhoid dysentery
T/D	treatment discontinued
TD50	median toxic dose
T & D	tetanus and diphtheria
Td	tetanus and diphtheria toxoids (adult type)
TDA	target-detection assay
	TSH-displacing antibody
TDB	third-degree burn
	Toxicology Data Bank
TDC	total dietary calories
TDCR	time-dose-cytotoxic relationship
TDD	telecommunication device for the deaf
	telephone device for the deaf
	tetradecadiene
	thoracic duct drainage
	toxic dose of drug
TDDM	toxic dose-dependent mechanism
TDE	tetrachlorodiphenylethane
	tissue dissociation enzyme
	total daily energy
T-dep	T-dependent
TDF	testis-determining factor (initiates differentiation of the gonad into a testis)
	thoracic duct flow
	tissue-damaging factor
TDH	threonine dehydrogenase
TDI	therapeutic donor insemination
	total dose infusion
	total dose insulin
	toluene diisocyanate
TDK	tardive dyskinesia
TDL	thymus-dependent lymphocytes
	toxic dose level
TDM	therapeutic drug management
	therapeutic drug monitoring
	thiamine deficency malnutrition (beriberi)
TDN	thoracodorsal nerve
	total digestible nutrients
tDNA	transfer deoxyribonucleic acid (DNA)
TDP	thoracic duct pressure
	thymidine diphosphate
	torsades de pointes [French] twisting of the points (on ECG)
	transdermal patch
TdP	*torsades de pointes* [French] twisting of the points (on ECG)
TdR	thymidine (ribonucleoside)
TDS	transduodenal sphincteroplasty
t.d.s.	*ter die sumendum* [Latin] to be taken three times a day
TDT	terminal deoxynucleotidyl transferase
	tumor doubling time
TdT	terminal deoxynucleotidyl transferase (cellular enzyme)
	terminal deoxytransferase
TDWB	touch-down weight bearing

TE echo time
expiratory time
tangential excision
tartar emetic
tennis elbow (lateral
humeral epicondylitis)
tetanus
therapeutically equivalent
thromboembolism
thyrotoxic exophthalmos
tick-borne encephalitis
tissue equivalent
tonsillectomy
tooth extraction
total ejaculate (number
of sperm)
total estrogen (excreted)
toxic epidermolysis
toxoplasmic encephalitis
trace element
tracheoesophageal
treadmill exercise

T & E testing and evaluation
trial and error

Te effective half-life
tellurium (a metalloid
element)
tetanus

TEA tetraethylammonium
thromboendarterectomy
total elbow arthroplasty
total endarterectomy

TEAB tetraethylammonium
bromide

TEAC tetraethylammonium
chloride

TEA CO₂ laser
transversely excited
atmospheric carbon
dioxide laser

TEB timed endometrial biopsy

TEBG testosterone-estradiol-
binding globulin

TeBG testosterone-binding
globulin

TEC total eosinophil count
transluminal extraction
catheter
transluminal extraction

coronary atherectomy

T & EC Trauma and Emergency
Center

tech technical

TECV traumatic epiphyseal coxa
vara

TED threshold erythema dose
thromboembolic disease
thyroid eye disease

TEDD total end-diastolic diameter

TED stockings
thromboembolic disease
stockings (antiembolism
stockings)

TEE total energy expenditure
transesophageal
echocardiography
(monitor)
transnasal endoscopic
ethmoidectomy

TEF tracheoesophageal fistula
trunk extension-flexion

Teff effective half-life

TEFS transmural electrical field
stimulation

TEG thromboelastogram

TEHIP Toxicology and
Environmental Health
Information Program

TEI total episode of illness

TEL telemetry
tetraethyl lead

Tel telemetry

TEM transepithelial movement
transmission electron
microscopy
triethylenemelamine
tuberculous meningitis

Temp temperature

temp temperature
temple

temp. dext.
tempori dextro [Latin] to
the right temple

temp. sinist.
tempori sinistro [Latin] to
the left temple

TEN total enteral nutrition
total excreted nitrogen

toxic epidermal necrolysis
TENPA triethylenethiophosphora-
mide (thiotepa)
TENS transcutaneous electrical
nerve stimulation
TEP thromboendophlebectomy
tracheoesophageal
puncture
transverse electrode
pacemaker
tubal ectopic pregnancy
TEPA triethylenethio-
phosphoramide
(thiotepa; generally
replaced by
cyclophosphamide as an
antineoplastic agent of
choice)
TEPP tetraethyl pyrophosphate
TER total elbow replacement
total endoplasmic
reticulum
transcapillary escape rate
term terminal
ter. sim. *tere simul* [Latin]
rub together
tert tertiary
TES tendon entrapment
syndrome
thoracic endometriosis
syndrome
thromboembolic stroke
transcutaneous electric
stimulation
transmural electric
stimulation
treatment emergent
symptoms
TESD total end-systolic diameter
TESS treatment emergent
symptoms scale
TEST tubal embryo stage transfer
TET total ejection time
transcutaneous
energy transfer
treadmill exercise test
tubal embryo transfer
Tet tetanus
TETD tetraethylthiuram disulfide

TETRAC tetraiodothyroacetic acid
Tet Tox tetanus toxoid
TEV talipes equinovarus (typical
clubfoot)
TF free thyroxine
tactile fremitus
term fetus
testicular feminization
tetrology of Fallot
(combination of
congenital cardiac
defects)
thymidine factor
tissue-damaging factor
to follow
tracheal fistula
transfemoral (amputation
above the knee)
transfer factor
transferrin
transverse foramen
trigger finger
tube feeding
tuning fork
typhoid fever
(enteric fever)
Tf transferrin (siderophilin)
TFA topical fluoride application
total fatty acids
typhus fever antibody
TFC triangular fibrocartilage
TFCC triangular fibrocartilage
complex
TFD target-film distance
TFd dialyzable transfer factor
TFE polytetrafluoroethylene
(Teflon)
Tf-Fe transferrin-bound iron
TFL talofibular ligament
tensor fasciae latae
TFM testicular feminization
male
TFPI tissue factor pathway
inhibitor
TFR total fertility rate
total flow resistance
TFS testicular feminization
syndrome
TFT thrombus formation time

thyroid function test
trifluorothymidine
(trifluridine)
TG tendon graft
testosterone glucuronide
thioglucose
thioglycolate
thioguanine
(antineoplastic agent)
thromboglobulin
thymus gland
thyroglobulin
thyroid gland
tophaceous gout
total gastrectomy
toxic goiter
trigeminal ganglion
triglyceride (the major
storage form of fatty acids
and is practically the
exclusive constituent of
adipose tissue)
Tg serum thyroglobulin
thioguanine
(antineoplastic agent)
thyroglobulin
TGA thyroglobulin activity
total gonadotropin actvity
transient global amnesia
transposition of great
arteries
tumor glycoprotein assay
TgAb thyroglobulin antibody
(titer)
TGAR total graft area rejected
TGB thyroglobulin
TGC thyroglossal cyst
time-varied gain control
TGCD thioglycolate-cysteine
disulfide
TGD thyroglossal duct
TGDC thyroglossal duct cyst
TGE transmissible
gastroenteritis
TGEF transabdominal thin-gauge
embryofetoscopy
TGF transforming growth factor
tumor growth factor
TGFA triglyceride fatty acid

TGF alpha
transforming growth
factor alpha
TGC thyroglossal cyst
TGDC thyroglossal duct cyst
TGF T-cell growth factor
transforming growth factor
tumor growth factor
TGFA triglyceride fatty acid
TGG trigeminal ganglion
(semilunar ganglion)

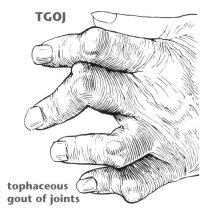

trigeminal ganglion TGG

turkey gamma globulin
TGI toxic gas inhalation
TGL triglyceride
TGOJ tophaceous gout of joints

TGOJ

tophaceous gout of joints

T. gondii *Toxoplasma gondii*
TGP tobacco glycoprotein
TGR tenderness, guarding
and rigidity
6-TGR 6-thioguanine riboside
TGS tincture of green soap
TGs triglycerides
TGSI thyroid growth-stimulating
immunoglobulin

TGSW tangential gunshot wound
TGT thromboplastin generation test
TGV thoracic gas volume
transposition of great vessels
TH tension headache
T helper (cell)
theophylline
thorax
thrombus
thyrohyoid
thyroid hormone
total hysterectomy
transhumeral (amputation above the elbow)
tyrosine hydroxylase
Th thenar
thigh
thoracic
thorax
thorium (A radioactive metallic element used to enhance visualization in roentgenography)
THA tetrahydroaminoacridine
total hip arthroplasty
traumatic hemolytic anemia
ThA thoracic aorta
THAA tetrahydroaminoacridine
Thal thalassemia
THAM tris(hydroxymethyl)amino-methane (tromethamine)
THAN transient hyperammon-emia of newborn
THB tetrahydrobiopterine
THb total hemoglobin
THBI thyroid hormone binding inhibitor
THBR thyroid hormone binding ratio
THC tetrahydrocannabinol
tetrahydrocortisol
transhepatic cholangiography
THCULT throat culture
THD teratologic hip dislocation

testicular hypothermia device
thyrotoxic heart disease
THDOC tetrahydrodeoxy-corticosterone
THE transhepatic embolization
THEO theophylline (smooth muscle relaxant, generally used as a diuretic)
ther therapy
therapeutic
ther ex therapeutic exercise
therm thermometer
THF tetrahydrofluorenone
tetrahydrofolate
thymic humeral factor
thyroid hyperfunction (thyrotoxicosis)
THFA tetrahydrofolic acid
Thg thyroglobulin (iodine-containing glycoprotein)
THGGI transient hypogammaglobulinemia of infancy (associated with increased susceptibility to infections)
THH telangiectasia hereditaria hemorrhagica
Thi thiamine (thiamin; vitamin B1)
THIO thiopental sodium (anesthetic)
thiotepa triethylenethiophos-phoramide
THL transverse humeral ligament
THM thyrohyoid membrane
thyrohyoid muscle
total heme mass
Thor thoracic
thorax
THP tissue hydrostatic pressure
total hip prosthesis
total hydroxyproline
trihexphenidyl hydrochloride
THPA tetrahydropteric acid

ThPP	thiamine pyrophosphate
THR	thyroid hormone resistance
	total hip replacement (total hip arthroplasty)
Thr	threonine (an essential amino acid)
THRA	total hip replacement arthroplasty
THRF	thyrotropic hormone releasing factor
thromb	thrombosis
THS	tetrahydrocompound S
	thrombohemorrhagic syndrome
	total hip system
THTH	thyrotropic hormone
THUG	thyroid uptake gradient
Thx	thromboxane
Thy	thymine (one of the pyrimidine bases commonly found in deoxyribonucleic acid)
	thymus
TI	terminal ileitis (Crohn's disease)
	terminal ileum
	terminal illness
	therapeutic index
	thymus-independent

thyrohyoid membrane   **THM**

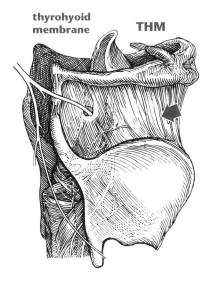

	time interval
	total iron
	translational inhibition
	tricuspid incompetene
	tricuspid insufficiency
	trauma index
	tubal insufflation
Ti	titanium (metallic element)
TIA	transient ischemic attack
	tumor-induced angiogenesis
TIA fistula	
	tracheo-innominate artery (brachiocephalic trunk) fistula
TIB	tibia
	time in bed
Tib	tibia
TIBC	total iron-binding capacity
TIC	Toxicology Information Center
	trypsin-inhibitory capacity
TICU	transplant intensive care unit
TID	therapeutic insemination, donor
	time interval difference
	titrated initial dose
	tubulointerstitial disease
t.i.d.	*ter in die* [Latin] three times a day
TIE	transient ischemic episode
TIF	thyrotropin-influencing factor
	tumor-inducing factor
	tumor-inhibiting factor
TIg	tetanus immune globulin
	tungsten inert gas
TIGR	The Institute of Genomic Research
TIH	therapeutic insemination, husband
	tumor-inducing hypercalcemia
TIIV	trivalent inactivated influenza vaccine
TIL	tumor-infiltrating leukocyte

tumor-infiltrating
  lymphocyte

tumor-infiltrating T
  lymphocyte

TILs tumor-infiltrating T
  lymphocytes

TILT tumor-infiltrating T
  lymphocytes therapy

TIM transthoracic intracardiac
  monitoring

TIMC tumor-induced marrow
  cytotoxicity

TIMI thrombolysis in myocardial
  ischemia

TIMP tissue inhibitor of
  metalloproteinase

TIN tissue infarction necrosis
  tubulointerstitial
  nephropathy

t.i.n. *ter in nocte* [Latin] three
  times nightly

tinc tincture

tinct tincture

T-ind T-independent

TINEM there is no evidence of
  malignancy

TIP terminal illness patient
  toxic interstitial
  pneumonitis
  Toxicology Information
  Program
  translation inhibiting
  protein

TIPS transjugular intrahepatic
  portosystemic shunts

TIS tetracycline-induced
  steatosis
  tumor *in situ*

TISS Therapeutic Intervention
  Scoring System

TIT thyroid iodide trap
  triiodothyronine
  tubal insufflation test

TITh triiodothyronine

Title XVIII
  Medicare

TIU trypsin-inhibiting unit

TIUP term intrauterine pregnancy

TIUV total intrauterine volume

TIV trivalent inactivated
  influenza vaccine
  Treponema
  immobilization volume

TIVC thoracic inferior vena cava

+tive positive

TJ tendon jerk (reflex test)
  thigh junction
  triceps jerk (reflex test)

TJA total joint arthroplasty

TJR total joint replacement

TK through knee (amputation
  or prosthesis)
  thymidine kinase

TKA total knee arthroplasty
  transketolase activity
  trochanter, knee
  and ankle

TKD thymidine kinase
  deficiency
  tokodynamometer

TKG tokodynagraph

TKNO to keep needle open

TKO technical knock-out
  (selection)
  to keep open (a vein to
  receive intravenous
  fluids)

TKP thermokeratoplasty
  total knee prosthesis

TKR total knee replacement

TKS turnkey system

TKVO to keep vein open

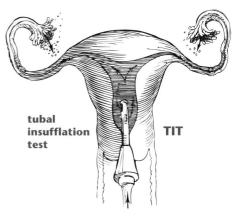

**tubal
insufflation
test**   **TIT**

TL	temporal lobe
	threat to life
	thymic lymphocyte
	thymic lymphoma
	time lapse
	total lipids
	total lung (capacity)
	total lymphocyte count
	tubal ligation
T-L	thymus-dependent lymphocyte
Tl	thallium (metallic element)
TLA	thymus leukemia antigen
	translaryngeal aspiration
	translumbar aortogram
	transluminal angioplasty
TLAA	T lymphocyte-associated antigen
TLam	thoracic laminectomy
TLB	transvenous liver biopsy
TLBS	tight low back syndrome
TLC	tender loving care
	theca lutein cyst
	thin-layer chromatography
	total lung capacity
	total lung compliance
	total lymphocyte count
TLCO	thoracolumbosacral orthosis
TLCs	theca lutein cysts
TLD	thermoluminescent dosimeter
	thoracic lymph duct
	tumor lethal death
	tumor lethal dose
TLE	temporal lobe epilepsy
	thin-layer electrophoresis
TLF	tumor-limiting factor
TLI	thymidine labeling index
	total lymph node irradiation
	total lymphoid irradiation
	trypsin-like immunoreactivity
TLm	median tolerance limit
TLNB	term living newborn
TLS	Tourette-like syndrome

	tumor lysis syndrome
TLSO	thoracolumbosacral orthosis
TLT	thrombolytic therapy
	tryptophan load test
TLV	threshold limit value
	total lung volume
TM	tectorial membrane
	telemedicine (World Wide Web at http://www 2. nas. edu/whatsnew/.
	temperature by mouth
	temporomandibular (joint)
	tender midline
	tendomyopathy
	teres major (muscle)
	teres minor (muscle)
	test meal (bland food, e.g., toast or crackers and tea given before analysis of stomach secretions)
	topical medication
	total mastectomy
	trademark
	traditional medicine
	transcendental meditation
	transitional mucosa
	transmembrane
	transmetatarsal (amputation)
	trapezius muscle
	tropical medicine
	tuberculous meningitis
	tympanic membrane (eardrum)
T & M	transients and migrants
	Trichomonas and Monilia
Tm	melting temperature
	thulium (rare metallic element)
	transport maximum
	tubular maximum excretory capacity of kidneys
TMA	tetramethylammonium
	thrombotic microangiopathy

thyroid microsomal
  antibody

transmetatarsal amputation

triceps muscle of arm

trimellitic anhydride

trimethoxyamphetamine

trimethylamine

TMAb thyroid microsomal
  antibody (titer)

TMAD temporomandibular
  articular disk

TMAS Taylor Manifest
  Anxiety Scale

T-MAX peak temperature

T$_{max}$ time of maximum
  concentration of a
  prescribed drug

TMB transient monocular
  blindness

TMC toxic megacolon

transmural colitis

triamcinolone (potent
  synthetic glucocorticoid)

TMCA trimethylcolchicinic acid

TMCD tectorial membrane of
  cochlear duct

TMD treating MD (physician)

TME transmural enteritis

TMET treadmill exercise test

TMF television-monitored
  fluoroscopy

TMG toxic multinodular goiter

TmG tubular maximum
  reabsorption of glucose

TMI transient myocardial
  ischemia (mild
  forerunner of
  heart attack)

transmandibular implant

TMIC Toxic Materials
  Information Center

TMIF tumor-cell migratory
  inhibition factor

TMJ temporomandibular joint

TMJD temporomandibular joint
  dysfunction

TMJP temporomandibular joint
  pain

TMJS temporomandibular joint

syndrome

TML tetramethyl lead

temporomandibular
  ligament

TMM torn medial meniscus

TMNG toxic multinodular goiter

TMP temporomandibular pain

thymine monophosphatase

trimethoprim
  (antibacterial agent)

trimethylpsoralen

TMPDS temporomandibular pain
  and dysfunction
  syndrome

TMPSMX

  trimethoprim-
  sulfamethoxazole (used
  to treat *P. carinii*
  pneumonia)

TMR trainable mentally retarded

TMRC tubular maximal
  reabsorption capacity

TMS temporomandibular joint
  syndrome

thallium myocardial

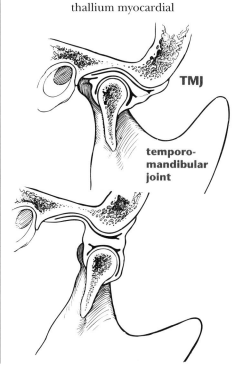

TMJ

temporo-
mandibular
joint

scintigraphy
TMST treadmill stress test
TMT tarsometatarsal (joint)
TMT angle
talometatarsal angle
TMTC too many to count
TMTX trimetrexate
TMV tobacco mosaic virus

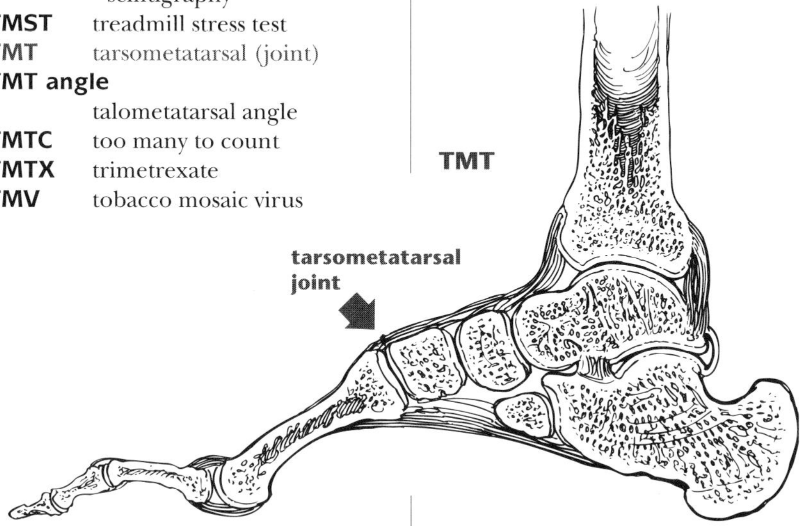

TMT

tarsometatarsal joint

TMX tamoxifen (a nonsteroidal oral antiestrogen)
TMZ temazepam (a minor tranquilizer)
transformation zone
TN temperature normal
thermal necrosis
thrombonecrosis
thyroid notch
toxic nephropathy
trigeminal nerve (5th cranial nerve)
trigeminal neuralgia (tic douloureux)
trigeminal nucleus
trochlear nerve (4th cranial nerve)
trochlear notch
trochlear nucleus
T&N tar and nicotine
tingling and numbness
T₄N normal serum thyroxine
Tn normal intraocular tension
TNB trigeminal nerve block
Tru-Cut needle biopsy
TNBP transurethral needle biopsy of prostate
TND Telecommunications Network for the Deaf
term normal delivery

transmissible neuro-degenerative disease
TNDS transdermal nicotine delivery system
tNE total norepinephrine
TNF tumor necrosis factor (capable of inducing hemorrhagic destruction of tumors)

TNF alpha
tumor necrosis factor-alpha
TNG transdermal nitroglycerin
tongue
trinitroglycerin
TNH transient neonatal hyperammonemia
TNI total nodal irradiation
TNM tumor size + regional node involvement + presence or absence of distant metastasis (for staging of cancer)
tumor-node-metastasis
TNMR tritium nuclear magnetic resonance
TNP transdermal nicotine patch trinitrophenol (picric acid)
TNR tonic neck reflex
TNS transcutaneous nerve stimulation

tumor necrosis serum
TNT trinitrotoluene
TNTC too numerous to count
(applied to bacteria in a
culture plate or blood
cells in a urine specimen)
TNV tobacco necrosis virus
TO target organ
telephone order
thoracic orthosis
tincture of opium
total obstruction
treatment outcome
turnover (numerical)
T(O) oral temperature
T&O tubes and ovaries
TOA time of arrival
tubo-ovarian abscess
TOB tobacco
TOC total organic carbon
tubo-ovarian complex
tubo-ovarian cyst
TOCS thoracic outlet
compression syndrome
TOD time of death
TODI transosteal dental implant
TODS toxic organic dust
syndrome
TOF tetralogy of Fallot
T of F tetrology of Fallot
TOGV transposition of the
great vessels
TOH transient osteoporosis
of hip
TOI transmission of infection (a
mechanism by which an
infectious agent is spread
to another person or
through the
environment)
TOL tolerated
trial of labor
Tolb tolbutamide (hypoglycemic
sulfonylurea)
TOM transcutaneous oxygen
monitor
tuberculous osteomyelitis
(Pott's disease)
tomo tomogram
tomography

TOMS tuberculous osteomyelitis
of spine
TOP termination of pregnancy
tobacco prevention
toxemia of pregnancy
TOPS take off pounds sensibly
TOPV trivalent oral polio vaccine
TORCH toxoplasmosis, other
infections, rubella,
cytomegalovirus infection
and herpes (simplex)
TORCHS toxoplasmosis, other
infections, rubella,
cytomegalovirus
infection, herpes
(simplex) and syphilis
(agents that can infect
the fetus or newborn)
TORP total ossicular (ear bones)
replacement prosthesis
TOS thoracic outlet syndrome
(neurovascular
compression syndrome)
TOT total operating time
Tot total
total PSA
total prostate-specific
antigen
Tot Bili total bilirubin
Tot Prot total protein
TOVO transoral vertical
osteotomy
tox toxic
toxicity
TOXICON toxicology information
conversational online
network
TOXLINE toxicology information
online
TOXLIT toxicology literature
(online)
TOXNET toxicology data network
(online)
Toxo toxoplasmosis
TP terminal phalanx
testosterone propionate
thallium poisoning

threshold potential
thrombocytopenic purpura
thrombophlebitis
thromboplastin
thrombopoietin
thymic polypeptide
tick paralysis (tick toxicosis)
Todd's paralysis
toilet paper
torsades de pointes [French]
  fringe of pointed tips
  (seen on the ECG as
  atypical rapid excessive
  contractions of the
  ventricular musculature
  with waxing and waning
  of amplitude of the QRS
  complexes)
total protein
toxoplasmosis (caused by
  Toxoplasma gondii)
Treponema pallidum (causes
  venereal syphilis)
trigger point
triphosphate
true positive
tryptophan (an essential
  amino acid)
tubal pregnancy
tuberculin precipitation
tuberculous pleuritis

TP-99 technetium-pertech-
  netate-99
T & P temperature and pressure
  temperature and pulse
Tp precursor T cells
TPA tissue plasminogen
  activator (enzyme crucial
  to the balance between
  clotting and bleeding)
  tissue polypeptide antigen
  total parenteral
  alimentation
  Treponema pallidum
  agglutination
  tumor polypeptide
  antigen
tPA tissue plasminogen
  activator (enzyme crucial

to the balance between
  clotting and bleeding)
  tissue-type plasminogen
  activator
TPAG total protein and albumin
  globulin
T. pallidum
  Treponema pallidum (causes
  venereal syphilis)
TPB tetraphenyl borate
TPBF total pulmonary blood flow
TPC thenar palmar crease
  thromboplastic plasma
  component
  total patient care
  total plasma
  catecholamines
  total plasma cholesterol
  total proctocolectomy
  Treponema pallidum
  complement (test)
  transvenous pacemaker
  catheter
TPCs third population cells
TPCV total packed cell volume
TPD temporary partial disability
  trichopoliodystrophy
  tumor-producing dose
TPE therapeutic plasma
  exchange
  total placental estrogens
  total protective
  environment
  tropical pulmonary
  eosinophilia (syndrome)
  two-photon excitation
  typhoid-parathyroid
  enteritis
TPECC transpapillary endoscopic
  cholecystotomy
TPES tooth pulp electric
  stimulation
TPF thymus permeability factor
  tibial plateau fracture
TPG transplacental gradient
TPH thromboembolic
  pulmonary hypertension
  transplacental (fetal)
  hemorrhage

tryptophan hydroxylase

TPHA *Treponema pallidum*
hemagglutination assay

TPI *Treponema pallidum*
immobilization (test)
triose phosphate isomerase

TPIA *Treponema pallidum*
immune adherence

TPIP tooth pulp
inflammatory pain

TPIT trigger point
injection therapy

TPL thromboplastin
transverse perineal
ligament

TPM temporary pacemaker
thrombophlebitis migrans
total passive motion

TPMT thiopurine
methyltransferase

TPN total parenteral nutrition
(parenteral
administration)
triphosphopyridine
nucleotide

TPNL total parenteral
nutrition line

TPO thyroid peroxidase
(thyroperoxidase, a
thyroid enzyme)
trial prescription order

TPP thiamine pyrophosphate
thyrotoxic periodic
paralysis
transpyloric plane

TP&P time, place and person

TPPase thiamine pyrophosphatase

TPPD thoracic-pelvic-phalangeal
dystrophy (Jeume
syndrome)
tuberculin purified
protein derivative

TPPN total peripheral
parenteral nutrition

TPR temperature, pulse
and respiration
testosterone
production rate
total peripheral resistance

total pulmonary resistance
tubular phosphate
reabsorption

TPRI total peripheral
resistance index

TPS transverse pelvic septum
tumor polysaccharide
substance

TPST true positive stress test

TPT tension pneumothorax
third-party transfusion
time-to-peak tension
traumatic pneumothorax
treadmill performance test
typhoid-paratyphoid
(vaccine)

TPUR transperineal urethral
resection

TPVR total peripheral vascular
resistance

TQ tourniquet

TQM total quality management

TR recovery time
rectal temperature
therapeutic radiology
thyroid hormone receptor
time recovery
(recovery time)
time release (release time)
time to repeat
total resistance
total response
toxic reaction
trace
transfusion reaction
transmission risk
tricuspid regurgitation
tuberculin residue
tubular reabsorption
Tumor Registry

T(R) rectal temperature

T & R teaching and research
treated and released

Tr trace
trypsin (an enzyme of the
hydrolase class)

tr tincture

TRA therapeutic recreation
associate

thyrotropin
  receptor antibody
total renin activity
transaldolase
tumor-resistant antigen

TRAb thyrotoxin receptor
  antibody

trach trachea
tracheal
tracheostomy

TRAIU thyroid radioactive iodine
  uptake

TRALI transfusion-related acute
  lung injury

TRAM flap
  transverse rectus
    abdominis muscle flap

Trans transverse

Trans D transverse diameter

transpl transplantation

Trans Rx transfusion reaction

TRAP tartrate-resistant acid
  phosphatase

Trap trapezius (muscle)

TRAPs thyroid hormone receptor
  auxiliary proteins

trau trauma

TRBF total renal blood flow

TRC tanned red cell
Telemedicine Research
  Center
total renin concentration
triradiate cartilage (located
  where the primary
  ossification centers of the
  ilium, ischium and pubis
  meet in the developing
  immature hipbone)

TRCV total red cell volume

TRD tubular reabsorptive defect

TRDN transient respiratory
  distress of newborn

TRE thyroid response element
true radiation emission

TREA triethanolamine (an
  alkanolamine resulting
  from ammonolysis of
  ethylene oxide)

TRF T cell replacing factor

thermal regulatory failure
thyroid-stimulating-
  hormone releasing factor
thyrotropin-releasing
  factor

trf transfer

TRFC total rosette-forming cell

TRFR tubular rejection
  fraction ratio

TRH thyrotropin-releasing
  hormone

trh thyrotropin-releasing
  hormone

TRHST thyrotropin-releasing
  hormone stimulation test

TRI Toxic Chemical Release
  Inventory (database)
trimester
tubuloreticular inclusion

TRI 1 first trimester

TRI 2 second trimester

TRI 3 third trimester

T$_3$RIA serum triiodothyronine
  level by
  radioimmunoassay

T$_4$RIA serum thyroxine level by
  radioimmunoassay

TRIAC triiodothyroacetic acid

TRIC trachoma inclusion
  conjunctivitis
Trichomonas (a genus of
  parasitic protozoan
  flagellates)

TRICB trichlorobiphenyl

TRICH trichinosis
Trichomonas

TRIFACTS
  Toxic Chemical Release
    Inventory Facts
    (database)

Trig triglyceride (the major
  storage form of fatty acids
  and is practically the
  exclusive constitutent of
  adipose tissue)

Tris tris(hydroxymethyl)amino-
  methane

TRISS Trauma Related Injury
  Severity Score

trit triturate

TRIX total rate imaging with x-rays

TRJ total replacement of joint

TRK transketolase (an enzyme of the transferase class)

TRLP triglyceride-rich lipoprotein

TRMSMX trimethoprim-sulfamethoxazole

tRNA transfer ribonucleic acid
transfer RNA
transport ribonucleic acid

TRNBP transrectal needle biopsy of the prostate

TRNG tetracycline-resistant *Neisseria gonorrhoeae*

TRO temporary restraining order

Troch troche (lozenge)

TROM total (entire) range of motion

TROP MED tropical medicine

TRP total refractory period
tubular reabsorption of phosphate

Trp tryptophan (an essential amino acid)

TRPA tryptophan-rich prealbumin

TrPl treatment plan

TRPT theoretical renal phosphorus threshold
transplant

TRR total respiratory resistance

TRS the real symptom

TRT thermoradiotherapy

trt treatment

TRU transrectal ultrasound
turbidity reducing unit

T₃RU T_3RU triiodothyronine resin uptake

TRUs terminal respiratory units

TRUS transrectal ultrasonography
transrectal ultrasound

TRUSGPNB transrectal ultrasound guided prostatic nerve blockade

TRUSP transrectal ultrasonography of prostate

TRX transsexual

trx traction

TRY tryptophan (an essential amino acid)

TRZ triazolam (tranquilizer)

TS Takayasu's syndrome
telesurgery
temperature sensitive
tensile strength
test solution
thoracic spine
thoracic surgery
thumb-sucking
thyroid storm (thyrotoxic crisis)
Tietze's syndrome (costochondritis)
Tinel's sign (pain elicited by percussion over volar surface of wrist)
tobacco smoke
toe sign
total solids
Tourette's syndrome (Tourette's disorder)
toxic substance
transitional sleep
transsexual
transverse section
transverse sinus
transverse tubular system
trauma score
travel sickness
tricuspid (right atrioventricular) stenosis
trisomy 13 syndrome (Patau syndrome)
trisomy 18 syndrome (Edwards's syndrome)
trisomy 21 syndrome (Down's syndrome)
tropical sprue (disease occurring in certain tropical areas,

characterized by
abnormal small bowel
structure and
malabsorption; caused by
vitamin deficiencies and/
or bacterial
contamination of the
intestines)
Trousseau sign
T suppressor (cell)
tubal sterilization
tuberculous salpingitis
tuberous sclerosis
(Bourneville's disease)
Turner's syndrome
(gonadal dysgenesis
caused by the absence
of a sex chromosome:
45XO)

T-S trimethoprim-
sulfamethoxazole (used
in the treatment of
urinary tract infections)

T&S type and screen
Ts suppressor T cells
ts temperature sensitive
TSA tissue-specific antigens
toluene sulfonic acid (test)
total shoulder arthroplasty
total solute absorption
total spinal anesthesia
toxic shock antigen
tumor-specific antigen
tumor-surface antigen
type-specific antibody

T₄SA thyroxine-specific activity
TSAb thyroid-stimulating
antibodies

TSAP toxic shock-associated
protein

TSAS total severity
assessment score

TSAT tube slide
agglutination test

TSB Taylor spinal brace
total serum bilirubin
typtone soy broth

TSBB transtracheal selective
bronchial brushing

TSC technetium sulfur colloid
theophylline serum
concentration
thumb spica cast
transverse spinal sclerosis
T suppressor cell
tryptose-sulfite
cyclosterone

TSCA Toxic Substances
Control Act

TSCI traumatic spinal cord
injury

TSD target-skin distance
Tay-Sachs disease (inborn
error of metabolism)

TSE targeted systemic exposure
testicular self-examination
total skin examination
transmissible spongiform
encephalopathy

TSEB total skin electron beam
T-sect transverse section
(cross section)

TSEM transmission scanning
electron microscopy

T-set tracheotomy set
TSF testicular feminization
syndrome
thrombopoietic
stimulating factor
triceps skinfold (test)
tympanosquamous fissure

TSGP tumor-specific glycoprotein
TSGs tumor suppressor genes
TSH thyroid-stimulating
hormone (thyrotropin)
thyrotropin-stimulating
hormone
transient synovitis of hip

TSH-RH thyroid-stimulating
hormone-releasing
hormone

TSI tendon sheath
inflammation
thyroid-stimulating
immunoglobulin
triple sugar iron (agar)
trypanosomal infection

tSIDS totally unexplained sudden

infant death syndrome

TSL   tobacco smoke level

toxic substances list
(compiledby the National
Institute of Occupational
Safety and Health)

TSNB   transsacral nerve block

TSP   tobacco smoke pollution

total serum protein

total suspended particulate

trisodium phosphate

tropical spastic paraparesis

tsp   teaspoon (approximate
5 ml measurement)

TSPAP   total serum prostatic acid
phosphatase

T-spine   thoracic spine

T. spiralis   *Trichinella spiralis* (causative
agent of trichinosis)

TSPP   tetrasodium
pyrophosphate

TSR   thyroid to serum ratio

total shoulder replacement

T/S ratio   thyroid/serum iodide ratio

TSS   total serum solids

toxic shock syndrome

transverse spinal sclerosis

TSSA   tumor-specific (cell)
surface antigen

TSSE   toxic shock syndrome
exotoxin

TSST-1   toxic shock syndrome
toxin-1

TST   terminal sulcus of tongue

tobacco smoke tar
(polycyclic hydrocarbons)

total sleep time

treadmill stress test

tuberculin skin test

tumor skin test

TSTA   tumor-specific
transplantation antigen

TSV   total stomach volume

TT   tactile tension

temper tantrum

tendon transfer

test tube

tetanus toxoid

theophylline toxicity

thoracic trunk

thrombin time

thrombolytic therapy

tibial torsion

tibial tubercle

tick toxicosis

tilt table

tine test

toilet tissue

toilet training

tolerance test

tongue-tied

total thyroxine

total time

transfusion therapy

transient tachypnea

transtibial (below-knee
amputation)

transtracheal

Trendelenburg's test

Trichuris trichiura
(whipworm)

tuberculin test

tympanic temperature

tympanostomy tube

typhoidal tularemia

TT$_2$ total diiodothyronine

TT$_3$ total triiodothyronine

TT$_4$ total thyroxine

T & T   time and temperature

touch and tone

TTA   tetanus toxoid antibody

total toe arthroplasty

transtracheal aspiration

TTAP   threaded titanium
acetabular prosthesis

TTB   test tube baby

TTC   thyrotoxic crisis

transtracheal catheter

triphenyltetrazolium
chloride

T-tube cholangiogram

TTD   temporary total disability

tissue tolerance dose

transient tic disorder

TTE   transthoracic
echocardiography

TTH   tension-type headache

thyrotropic hormone

tritiated thymidine

TTI tension-time index

TTJ transverse tarsal joint
(Chopart's joint)

TTJV transtracheal jet ventilation

TTL total thymus lymphocytes

TTLC true total lung capacity

TTM tensor tympani muscle

TTN transient tachypnea
of newborn

TTNA transthoracic needle
aspiration

TTNB transient tachypnea
of newborn
transthoracic needle biopsy

TTO to take out

TTOT transtracheal oxygen
therapy

TTP thrombotic
thrombocytopenic
purpura
thymidine triphosphate
time to peak
transtubercular plane

TTPA triethylene
thiophosphoramide

TTR triceps tendon reflex

T. trichiura
Trichuris trichiuria
(whipworm)

TTS tarsal tunnel syndrome
(entrapment neuropathy
of posterior tibial nerve
at ankle beneath the
flexor retinaculum)
temporary threshold shift
through the skin
transdermal therapeutic
system
twin transfusion syndrome

TTT tilt table test
tolbutamide tolerance test
total tourniquet time
tuberculin time test
two-tail test (to determine
any difference between
the variable)

TTTS twin-twin
transfusion syndrome

TTTT test tube turbidity test

T tube tracheostomy tube

TTUGP transabdominal/
transvesical ultrasonically
guided puncture

TTV transfusion-transmitted
virus

TTVP temporary transvenous
pacemaker

TTWB toe touch weight bearing

TTx tetrodotoxin (lethal
neurotoxic substance
found in puffer fish
and newts)

TTYs teletypewriters
text telephones

TU thiouracil
thyroid uptake
toxic unit
transurethral
tuberculin unit

TUBD transurethral balloon
dilatation

tub lig tubal ligation

TUD total urethral discharge

TUE transurethral extraction

TUER transurethral
electroresection

TUI transurethral incision

TUIBN transurethral incision of
the bladder neck

TUIP transurethral incision of
prostate

TULIP transurethral ultrasound-
guided laser-induced
prostatectomy

TUMT transurethral microwave
thermotherapy (causes
diminution of overgrown
prostate)

TUNA transurethral needle
ablation

T$_3$UP triiodothyronine uptake

TUR transurethral resection

T$_3$UR triiodothyronine uptake
ratio

TURB transurethral resection
of bladder

turb turbidity

TUR-BN transurethral resection bladder neck

TUR-BT transurethral resection bladder tumor

TURP transurethral resection of the prostate

turp turpentine

tus. *tussis* [Latin] a cough

TUU transurethroureterectomy

TUV transurethral valve

TUWB timed uterine-wall biopsy

TV talipes varus (foot deformity)

tibia valga (bowing of the leg)

tibia vara (Blount's disease)

tickborne virus

tidal volume

total volume

transport vesicle

transvestite

trial visit

tricuspid (right atrioventricular) valve

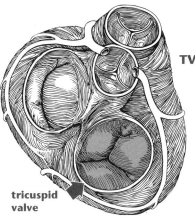

TV

tricuspid valve

true vertebra

tuberculin volutin

T. vaginalis

Trichomonas vaginalis (causative agent of inflammation in the urinary tract of men and in the vagina of women)

TVC timed vital capacity

total vital capacity

total volume capacity

transvaginal cone

triple-voiding cystogram

true vocal cord

TVCs tricuspid (right atrioventricular)-valve cusps

TVD transmissible virus dementia

TVF tactile vocal fremitus

TVH total vaginal hysterectomy

transvaginal hysterectomy

turkey viral hepatitis

TVI tricuspid (right atrioventricular)-valve insufficiency

TVP tensor veli palatini (muscle)

transvenous pacemaker

tricuspid (right atrioventricular)-valve prolapse

TVPM tensor veli palatini muscle

TVR total vascular resistance

tricuspid valve replacement

TVS transvaginal sonography

TVT tunica vaginalis testis

TVU total volume of urine (passed in 24 hours)

TVUS transvaginal ultrasonography

TVV transmissable venereal virus

TW tapeworm (segmented worm)

tapwater

threadworm (*Strongyloides stercoralis*)

total body water

trichina worm (*Trichinella spiralis*)

TWA time-weighted average

T wave an upward deflection of the ECG cycle from the end of the S-T segment to the beginning of the U wave

TW

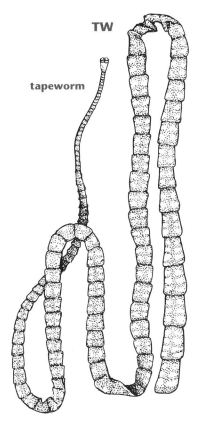

tapeworm

TWBC	total white blood count
TWD	tobacco workers' disease
	total white and differential count
TWE	tapwater enema
TWG	total weight gain
TWiST	time without symptoms of toxicity
TWR	total wrist replacement
TWS	tranquilizer withdrawal syndrome
TWWD	tap water wet dressing
TWZ	triangular working zone
T & X	type and crossmatch

TX	therapy
	thromboxane (compound isolated from platelets; related to the prostaglandins, but more potent in some biologic activities, such as smooth muscle contraction and platelet aggregation)
	traction
	transplant
	treatment
	tuberous xanthoma
	tympanostomy
tx	traction
TxA	thromboxane (compound isolated from platelets; related to prostaglandins, but more potent in some biologic activities, such as smooth muscle contraction and platelet aggregation)
TXA$_2$	thromboxane A$_2$
TXB$_2$	thromboxane B$_2$
TXDS	qualifying toxic dose
TXN	traction
Ty	typhoid
Tyl	tylenol
	tyloma (a callus)
Tylenol #3	
	Tylenol with 30 mg of codeine
Tymp	tympanic
TY-NEG	tyrosinase-negative
typ	typical
TY-POS	tyrosinase-positive
Tyr	tyrosine (an essential amino acid)
TyRIA	thyroid radioisotope assay
TZ	transition zone

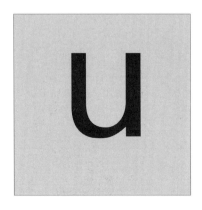

U congenital limb absence
ulcer
ulna
umbilicus
unerupted
unit (international)
unknown
upper
uracil
uranium (radioactive
  metallic element)
urea
ureter
urethra

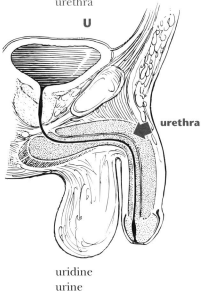

U

urethra

uridine
urine
uterus

utricle
uvula

U/1 one finger breadth below
  the navel (umbilicus)
1/U one finger breadth above
  the navel (umbilicus)
u atomic mass unit
  unit
UA ultrasonic arteriography
  umbilical artery
  unaggregated
  uncertain about
  unstable angina
  uremic acidosis
  uric acid
  urinalysis
  urinary aldosterone
  urine amylase
  upper airway
  upper arm
  uterine aspiration
U/A urinalysis
UAB upper airway burns
UAC umbilical artery
  catheterization
  upper airway congestion
  uric acid
UA/C uric acid to
  creatinine (ratio)
UAD upper airway disorder
UAE unilateral absence
  of excretion
  urinary albumin excretion
UAN uric acid nephropathy
UAO upper airway obstruction
UAP unstable angina pectoris
  urinary acid phosphatase
  urinary alkaline
  phosphatase
UAR upper airway resistance
UAS uric acid stone
UASD uric acid stone disease
UAT up as tolerated
UAV umbilical artery
  velocimetry
UAVC univentricular
  atrioventricular
  connection
UB urinary bladder

UBA	undenatured bacterial antigen
UBC	University of British Columbia (orthopedic brace)
UBF	uterine blood flow
UBG	urobilinogen (formed in the intestines by the reduction of bilirubin; found in large amounts in feces and in small amounts in urine)
UBI	ultraviolet blood irradiation
UBL	undifferentiated B-cell lymphoma
UBM	ultrasound biomicroscopy
UBO	unidentified bright object (cerebral)
UBSL	unilateral brainstem lesion
UBT	urea breath test uterine balloon therapy
UBW	usual body weight
UC	ulcerative colitis umbilical cord unchanged

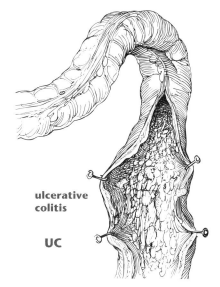

ulcerative colitis

UC

unclassifiable
unsatisfactory condition
urea clearance
uremic syndrome
ureteral colic
urethral catheterization
urethrocele

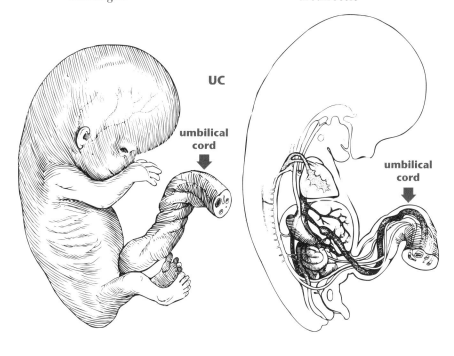

UC

umbilical cord

umbilical cord

urinary calculi
urinary catheter
urine creatinine
urine culture
uterine contraction
U&C usual and customary
u cats urinary catecholamines
UCB umbilical cord blood
(fetal blood)
unconjugated bilirubin
UCBC umbilical cord blood
culture
UCC umbilical cord clamp
UCD urine collection device
usual childhood diseases
UCG unilateral congenital
glaucoma
urinary chorionic
gonadotropin (test
for pregnancy)
UCHD usual childhood diseases
UCHI usual childhood illnesses
UCI umbilical coiling index
unusual childhood illness
urethral catheter in
UCL ulnar collateral ligament
(connects the styloid
process of the ulna to the
carpal bones of the wrist)
uncomfortable loudness
(level)
urea clearance (test)
UCLS ulnar collateral ligament
sprain
UCO urinary catheter out
UCOD underlying cause of death
UCP urethral closure pressure
urinary coproporphyrin
urinary C-peptide
UCPA United Cerebral Palsy
Association
UCPT urinary coproporphyrin
test
UCR unconditioned reflex
unconditioned response
usual, customary and
reasonable (applied to
plans and fees)
UCRE urine creatinine

UCS unconditioned stimulus
unconscious
unicoronal synostosis
uterine compression
syndrome
ucs unconscious
uCTD undifferentiated
connective tissue disease
UD ulcerative dermatosis
ulnar deviation
undetermined
unit dose
urethral dilatation
urethral discharge
urethral diverticulum
uridine diphosphate
uroporphyrinogen
decarboxylase
uterine distention
u.d. *ud dictum* [Latin]
as directed
UDC usual diseases of childhood
UDCA ursodeoxycholic acid
UDD ulnar drift deformity
UDDA Uniform Determination of
Death Act
UDE undetermined etiology
UDMH unsymmetrical dimethyl
hydrazine
UDN ulcerative dermal necrosis
UDO undetermined origin
UDP uridine diphosphate (a
nucleotide that serves as
a carrier in the synthesis
of glycogen,
glycoproteins and
glycosaminoglycans)
UDPG uridine diphosphoglucose
UDPGA uridine diphospho-
glucuronic acid
UDP-Gal uridine diphospho-
galactose
UDP-galactose
uridine diphospho-
galactose
UDP-Glc uridine diphosphate
glucose
UDP-glucose
uridine diphosphoglucose

UDP-glucuronate
    uridine diphospho-
      glucuronate
UDP-Gly uridine
    diphosphoglycogen
UDP-glycogen
    uridine diphospho-
      glycogen
UDPG p'tase
    uridine diphosphoglucose
      pyrophosphatase
UDPGT uridine diphospho-
    glucuronyl transferase
UDRP urine diribose phosphate
UDS ultra-Doppler sonography
    unconditioned stimuli
UDSD urinary-detrusor-sphincter
    dyssynergia
UDSMR uniform data system for
    medical rehabilitation
UDT undescended testicle
UDV under direct vision
UE uncertain etiology
    upper esophagus
    upper extremity
UEES upper extremity
    entrapment syndrome
UEG ultrasonic
    encephalography
UEO ureteroenterostomy

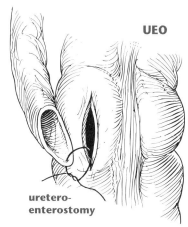

UEO

uretero-
enterostomy

UEP uremic encephalopathy
UES upper esophageal
    sphincter

UEV urinary extravasation
u/ex upper extremity
UF ultrafiltration
    ultrasonic frequency
    unexplained fever
    unknown factor
    urinary frequency
UFA unesterified (free)
    fatty acid
UFB urinary fat bodies
UFCT ultrafast computed
    tomography (scan)
UFCTEBT
    ultrafast CT electron beam
    tomography
UFD unilateral facet dislocation
UFF unusual facial features
UFH unfractionated heparin
UFN until further notified
UFR ultrafiltration rate
    urine filtration rate
UFS ultraflex stent
uFSH urinary follicle-stimulating
    hormone
UFV ultrafiltration volume
UG until gone
    urogenital (genitourinary)
UGA under general anesthesia
UGCC ultrasound-guided
    compression closure
UGD urogenital diaphragm
UGF urinary gonadotropin
    fragment
    urinary gonadotropin
    factor
UGH upper gastrointestinal
    hemorrhage
    uveitis, glaucoma and
    hyphema (syndrome)
UGI upper gastrointestinal
    (tract)
UGI bleeding
    upper gastrointestinal
    bleeding
UGI series
    upper gastrointestinal
    series
UGIB upper gastrointestinal
    bleeding

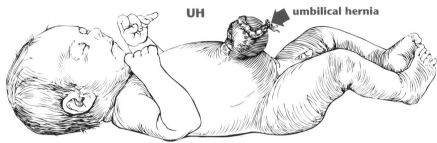

UH — umbilical hernia

UGIH	upper gastro-intestinal hemorrhage
UGIS	upper gastrointestinal series
UGS	urogenital sinus
UGT	ulceroglandular tularemia
	urogenital tuberculosis
UH	umbilical hernia
	upper half
U24H	24 hour urine specimen
UHD	unstable hemoglobin disease
UHDDS	Uniform Hospital Discharge Data Set
UHF	ultra high frequency
UHMWP	ultra high molecular weight
UHT	ultra high temperature
UI	unidentified
	urge incontinence
	urinary incontinence
	uroporphyrin isomerase
U/I	unidentified
UIBC	unbound iron-binding capacity
	unsaturated iron-binding capacity
UICC	International Union against Cancer (Geneva)
u.i.d.	*uno in die* [Latin] once every day
UIF	undegraded insulin factor
UIP	usual interstitial pneumonitis
UIQ	upper inner quadrant
UIS	uroporphyrinogen I synthetase
UK	unknown
	urokinase
UKa	urinary kallikrein

	(proteolytic enzyme that cleaves kininogens to form kinins and activates plasminogen; found in various body fluids including urine)
UL	ultrasonic
	Underwriters Laboratories
	undifferentiated lymphoma
	upper lid (eyelid)
	upper limb
	upper lobe
U/L	upper and lower
U & L	upper and lower
ULBW	ultra low birth weight
ULC	ulnar longitudinal crease (of palm)
ULDH	urinary lactate dehydrogenase
ULFUSW	ultra low-frequency ultrasound waves
ULL	uncomfortable loudness level
ULLE	upper lid of left eye
ULN	upper limits of normal
	ureteral lymph node
uln	ulna
ULNS	upper limits of normal size
ULPE	upper lobe pulmonary edema
ULQ	upper left quadrant (of breast)
ULRE	upper lid of right eye
ULSB	upper left sternal boder
ULT	ultra high temperature
ult. praes.	
	ultimum praescriptus [Latin] last prescribed
UM	unmarried

uracil mustard

UMA urinary muramidase
(lysozyme) activity

Umax maximum urinary
osmolality

Umb umbilical
umbilicus

Umb A umbilical artery

Umb V umbilical vein

UMCD uremic medullary
cystic disease

UMI unstable myocardial
ischemia
urinary meconium index

UML unmedicated labor

UMLS United Medical
Language System

UMN upper motor neuron

UMNB upper motor neurogenic
bladder

UMNL upper motor neuron lesion

UMP uridine monophosphate

UMPK uridine monophosphate
kinase

UN ulnar nerve
undernourished
unilateral neglect
urate nephropathy
urea nitrogen

UNA urinary nitrogen
appearance

UNa sodium excretion in urine

UNCOR uncorrected

undet undetermined

UNES ulnar nerve entrapment
syndrome

UNESCO United Nations
Educational, Scientiic,
and Cutural Organization

UNG uracil-N-glycosylase

ung. *unguentum* [Latin] ointment

UNICEF United Nations
International Children's
Emegency Fund

UNID unidentified

unil unilateral

unilat unilateral

UNIV university

univ universal

university

UNK unknown

unk unknown

UNL upper normal limit

UNOS United Network for
Organ Sharing

UNP ulnar nerve palsy

UNRRO United Nations Relief
and Rehabilitation
Organization

uns unsatisfactory

unt untreated

UNX uninephrectomy

UO under observation
ureteral orifice
urinary obstruction
urine output

U/O urine output

u/o under observation

UOA United Ostomy Association

UOD ulnar oligodactyly

UOP urinary output

UOQ upper outer quadrant (of
breast)

Uosm urinary osmolality

UP ulcerative proctitis
unipolar
upright position
upright posture
uremic pleuritis
uremic pneumonitis
urethral prolapse
uridine phosphorylase
uroporphyrin
urticaria pigmentosa
uterine prolapse
uteropelvic

U/P ratio of urine to plasma

UPB Unna's paste boot (a rigid
dressing for varicose
ulcers)

UPC unipolar cell

UPEP urine protein
electrophoresis

UPF upper palpebral furrow
uveoparotid fever

upf universal proximal femur
(prosthesis)

UPG uroporphyrinogen

upper palpebral furrow **UPF**

UPI	uteroplacental insufficiency
	uteroplacental ischemia
UPJ	ureteropelvic junction
UPL	unusual position of limbs
UPOR	usual place of residence
UPP	urethral pressure profile
	uvulopalatoplasty
UPPP	uvulopalatopharyngoplasty
U/P ratio	
	urine-to-plasma concentration ratio
UPS	ureteropelvic stenosis
UPT	urine pregnancy test
UQ	upper quadrant
UR	unconditioned reflex
	unconditioned response
	upper respiratory
	uridine (a ribonucleoside containing uracil)
	urinal
	urinary retention
	urine
	utilization review
Ur	urine
Ura	uracil (pyrimidine component seen in nucleic acid)
URAC	uric acid
URAP	urinary retention with acute pain
URC	utilization review committee
URD	undifferentiated respiratory disease
	upper respiratory disease
Urd	uridine (a ribonucleoside containing uracil)
Ureth	urethra
URF	uterine-relaxing factor (relaxin)
urg	urgent
URI	upper respiratory (tract) infection
URL	Uniform Resource Locator (World Wide Web browser to open the Internet Grateful Med)
url	unrelated
URO	urology
	uroporphyrin (a porphyrin, usually found in small amounts in the urine)
	uroporphyrinogen
Uro-Gen	urogenital
Urol	urology
URQ	upper right quadrant
URR	urea reduction ratio
URS	ultrasonic renal scanning
URSB	upper right sternal border
URT	upper respiratory tract
URTI	upper respiratory tract infection
URV	urine residual volume
US	ultrasonography
	ultrasound
	unconditioned stimulus
	unique sequence
	ureteric stone
	urethral stent (to treat recurrent bulbomembranous urethral strictures)
	urethral stricture
	urinary space
	urinary sugar
	Usher syndrome
U/S	ultrasound
USAH	United States Army Hospital
USAN	United States Adopted Name (Council)
USAP	unstable angina pectoris
USB	unsafe sexual behavior
	upper sternal border

USBS	United States Bureau of Standards	**USW**	ultrashort waves
USC	usual states of consciousness	**UT**	undescended testis untreated
USCC	ulcerated squamous cell carcinoma		urinary tract uterine tube
USDA	United States Department of Agriculture		uterus
USDHHS	United States Department of Health and Human Services	**Ut**	uterus
		uT	unbound testosterone
		UTBG	unbound thyroxine-binding globulin
USE	ultrasonic echography	**UTC**	upper thoracic compression
USG	ultrasonography		urinary tract calculus
USGB	ultrasound-guided biopsy	**UTD**	up-to-date
USGC	urinary space of glomerular capsule	**ut dict.**	*ut dictum* [Latin] as directed
USI	urinary stress incontinence	**UTF**	usual throat flora
USL	uterosacral ligament	**utend.**	*utendus* [Latin] to be used
USLT	uterosacral ligament transection	**UTI**	urinary tract infection
		UTJ	uterotubal junction
USMLE	United States Medical Licensing Examination	**UTO**	unable to obtain urinary tract obstruction upper tibial osteotomy
USN	ultrasonic nebulizer		
USNH	United States Naval Hospital	**UTP**	unilateral tension pneumothorax
USO	unilateral salpingo-oophorectomy		uridine triphosphate (a nucleotide required for RNA synthesis)
USP	*United States Pharmacopeia*		
USPC	United States Pharmacopeial Convention	**UTS**	ulnar tunnel syndrome (pressure on the ulnar nerve within Guyon's canal at the wrist)
USPDI	United States Pharmacopeia Drug Information		
			ultimate tensile strength
USPHS	United States Public Health Service	**ut supr.**	*ut supra* [Latin] as above
		UTV	unable to void
USP PRN		**UU**	urinary urgency urine urobilinogen
	United States Pharmacopeia Practitioners' Reporting Network	**UUN**	urinary urea nitrogen
		UUO	unilateral ureteral obstruction
USPTA	United States Physical Therapy Association	**UUP**	urinary uroporphyrin
USR	unheated serum reagin (test)	**UV**	ultraviolet light (portion of spectrum between 10 and 400 nm)
USRDR	US Renal Disease Registry		umbilical vein
USS	ultrasound scanning		Uppsala virus
UST	ultrasound therapy		urine volume
USVMD	urine specimen volume measuring device	**UVA**	ultraviolet light A (portion of spectrum

	between 320 and 400 nm)
	ureterovesical angle
UVB	ultraviolet light B (portion of spectrum between 290 and 320 nm) (sunburn spectrum)
UVC	ultraviolet light C (portion of spectrum between 10 and 290 nm)

	umbilical vein catherization
UVF	urethrovaginal fistula uterovaginal fascia
UVJ	ureterovesical junction
UVL	ultraviolet light
UVP	ultraviolet photometry
UVR	ultraviolet radiation
UWB	unit of whole blood
UWD	Urbach-Wiethe's disease

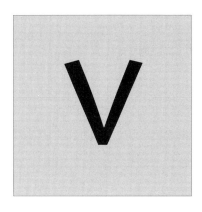

V gas volume
vagina
valine (an essential
amino acid)
vanadium (a rare metallic
element)
variable (any event,
phenomenon, or
attribute that can have
different values)
velocity
ventilation
ventral
verbal
vertex
vinyl
virgin
virus
vision
voice
volt
voltage
volume (measurement)
vomer
vomiting

V₁ ECG placement of
precordial chest lead at
right sternal border (4th
intercostal space)

V₂ ECG placement of
precordial chest lead at
left sternal border (4th
intercostal space)

V₃ ECG placement of

precordial chest lead
between V2 and V4

V₄ ECG placement of
precordial chest lead at
midclacivular line (5th
intercostal space)

V₅ ECG placement of
precordial chest lead at
anterior axillary line

V₆ ECG placement of
precordial chest lead at
midaxillary line

3rd V third ventricle
4th V fourth ventricle

v valve
vein
velocity
ventilation
ventral
ventricular
vision
vitamin
voice
volt
volume (measurement)
vomiting

v. *vena* [Latin] vein
vide [Latin] see

VA vacuum aspiration
valproic acid
variant angina
(Prinzmetal's angina)
vasodilator agent
ventricular aneurysm
ventricular arrest
ventricular arrhythmia
ventriculoatrial
vertebral artery
Veterans Administration
vinca alkaloids
viral antigen
viral arthritis
visual acuity

V-A ventriculoatrial

Vₐ alveolar gas volume
alveolar ventilation

VAA Vaccination Assistance Act
visual associated area

VAB vinblastine + actinomycin

D (dactinomycin) + bleomycin (combination chemotherapy)

violent antisocial behavior

VAC vincristine + actinomycin D (dactinomycin) + cyclophosphamide (combination chemotherapy)

vincristine + Adriamycin (doxorubicin) + cyclophosphamide (combination chemotherapy)

vac vacant (beds)

vacuum

vacc vaccination

VAC EXT vacuum extractor

VACTERL vertebral, anal, cardiac. tracheal, esophageal, renal and limb (a pattern of associated congenital anomalies)

VAD venous access device

ventricular assist device

vincristine + Adriamycin (doxorubicin) + dexamethasone (combination chemotherapy)

vitamin A deficiency

VAE venous air embolism

Vag vagina

vaginal

VAG HYST

vaginal hysterectomy

VAH vertebral ankylosing hyperostosis

Veterans Administration Hospital

VAIN vaginal intraepithelial neoplasm

Val valine (an essential amino acid)

Valium (tranquilizer diazepam)

VALE visual acuity, left eye

VAM ventricular arrhythmia monitor

VAMP vincristine + actinomycin D (dactinomycin) + methotrexate + prednisone (combination chemotherapy)

VAMC Veterans Affairs Medical Center

VAMP vincristine + actinomycin D (dactinomycin) + methotrexate + prednisone (combination chemotherapy)

VAN vulvar acanthosis nigrans

VAP variant angina pectoris

ventilator-associated pneumonia

vincristine + Adriamycin + prednisone (combination chemotherapy)

VAPE vincristine + Adriamycin + prednisone + etoposide (combination chemotherapy)

VAPP vaccine-associated paralytic poliomyelitis

VAPSV volume-assured pressure support ventilation

var variant

varicose

VARE visual acuity, right eye

VAS valvular aortic stenosis

vas deferens (deferent duct)

video assisted surgery

viral arthritis syndrome

vas vas deferens (deferent duct)

vasectomy

VASC Verbal-Auditory Screen Test for Children

Visual-Auditory Screen Test for Children

vasc vascular

VAS RAD vascular radiology

vas x vasectomy

VAT variable antigen type

video-assist thoracoscopy

visual apperception test

vocational

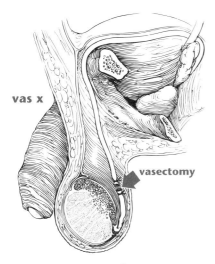

vas x

vasectomy

apperception test
voice-activated
transcription

VATER vertebral defects, anal
atresia,
tracheoesophageal fistula,
esophageal atresia, renal
anomalies (a pattern of
associated congenital
anomalies)

VATH vinblastine + Adriamycin
(doxorubicin) + thiotepa
+ halotensin
(combination
chemotherapy)

VATS video-assisted thoracic
surgery

VAV vegetations on aortic valve

VAVP valine arginine vasopressin

VB valence bond
van Buren (catheter)
Velpeau bandage
venous blood
vertebral body
ventricular bradycardia
ventrobasal (complex)
viable birth
vinblastine (antineoplastic
agent)
vitreous body
voided bladder

VB₁ first voided urine specimen

VB₂ second midstream
urine specimen

VBAC vaginal birth after
(previous) Cesarean
section

VBAP vincristine + BCNU
(carmustine) +
Adriamycin
(doxorubicin) +
prednisone (combination
chemotherapy)

VBC Verbrugge bone clamp (to
facilitate acetabular
fracture repair)
vincristine + bleomycin +
cisplatin (combination
chemotherapy)

VBD vector-borne disease

VBG venous blood gas
venous bypass graft
vertical banded
gastroplasty

VBI vector-borne infection
vertebrobasilar
insufficiency

Vbl vinblastine (antineoplastic
agent)

VBM vinblastine + bleomycin +
methotrexate
(combination
chemotherapy)

VBP ventricular premature beat
vinblastine + bleomycin +
Platinol (cisplatin)
(combination
chemotherapy)

VBS veronal-buffered saline
vertebrobasilar system

VC color vision
vascular claudication
vasoconstriction
vena cava
ventilatory capacity
ventricular contraction
vertebral canal
vertebral column
videocassette
vincristine
(antineoplastic agent)

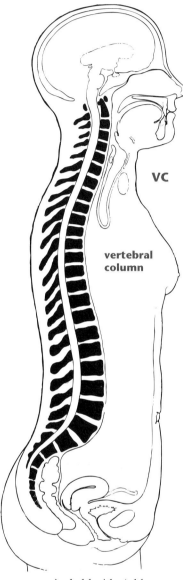

VC

vertebral column

blood volume

VCA vasoconstrictor assay
viral capsid antibody
viral capsid antigen

VCAM-1 vascular cell adhesion
molecule 1 (enhances
leukocyte adhesion to
wall of blood vessel)

VCAP vincristine +
cyclophosphamide
+Adriamycin
(doxorubicin) +
prednisone (combination
chemotherapy)

vCBF venous cerebral blood flow

VCDF volume-cycled
decelerating-flow
(ventilation)

VCF vaginal contraceptive film

VCG vectorcardiogram
vectorcardiography
voiding cystography

V. cholerae
Vibrio cholerae (a comma-
shaped bacterial rod
causing Asiatic cholera)

VCM vertebrocostal muscle

VCMP vincristine +
cyclophosphamide +
melphalan + prednisone
(combination
chemotherapy)

VCN vestibulocochlear nerve
(8th cranial nerve)
Vibrio cholerae
neuraminidase

V_{CO_2} carbon dioxide output

VCP vincristine +
cyclophosphamide +
prednisone (combination
chemotherapy)

VCR videocassette recorder

Vcr vincristine sulfate
(leurocristine)

VCS vincristine sulfate
(leurocristine)

VCSA viral cell surface antigen

VCSF ventricular cerebrospinal fluid

vinyl chloride (old name
for chloroethene)
visual cortex
vital capacity
vitamin capsule
vocal cords
Volkmann's contracture
vomiting center
vulvar carcinoma

Vc pulmonary capillary

VCT	venous clotting time
VCU	voiding cystourethrogram
	voiding
	cystourethrography
VCUG	voiding cystourethrogram
	voiding
	cystourethrography
VD	vaginal delivery
	vasodilation
	vasodilator
	venereal disease
	Venn diagram (graphical
	representation of the
	extent to which two or
	more quantities or
	concepts are mutually
	inclusive and mutually
	exclusive)
	venous distention
	ventricular dilator
	vertical deviation
	vestibular dysfunction
	Vigilon dressing
	(polyethylene occlusive
	dressing)
	Vincent's disease
	(trench mouth)
	viral diarrhea
	voided
	voiding dysfunction
	Volkman deformity
	volume of distribution
	vulvar dysplasia
V&D	vomiting and diarrhea
VD	volume of dead air space
	volume of distribution
Vd	voided
VDA	venous digital angiogram
	visual discriminatory acuity
VDBR	volume of distribution of
	bilirubin
VDAC	vaginal delivery after
	Cesarean section
	voltage-dependent anion
	channel
VDD	vitamin D deficiency
VDDR	vitamin D-dependent
	rickets
VDF	ventricular diastolic

	fragmentation
VDG	venereal disease –
	gonorrhea
Vdg	voiding
VDH	valvular disease of
	the heart
	vascular disease of
	the heart
VD HL	Venereal Disease Hotline
	(800) 227-8922
VDL	vasodepressor lipid
	visual detection level
VDM	vasodepressing material
VDP	ventricular demand
	pacemaker
VDRL	Venereal Disease Research
	Laboratory (test) for
	syphilis
VDRR	vitamin D-resistant rickets
VDS	venereal disease –
	syphilis vindesine
	(antineoplastic agent)
VDT	video display terminal
VDV	ventricular end-diastolic
	volume
VE	vaccine efficacy
	vaginal examination
	vallecula epiglottica
	Venezuelan encephalitis
	ventilatory equivalent
	vertex
	viral encephalitis
	visual efficiency
	volumic ejection
VE	minute volume
	(expired air)
Ve	ventilation
VEA	vaccine efficacy analysis
	ventricular ectopic
	arrhythmia
VEB	ventricular ectopic beat
VEC	vaginal estrogen cream
VECG	vector electrocardiogram
VED	vacuum erection device
	vacuum extraction delivery
VEDV	ventricular end-diastolic
	volume (preload)
VEE	Venezuelan equine
	encephalitis

	Venezuelan equine encephalomyelitis
VEEV	Venezuelan equine encephalomyelitis virus
VEF	visually evoked field
VEGAS	ventricular enlargement with gait apraxia syndrome
VEGF	vascular endothelial growth factor
vel	velocity
VEM	vaso-exciting material
VENT	ventilator
	ventral
	ventricular
vent	ventral
	ventricle
	ventricular
vent fib	ventricular fibrillation
VEP	visually evoked potential
VER	ventricular escape rhythm
	visual-evoked response
	visually evoked response
vert	vertebra
VES	ventricular extrasystole
	vesicular
	viscoelastic substance
vesic.	*vesicula* [Latin] blister
VET	vacuum erection technology
	veteran
Vet	veterinarian
VF	unipolar left leg (electrocardiographic lead)
	ventricular fibrillation
	ventricular flutter
	vertebral foramen
	visual field
	vitreous fluorophotometry
	vocal fremitus
	Volkman fracture
vf	visual field
VFA	volatile fatty acid
VFD	visual fields
VFF	valley fever fungus
VFI	visual fields intact
VFI	ventricular flutter
VFIB	ventricular fibrillation

VFL	ventricular flutter
VFP	ventricular fluid pressure
VFR	voiding flow rate
VFS	vascular fragility syndrome
VFT	venous filling time
VG	vein graft
	ventricular gallop
	very good
	viral gastroenteritis
	volume of gas
vGD	von Gierke's disease (glycogen storage disease)
VGE	viral gastroenteritis
VGH	very good health
VGM	venous graft myringoplasty
VH	vaginal hysterectomy
	vascular headache
	venous hematocrit
	ventricular hypertrophy
	viral hepatitis
	visually handicapped
	vitreous humor
VHA	Veterans Health Administration
VHD	valvular heart disease
VHDL	very high density lipoprotein
VHF	very high frequency
	viral hemorrhagic fever
VHL gene	
	von Hippel–Lindau gene
VHS	viral hemorrhagic septicemia
VI	vaginal irritation
	valvular insufficiency
	variable interval
	vascular insufficiency
	viral infection
	virtual image
	virulent
	viscosity index
	visual impairment
	volume index
Vi	virulent
VIA	viral inactivating agent
vib	vibration
VIBS	Victim's Information Bureau Services

vic.	*vices* [Latin] times
VICA	velocity (of blood in) internal carotid artery
VI-CTS	vibration-induced carpal tunnel syndrome
VID	videodensitometry
VIEN	vaginal intraepithelial neoplasia
	vulvar intraepithelial neoplasia
VIF	virus-induced interferon
VIG	vaccinia immune globulin
VIM	video intensification microscopy
VIN	vaginal intraepithelial neoplasia
	vulvar intraepithelial neoplasia
VIN I	vulvar intraepithelial neoplasia, mild (with mild dysplasia)
VIN II	vulvar intraepithelial neoplasia, moderate (with moderate dysplasia)
VIN III	vulvar intraepithelial neoplasia, severe (with severe dysplasia)
vin.	*vinum* [Latin] wine
VIP	vasoactive intestinal peptide
	vasoactive intestinal polypeptide
	vasoinhibitory peptide
	vasointestinal peptide

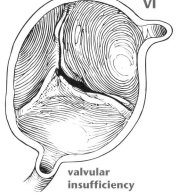

VI

valvular
insufficiency

	venous impedance plethysmography
	very important patient
	very important person
	vinblastine + ifosfamide + Platinol (cisplatin) (combination chemotherapy)
	voluntary interruption of pregnancy
VIPoma	vasoactive intestinal peptide apudomas (pancreatic cholera)
VIQ	verbal intelligence quotient
	verbal IQ
VIR	virology
Vir	virus
VIS	vaginal irrigation smear
	Vegetarian Information Service
	venous insufficiency syndrome
	visual information storage
vis	vision
VISC	vitreous infusion suction cutter
visc	viscera
VISI	volar-flexed intercalated segment instability
VISN	Veterans Integrated Service Network
VIT	venom immunotherapy
Vit	vitamin
vit	vital
	vitamin
vit B$_1$	vitamin B$_1$ (thiamin)
vit B$_2$	vitamin B$_2$ (riboflavin)
vit B$_3$	vitamin B$_3$ (niacin)
vit B$_6$	vitamin B$_6$ (pyridoxine)
vit B$_{12}$	vitamin B$_{12}$ (cyanocobalamin)
vit C	vitamin C (ascorbic acid)
vit D	vitamin D (calciferol)
vit D$_2$	vitamin D$_2$ (ergocalciferol)
vit D$_3$	vitamin D$_3$ (cholecalciferol)
vit E	vitamin E (alpha-tocopherol)

vit G	vitamin G (vitamin B$_2$; riboflavin)
vit H	vitamin H (biotin)
vit K	vitamin K (has critical role in clotting of blood)
vit K$_1$	vitamin K$_1$ (phytonadione)
vit K$_2$	vitamin K$_2$ (menaquinone)
vit K$_3$	vitamin K$_3$ (menadione)
vit M	vitamin M (folic acid)
vit PP	vitamin PP (nicotinic acid)
VIU	visual internal urethrotomy
viz	*videlicet* [Latin] namely
VKC	vernal keratoconjunctivitis
VKH	Vogt-Koyanagi-Harada (syndrome)
VL	left arm unipolar (electrocardio-graphic lead)
	ventrolateral
	vestibular labyrinth
	vial
	visceral leishmaniasis
VLA	very late activation (antigen)
	very late antigen
	virus-like agent
VLAP	video laser ablation of prostate
VLBW	very low birth weight
VLCD	very low calorie diet
VLD	very low density
VLDL	very low-density lipoprotein (densities of 0.95–1.006)
VLF	very low frequency
VLH	ventrolateral nucleus of hypothalamus
VLM	visceral larva migrans (toxocariasis)
VLP	virus-like particle
VLS	vascular leak syndrome
VM	Valsalva maneuver
	vasomotor
	Venturi mask
	vestibular membrane
	viomycin (antibiotic)
	viral myalgia
	viral myositis
	voluntary muscle

VM 26	teniposide
VMA	vanillylmandelic acid (vanilmandelic acid; vanyl mandelic acid)
	Veterinary Medical Association
VMAT	vanillylmandelic acid test
V max	maximum velocity (in an enzymatic reaction)
VMCD	vestibular membrane of cochlear duct
VMCP	vincristine + melphalan + cyclophosphamide + prednisone (combination chemotherapy)
VMD	Doctor of Veterinary Medicine
	vitelliruptive macular degeneration
VMF	VP-16 (etoposide) +methotrexate + fluorouracil (combination chemotherapy)
VMH	ventromedial nucleus of hypothalamus
VMI	visual-motor integration
VMIT	visual-motor integration test
VMN	ventromedial nucleus
VMR	vasomotor rhinitis
VMS	Verner-Morrison syndrome
	vertical mattress suture
	visual memory span
VMST	visual motor sequencing test
VMT	ventilatory muscle training
VN	vagus nerve (10th cranial nerve)
	vesical neck
	Virchow's nodes (signal node; sentinel node)
	virus-neutralizing
	visiting nurse
	vocational nurse
VNA	Visiting Nurse Association
VNB	vagus nerve block
VNC	vesicle neck contracture
	vomeronasal cartilage

VNH	Victims National Hotline (518) 372-0034
VNN	vagus nerve neuralgia
VNT	visual neglect test
VNTR	variable number tandem repeat
VO	verbal order
VO$_2$	oxygen consumption
Vo	standard volume
VOA	Volunteers of Ameica
VOB	ventricle of brain
VOCs	volatile organic compounds
VOD	veno-occlusive disease
	venous occlusive disease
v.o.d.	*visio oculus dextra* [Latin] vision of right eye
VOE	vascular occlusive episode
VOF	vesicular ovarian follicle
VOG	viral oncogene
VO$_2$I	oxygen consumption index
VOL	volume
vol	volar
	voluntary
VOM	ventricular osteomyelitis
vom	vomited
V-ONC	viral oncogene
VOP	venous occlusion plethysmography
VOR	vestibulo-ocular reflex
VOSMA	Vicon optoelectric system for movement analysis (automatically records gait kinematic parameters)
VP	vallate papilla (on tongue)
	variegate porphyria
	vasa previa
	vascular permeability
	vasopressin
	velopharyngeal
	venipuncture
	venous pressure
	ventricular premature (beat)
	ventriculo-peritoneal
	vincristine + prednisone (chemotherapeutic regimen)
	viral proteins

	(structural proteins)
VP1	virus-specific 1
VP$_1$	principal (75%) capsid protein of the virion
VP$_2$	minor capsid protein of the virion
VP$_3$	minor capsid protein of the virion
VP16	etoposide (antineoplastic agent)
V/P	ventilation/perfusion ratio
V & P	vagotomy and pyloroplasty
Vp	peak voltage
vp	vapor pressure
VPA	valproic acid
VPB	ventricular premature beat
VPC	vapor-phase chromatography
	ventricular premature complex
	ventricular premature contractions
	volume percent
VPD	vaccine-preventable disease
	ventricular premature depolarization
VPF	vascular permeability factor
	Vulvar Pain Foundation
VPGSS	venous pressure gradient support stockings
VPI	velopharyngeal incompetence
	velopharyngeal insufficiency
VPL	ventral posterolateral (nucleus)
VPM	ventilator pressure manometer
	ventral posteromedial (nucleus)
VPMI	Vanderbilt Pain Management Inventory
VPO	velopharyngeal opening
VPR	volume pressure response
VPRC	volume of packed red cells
VPS	valvular pulmonic stenosis
	ventilation/perfusion scanning
	ventriculo-peritoneal shunt

	volume perfomance standards
VPT	vibratory perception threshold
V/Q	ventilation-perfusion ratio
VR	unipolar right arm (electrocardiographic lead)
	valsalva retinopathy
	valve replacement
	vascular resistance
	venous reflux
	ventilation ratio
	ventral root
	ventricular rhythm
	Vicryl Rapide (synthetic rapid absorbable suture)
	visible radiation (light)
	vital records (certificates of birth, marriage, divorce and death required for legal and demographic purposes)
	vocal resonance
	vocational rehabilitation
VRBC	red blood cell volume
VRC	cervical ventral root (spinal nerve)
	venous renin concentration
VRD	ventricular radial dysplasia
	von Recklinghausen's disease (neurofibromatosis)
VRE	vancomycin-resistant enterococci
VRGs	ventral respiratory groups
VRI	viral respiratory infection
VRL	lumbar ventral root (spinal nerve)
	vinorelbine
VRM	valve-related mortality
VRML	virtual reality modelling language (allows the presentation and manipulation of three-dimensional environments)
vRNA	viral ribonucleic acid
VROM	voluntary range of motion

VRP	very reliable product
	vocational rehabilitation program
VRR	ventral root reflex
VRS	verbal rating scale
VRT	thoracic ventral root (spinal nerve)
VRV	ventricular residual volume
VS	vaccination scar
	vaginal spermicide
	vaginal sponge
	vagal stimulation
	vasospasm
	vein stripper
	vein stripping
	venisection (phlebotomy)
	ventricular septum
	verbal scales
	Vernet's syndrome (jugular foramen syndrome)
	versus
	visceral sepsis
	vesicular sound
	vesicular stomatitis
	vestibular schwannoma
	visited
	vital signs (temperature, pulse and respiration)
	vital statistics (registered records concerning births, marriages, separations, divorces and deaths)
	volumetric solution
	voluntary sterilization
vs	versus
v.s.	*vide supra* [Latin] see above
VSA	variant-specific surface antigen
VSBE	very short below elbow (amputation or cast level)
VSCs	volatile sulfa compounds
VSCT	ventral spinocerebellar tract
VSD	ventricular septal defect
	virtual safe dose
VSFP	venous stop flow pressure
VSG	variable surface glycoprotein
VSHD	ventricular septal

	heart defect
VSI	very seriously ill
VSINC	Virus Subcommittee of the International Nomenclature Committee
VSL	very serious list
VSN	vital signs normal
VSNG	vertical supranuclear gaze
VSOK	vital signs okay (normal)
VSR	venous stasis retinopathy
VSS	vital signs stable
VST	vapocoolant spray therapy
	ventral spinothalamic tract
	vestibulospinal tract
VSULA	vaccination scar, upper left arm
VSV	vesicular stomatitis virus
VSW	ventricular stroke work
VT	valve thrombosis
	venous thrombosis
	ventricular tachycardia
	vestibular toxicity
	vitality test
V$_T$	tidal volume
	total ventilation
V tach	ventricular tachycardia
VTE	venous thromboembolism
VTED	venous thromboembolic disease
VTEX	verotoxin-producing *E.coli*
VTF	vertical tripod fixation
VTI	vertically transmitted infection
VTM	mechanical tidal volume
VT-NS	ventricular tachycardia-not sustained
VTR	variable tandem repeats
VT-S	ventricular tachycardia sustained
VT/VF	ventricular tachycardia/ ventricular fibrillation
VTX	vertex
VU	varicose ulcer
	very urgent
	volume unit
VUI	vertical uterine incision
VUR	vesicoureteral reflux
VV	varicose veins

	verrucae vulgaris (common warts)
	vesicovaginal
	viper venom
	vulvovaginitis
V & V	vulva and vagina
vv	veins
vvs	varicose veins
	vice versa
vv.	*venae* [Latin] veins
v/v	volume of solute to volume of solvent (ratio)
VVA	vasovasostomy approximator
	volume ventilator adult
VVC	vulvovaginal candidiasis
VVD	vaginal vertex delivery
VVF	vesicovaginal fistula
VVFR	vesicovaginal fistula repair
VVI	vocal velocity index
VVO	vasovasostomy
VVOR	visual-vestibulo-ocular reflex
VVR	vasovagal reflex
VVS	vulvar vestibulitis syndrome
VVs	varicose veins
VVT	ventricular triggered (pacemaker)
VW	venereal warts (condylomata acuminata)
	vessel wall
vWD	von Willebrand's disease (most common inherited bleeding disorder)
VWF	vibratory white finger (vibration-induced white finger)
vWF	von Willebrand's factor
VWM	ventricular wall motion
vWS	von Willebrand syndrome
VWSP	vaginal wall sling procedure
Vx	vertex
VYI	vaginal yeast infection
VZ	varicella zoster (virus)
VZIG	varicella-zoster immune globulin
	varicella-zoster immunoglobulin
VZV	varicella zoster virus

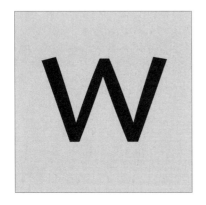

W energy
tryptophan
tungsten (wolfram)
ward
water
watt
wedge pressure
week
weight
white
widow
widower
width
wife
work
W. *wolfram* [German]
tungsten
w water
watt
week
weight
white
wife
with
work
WA Wernicke's aphasia
when awake
while awake
wrist arthrodesis
W/A while awake
W & A weakness and atrophy
WAF weakness, atrophy and
fasciculation
white adult female

WAI whole-abdomen irradiation
WAIS Wechsler Adult Intelligence
Scale
Wide Area Information
Servers (network-based
information retrieval)
WAP wandering atrial
pacemaker
WAR Wasserman antigen
reaction
whole abdominal
radiotherapy
WARDS Welfare of Animals Used
for Research in Drugs and
Therapy
WARF warfarin (Wisconsin
Alumni Research
Foundation)
WAS Wiskott-Aldrich syndrome
(X-linked genetic disease)
World Association
for Sexology
WASO wakefulness after
sleep onset
WAT word association test
WB water balance
water bottle
weber
weight bearing
well baby
Western blot
whole blood
whole body
William's brace (a
lumbosacral extension-
lateral control orthosis)
Wb weber
WBA Western blot assay
W. bancrofti
Wuchereria bancrofti
(filarial worm)
WBAPTT whole blood activated
partial thromboplastin
time
WBAT weight-bearing as tolerated
WASS Wasserman test
(for syphilis)
WBC weight-bearing cast
well baby clinic

	white blood cell
	white blood (cell) count
wbc	white blood cell
WBCT	whole blood clotting time
WBE	weight-bearing exercise
	whole blood extract
WBH	whole blood hematocrit
	whole body hypothermia
WBI	will be in
WBN	whole blood nitrogen
WBPTT	whole blood partial thromboplastin time
WBR	whole body radiation
	whole brain radiation
WBR-N	whole body responses, neonate
WBRT	whole blood recalcification time
WBS	whole blood serum
	Williams-Beuren syndrome
	whole body scan
	whole body shower
	withdrawal body shakes
WC	walking cast
	warm compress
	water closet
	wedged catheter
	wheelchair
	when called
	white (blood) cell
	white (blood cell) count
	whooping cough
	will call
	work capacity
	worker's compensation
	writer's cramp
WC'	whole complement
w/c	wheelchair
WCA	work capacity assessment
WCB	will call back
WCBA	woman of childbearing age
WCC	white (blood) cell count
WCD	Weber-Christian disease (mesenteric panniculitis)
WCE	work capacity evaluation
WCGTC	World Council for Gifted and Talented Children
WCL	whole cell lysate
WCM	Watson-Crick model

	whole cow's milk
WCP	weight-control program
WCPV	whole-cell pertussis vaccine
WCS	white clot syndrome
	Williams-Campbell syndrome
WD	wallerian degeneration
	warm and dry
	watery diarrhea
	Weil's disease
	well developed
	Wernicke's disease (encephalopathy)
	wet dressing
	Whipple's disease (intestinal lipodystrophy)
	Wilson's disease (hepatolenticular degeneration)
	with disease
	wound

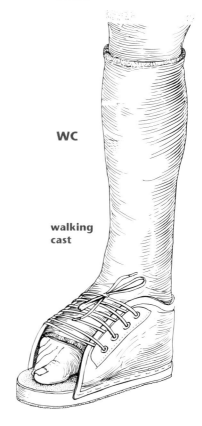

WC

walking cast

wrist disarticulation
wrist dislocation
wrist drop
W/D warm and dry
withdrawal
wd well developed
w/d wound debridement
WDCC well-developed collateral circulation
WDD wet-to-dry dressing
WDHA watery diarrhea, hypokalemia and achlorhydria (syndrome)
watery diarrhea with hypokalemic alkalosis (syndrome)
WDHAS watery diarrhea, hypokalemia and achlorhydria syndrome
WDHH watery diarrhea, hypokalemia and hypochlorhydria (syndrome)
WDHHS watery diarrhea, hypokalemia and hypochlorhydria syndrome
WDLL well-differentiated lymphocytic lymphoma
WDMF wall-defective microbial forms
WDN well-developed and nourished
WDS watery diarrhea syndrome
withdrawal symptoms
wrongful death statute
WDWN well developed, well nourished
WE weekend
Wernicke's encephalopathy
Western encephalitis
Western encephalomyelitis
W/E wound of entry (of a bullet)
We weber
WEE western equine encephalitis

western equine encephalomyelitis
WEEV western equine encephalomyelitis virus
WEM wire ether mask
WEP Wernicke's encephalopathy
WER wheal erythema reaction
WESR Westergren erythrocyte sedimentation rate
Wintrobe erythrocyte sedimentation rate
WES sign wall-echo-shadow sign
WEST work evaluation systems technology
WF white female
W/F weakness and fatigue
WFD whitefinger disease
WFE Williams flexion exercise
WFI water for injection
WFL within functional limits
WFOT World Federation of Occupational Therapists
WFR wheal-and-flare reaction
WFS Waterhouse-Friderichsen syndrome
wheat flour sensitivity
whistling face syndrome (craniocarpotarsal dystrophy)
WG Wright-Giesma (histologic stain)
WGA wheat germ agglutinin (vitamin-rich embryo of the wheat kernel)
WGI wheat gluten intolerance
wgt weight
WH walking heel (cast)
well healed
well hydrated
white
WHA warm and humid air
WHC Witch Hazel compress
wh ch wheelchair
WHCOA White House Conference on Aging
WHE Wernicke's hemorrhagic encephalopathy

WHO	World Health Organization
	wrist-hand orthosis
WHO GU LA	
	whole gut lavage
WHO ICD	
	World Health Organization's
	International Classification
	of Diseases
whp	whirlpool
whpb	whirlpool bath
WHR	waist to hip
	(circumference) ratio
WHRC	World Health
	Research Center
WHS	well-healed scar
WHV	woodchuck hepatic virus
WHVP	wedged hepatic venous
	pressure
WI	whiplash injury
	Whiteley Index (of
	hypochondriasis)
	wound infection
W & I	wounds and injuries
WIA	wounded in action
WIC	women, infants and
	children
WIMC	walk-in medical center
WIS	Wechsler Intelligence Scale
WISC	Wechsler Intelligence Scale
	for Children
wk	weak
	week
	work
WKD	Wilson-Kimmelstiel disease
WKS	Wernicke-Korsakov
	(Korsakoff) syndrome
WL	waiting list
	water loss
	wavelength
	weight loss
	wet lung
	whiplash (violent force on
	the cervical spine, first in
	one direction and then
	suddenly in the opposite
	direction)
	withdrawal
wl	wavelength
WLF	whole lymphocytic fraction

WLI	whiplash injury

WLI

whiplash
injury

WL & M	weight loss and
	maintenance
WLS	wet lung syndrome
WLT	water-loading test
	waterload test
WM	Waldenström's
	macroglobulinemia
	warm and moist
	white male
	whole milk
WMA	World Medical Association
WMF	white, middle-aged female
WMG	Waldenström's
	macroglobulinemia
WMM	white, middle-aged male
WMMR	CDC's *Weekly Morbidity and*
	Mortality Report
WMP	warm moist packs
	weight management
	program
WMR	work metabolic rate
WMS	Wechsler Memory Scale
WMX	whirlpool, massage and
	exercise
WN	well nourished
	wry neck (torticollis)
WND	wound
WNF	well-nourished female
WNL	within normal limits
WNM	well-nourished male
WNOS	Waddel non-organic signs
WNPW	wide, notched P wave
WNV	West Nile virus
WO	wide open
	without
	wrist orthosis

written order
wo weeks old
w/o without
WOB work of breathing
WOP without pain
WORD Weber-Osler-Rendu disease
WOWS weak opiate
withdrawal scale
WP weakly positive
wedge pressure
whirlpool
word processor
W/P water-powder ratio
WPB whirlpool bath
WPk wet pack
WPPSI Wechsler Preschool
Primary Scale of
Intelligence
WPW Wolff-Parkinson-White
(syndrome)

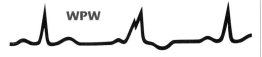

Wolff-Parkinson-White (syndrome)

WPWS Wolff-Parkinson-White
syndrome
WR waiting room
washroom
Wassermann reaction
water retention
weakly reactive
weak response
wr wrist
WRAMC Walter Reed Army
Medical Center
WRAML Wide Range Assessment of
Memory and Learning
WRAT Wide Range
Achievement Test
WRBC washed red blood cells
WRC water retention coefficient
WRE whole ragweed extract
WRVP wedged renal vein pressure
WS Waardenburg's syndrome
Wallenberg syndrome
(low brain infarct)

wasting syndrome
water soluble
Weil's syndrome
Welt's syndrome
Wernicke's syndrome
Westphal's sign (loss of the
knee jerk reflex)
West syndrome
Wickham's striae
Winchester syndrome
(mucopolysacchar-
idosis VII)
withdrawal symptoms
Wolfram syndrome
wrist splint

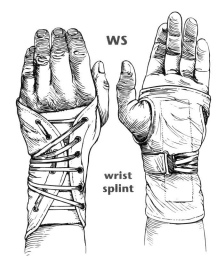

WS

wrist splint

WSA water-soluble antibiotic
WSD wool sorters' disease
WSDF water-soluble dietary fiber
w-sec watt-second
WSF white single female
WSM white single male
WSP withdrawal seizure prone
WSR withdrawal seizure resistant
WSS warm saline solution
WSWS windshield wiper sign
(to-and-fro movement of
an implant)
WT Wada test
walking tank
wall thickness

Warthin's tumor

Weber test (for differentiating between hearing impairment of conductive or sensorineural origin)

weight

whistletip (catheter)

white

Wilms' tumor

wisdom teeth (3rd molars)

wt weight

WtB weight bearing

WTF weight transferral frequency

WTHR waist-to-hip ratio

W/U work up

WUE warm-up exercise

WV whispered voice

w/v weight of solute to volume of solvent (ratio)

WVEIS whole-virus enzyme immunoassay screen

WVIL written and verbal informed consent

WVPOI written and verbal pre/post operative instruction

WW watchful waiting

Weight Watchers

wheeled walker

whipworm (*Trichuris trichiura*)

W/W weight of solute to weight of solution (ratio)

WWAC walk with aid of cane

WWB warm water bath

WW Brd whole wheat bread

WWE warm water enema

W/wo with or without

WWW World Wide Web

W/X wound of exit (of a bullet)

WxB wax bite

WxP wax pattern (of dental restoration)

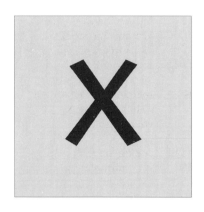

X   x-ray
break
crossbite
cross-section
crossed with
except
exophoria
extra
female sex chromosome
ionization exposure rate
Kienbock's unit of x-ray
exposure
magnification sign
multiplied by
number of times
reactance
removal
respirations
start of anesthesia
ten
times
translocation between two
X chromosomes
transverse
xanthine (derivatives
include caffeine,
theobromine and
theophylline)
xanthosine (a nucleoside
which on hydrolysis yields
xanthine and ribose)
xylene (an antiseptic
hydrocarbon)
Xylocaine (lidocaine)

X²   chi-squared (statistics)
x   abscissa
axis (of cylindric lens)
except
mole fraction
roentgen (ray)
unknown factor
XA   xanthurenic acid (a minor
catabolite of tryptophan)
X & A   xylene and alcohol
Xa   chiasma
Xaa   unknown amino acid
Xam   examination
Xan   xanthine (derivatives
include caffeine,
theobromine and
theophylline)
Xanth   xanthomatosis
Xao   xanthosine (a nucleoside
which on hydrolysis yields
xanthine and ribose)
XBT   xylose breath test
X & D   examination and diagnosis
XC   excretory cystogram
excretory cystography
XCCE   extracapsular cataract
extraction
X-CGD   X-linked variety of chronic
granulomatous disease
XCT   x-ray computed
tomography
X2d   two times a day
XDH   xanthine dehydrogenase
XDP   xanthine diphosphate
xeroderma pigmentosum
Xe   xenon (an unreactive
gaseous element)
XeCT   xenon-enhanced
computed tomography
XES   x-ray energy spectrometer
x-ray energy spectrometry
XF   xerophthalmic fundus
XGP   xanthogranulomatous
pyelonephritis
(also XPN)
XGPN   xanthogranulomatous
pyelonephriris
XGR   x-gene reactivation
XIP   x-ray-induced polypeptide

	x-ray in plaster of Paris
XKO	not knocked out
XL	excess lactate
	extra large
	X-linked
XLA	X-linked agammaglobulinemia
X-LAG	X-linked agammaglobulinemia
XLD	xylose, lysine, deoxycholate (agar)
X-LD	X-linked disease
XLH	X-linked hypophosphatemia
XLI	X-linked ichthyosis
XLIH	X-linked infantile hypoparathyroidism
XLJR	X-linked juvenile retinoschisis
XLLS	X-linked lymphoproliferative syndrome
XLMR	X-linked mental retardation
XLP	X-linked lymphoproliferative (syndrome)
XLR	X-linked recessive
XLSA	X-linked sideroblastic anemia
XLSCID	X-linked severe combined immunodeficiency
xma	chiasma
X match	crossmatch
XMP	xanthosine monophosphate
XO	extraction of xanthine oxidase
XOP	x-ray out of plaster of Paris
XP	xeroderma pigmentosum
Xp	short arm of chromosome X
Xp-	deletion of short arm of chromosome X
XPN	xanthogranulomatous pyelonephritis (also XGP)
X-Prep	bowel evacuation in preparation for radiology

XPS	xiphoid process of sternum
	x-ray photoemission spectroscopy
Xq	long arm of chromosome X
Xq-	deletion of long arm of chromosome X
XR	roentgen ray
	x-ray
x-rays	roentgen rays
XRD	x-ray diffraction
	x-ray dose
XRF	x-ray fluorescence (spectrometry)
XRMR	X-linked recessive mental retardation
XRS	x-ray sensitivity
XRT	external radiation therapy
	x-ray technician
	x-ray therapy
XS	cross section
	excessive
	xiphisternum
xs	excess
	excessive
X-sect	cross-section
XSLR	crossed straight leg raising (sign)
XSP	xanthoma striatum palmare
XT	exotropia
X²t	chi-square test
Xta	chiasmata
XTE	xeroderma, talipes and enamel syndrome
XTM	xanthoma tuberosum multiplex
XTP	xanthosine triphosphate
XU	excretory urogram
XuMP	xylulose monophosphate
3x/wk	three times a week
XX	homogametic sex chromosomes for female (normal female chromosome type)
46XX	normal number of female chromosomes
XX/XY	normal sex karyotypes
47XXY	XXY syndrome (1 Y and 2

X chromosomes)

XY   heterogametic sex chromosomes for male (normal male chromosome type)

46XY   normal number of male chromosomes

Xyl   xylose (a diagnostic aid in determining intestinal function)

Xylo   Xylocaine (lidocaine hydrochloride)

47XYY XYY syndrome (1 X and 2 Y chromosomes)

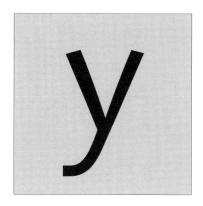

Y male sex chromosome
tyrosine (a precursor of
thyroid hormones)
year
yellow
yttrium (rare
metallic element)

y ordinate
year

YAC yeast artificial chromosome

YACP young adult chronic
patient

YADH yeast alcohol
dehydrogenase

YAG laser
yttrium-aluminum-
garnet laser

Yb ytterbium (rare metallic
element)

YCOSA Young Children of
Substance Abusers

yd yard

YDV yeast-derived
hepatitis B vaccine

YEI *Yersinia enterocolitica*
infection

Y. enterocolotica
Yersinia enterocolitica

(cause of acute
gastroenteritis and
mesenteric lymphadenitis
in children)

YF yellow fever

YFI yellow fever immunization

YFMD yellow fever membrane
disease

YHMD yellow hyaline
membrane disease

YJV yellow jacket venom

YLC youngest living child

YM yellow marrow (bone)

YMC young male Caucasian

Y/N yes/no

YNS yellow nail syndrome

YO years old

y/o years old

YOB year of birth

YORA younger-onset
rheumatoid arthritis

YP *Yersinia pestis*
(causes plague)

Y. pestis *Yersinia pestis*
(causes plague)

YPLL years of potential life lost
(before age 65)

yr(s) year(s)

YRD Yangtze River disease

Y rings Yoon rings (for fallopian
tube ligation)

YS yellow spot
yolk sac

YSC yolk sac carcinoma

YST yeast
yolk sac tumor

YTD year to date

YTDY yesterday

Yu yusho (acneform skin
eruptions)

YV youth violence

YVS yellow vernix syndrome

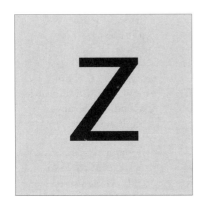

Z	acoustic impedance
	atomic number
	band or disk that separates
	sarcomeres
	contraction
	impedance
	ionic charge number
	proton number
	standardized deviate
	standard score
	zero
	Z-line
	zone
Z′, Z″	increasing degrees
	of contraction
z	atomic number
	standardized device
	standard normal deviate
	zero
	zone
ZA	zygomatic arch
ZAP	zymosan-activated-plasma
ZAS	zymosan-activated
	autologous serum
ZB	zygomatic bone
ZCFS	zero-calorie fat substitute
ZCP	zinc chloride poisoning
ZD	Zenker's degeneration
	Zenker's diverticulum
	(mucosal diverticulum
	between the pharynx and
	esophagus that may trap
	some food when
	swallowed)

	zero defects
	zinc deficiency
ZDDP	zinc
	dialkyldithiophosphate
Z DNA	Z deoxyribonucleic acid
	(DNA twisted in the
	opposite direction from
	the usual DNA; may play
	a role in gene
	expression)
ZDS	zinc depletion syndrome
ZDV	zidovudine
ZEEP	zero end-expiratory
	pressure
ZES	Zollinger-Ellison syndrome
ZESR	zeta erythrocyte
	sedimentation rate
Z-E syndrome	
	Zollinger-Ellison syndrome
	(caused by excessive
	production of gastrin)
ZET	Zollinger-Ellison tumor
ZF	zero frequency
ZFF	zygomaticofacial foramen
ZFN	zygomaticofacial nerve
ZFP	zinc finger protein
ZFS	zero-calorie fat substitute
ZIFT	zygote intrafallopian
	(tube) transfer
ZIg	zoster immune globulin
	(vaccine)
	zoster immunoglobulin
	(vaccine)
ZIM	zimelidine (an
	antidepressant)
ZIP	zoster immune plasma
ZLS	Zimmerman-Laband
	syndrome
ZN	Zickel nail (intramedullary
	femoral nail)
Zn	zinc (necessary in trace
	amounts in diet)
ZnO	zinc oxide
ZnO₂	zinc peroxide
ZnOE	zinc oxide and eugenol
	(white zinc)
ZO	Zuckerkandl's organ
ZOE	zinc oxide and eugenol
	(white zinc)

ZP	zona pellucida
ZPA	zone of polarizing activity
ZPD	zona pellucida partially dissected
ZPG	zero population growth
ZPJs	zygapophyseal joints (paired synovial joints articulating between the lower aspect of the superior vertebra and the upper aspect of the inferior vertebra)
ZPO	zinc peroxide
ZPP	zinc protoporphyrin
ZR	zero risk zona reticularis
Zr	zirconium (rare metallic element)
ZS	Zieve's syndrome
ZSB	zero stools since birth
ZSCD	Zickel supracondylar

	device (for fixation of supracondylar fracture of femur)
ZSR	zeta sedimentation rate zeta sedimentation ratio
ZST	zinc sulfate turbidity (test)
ZT	zidovudine therapy zolpidem tartrate
ZTL	zinc throat lozenges
ZTN	zygomaticotemporal nerve
ZTS	zymosan-treated serum
ZTT	zinc turbidity test
Zy	zygion (a craniometric landmark located on the most lateral point of the zygomatic arch)
zyg	zygotene (a meiotic stage in which the chromosomes undergo pairing)
Zz.	*zingiber* [Latin] ginger